MUSHROOM PHARMACY

MUSHROOM PHARMACY

A Practical Guide to Psychedelic Mushrooms

Stacey Simmons, MA, PhD, LMFT

Illustrated by Paula Schultz

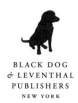

BLACK DOG
& LEVENTHAL
PUBLISHERS
NEW YORK

Black Dog & Leventhal Publishers
Hachette Book Group
1290 Avenue of the Americas, New York, NY 10104
www.blackdogandleventhal.com
 BlackDogandLeventhal   @BDLev

First Edition: February 2025

Published by Black Dog & Leventhal Publishers, an imprint of Hachette Book Group, Inc.
The Black Dog & Leventhal Publishers name and logo are trademarks of Hachette Book Group, Inc.

The Hachette Speakers Bureau provides a wide range of authors for speaking events. To find out more, go to hachettespeakersbureau.com or email HachetteSpeakers@hbgusa.com.

Black Dog & Leventhal books may be purchased in bulk for business, educational, or promotional use. For more information, please contact your local bookseller or the Hachette Book Group Special Markets Department at Special.Markets@hbgusa.com.

The publisher is not responsible for websites (or their content) that are not owned by the publisher.

Print book cover and interior design by Katie Benezra

Library of Congress Cataloging-in-Publication Data
Names: Simmons, Stacey, author.
Title: Mushroom pharmacy : a practical guide to psychedelic mushrooms / Stacey Simmons.
Description: New York : Black Dog & Leventhal, [2024] | Includes bibliographical references and index. | Summary: "The go-to, illustrated reference guide for all things related to mushrooms and psilocybin, Mushroom Pharmacy is a comprehensive and approachable guide to psychedelic mushrooms, including information on varietals, delivery, dosing, and treatable conditions"—Provided by publisher.
Identifiers: LCCN 2023054068 (print) | LCCN 2023054069 (ebook) | ISBN 9780762487981 (trade paperback) | ISBN 9780762487998 (ebook)
Subjects: LCSH: Hallucinogenic drugs—Therapeutic use. | Mushrooms, Hallucinogenic—Therapeutic use. | Hallucinogenic plants—Therapeutic use.
Classification: LCC RM324.8 .S56 2024 (print) | LCC RM324.8 (ebook) | DDC 615.7/883—dc23/eng/20240411
LC record available at https://lccn.loc.gov/2023054068
LC ebook record available at https://lccn.loc.gov/2023054069

ISBNs: 978-0-7624-8798-1 (paperback), 978-0-7624-8799-8 (ebook)

Printed in China

APS

10 9 8 7 6 5 4 3 2 1

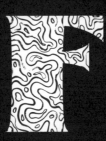

For my clients, who have taught me so much, and for my teachers, who have given me the gift of their learning.

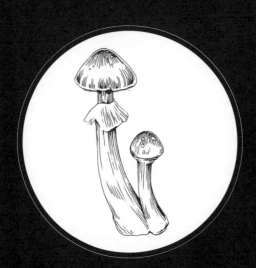

GOLDEN TEACHER

CONTENTS

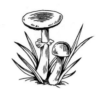

CHAPTER 1:

A Brief History of Mushrooms and Psychedelics, 1

CHAPTER 2:

Mushrooms as Medicine, 9

CHAPTER 3:
Mushroom Anatomy, 39

CHAPTER 4:

Mushroom Environments, 53

CHAPTER 5:

Working with Mushrooms, 67

CHAPTER 6:

Varieties of Mushrooms, 93

CHAPTER 7:
Medicinal Uses for Mushrooms, 133

CHAPTER 8:

Mushrooms, Psychedelics, and the Law, 175

FOREWORD

WHEN DR. STACEY SIMMONS asked me to write this foreword to *Mushroom Pharmacy*, I was delighted. Stacey possesses a deep knowledge and curiosity about the science of psychedelics and their ability to heal the body and mind. We met a few years ago when she enrolled in the year-long psychedelic-assisted therapy training program we offer at the Integrative Psychiatry Institute. I was immediately impressed with her astute ability to integrate the esoteric with the scientific; exactly the skills required of a medical professional in the field of research and application of psilocybin for health and healing.

As one of the co-founders of the leading institute for training in psychedelic-assisted therapy, I believe that the publication of *Mushroom Pharmacy* is both timely and profoundly essential. There is nothing else like this book available to readers who are looking for trustworthy, well-researched guidance on the use of mushrooms as medicine.

Interest, particularly in the mental health benefits of mushrooms, has skyrocketed in recent years, and for good reason. First, the conventional FDA-approved treatments for depression, anxiety, PTSD, eating disorders, and so many other types of emotional suffering simply do not work for far too many people. Second, the challenges we face as a species are much more complex now than even five years ago.

Fortunately, the protocol for mental health treatment is experiencing a much-needed update and mushrooms are playing a starring role in this revolution. It's important to understand just how serious the mental health calamity is that we are facing on our planet. The situation was dire before the COVID-19 pandemic and worsened during in the quarantines of 2020 and 2021. Although COVID-19 infection rates have tapered off, mental health diagnoses continue to rise. U.S. Surgeon General Vivek Murthy has called mental health "the defining public health crisis of our time." Here are a few statistics that we all should know about:

- According to the World Health Organization, 280 million folks on the planet are dealing with depression, one of the top causes of disability globally.
- One-third of people who undergo currently approved treatments for depression get no long-term benefits.
- Approximately 25% of American girls ages 12 to 17 had at least one episode of depression in 2020.
- More than 48 million Americans above the age of 12 are addicted to a substance.
- The National Institute of Mental Health reported that 57.8 million U.S. adults lived with a mental illness in 2021—more than one in five.

I spent almost twenty years as a psychiatrist searching for better tools to help my patients overcome deep suffering. At times I struggled with the limited toolkit of medications and psychotherapy that medical training put in my hands, which achieved only minimal or partial results at best. The depth of healing that is possible in psilocybin-assisted therapy is profound. No longer do folks with depression, PTSD, substance dependency, and other mental health challenges need to settle for treatments that cannot achieve a cure. Research projects, treating such conditions with psilocybin-assisted therapy, are revealing that benefits of even one or two psilocybin experiences, with skillful guidance, can last for months or years.

My search for better answers to my patients' problems led to getting involved in clinical trials of psychedelic-assisted therapy (PAT). I saw chronic treatment-resistant PTSD melt away in just a few PAT sessions. In one of these studies, our subjects entered with, on average, 29.4 years of PTSD symptoms and at twelve-month follow-up, fully two-thirds still did not meet criteria for PTSD. Although I knew that shamans and psychedelic guides

had been working in the underground for decades—some with impeccable integrity, and others more than a little shady—I recognized my calling when I realized how much training psychedelic therapists would need to provide responsible care and deliver what these medicines are capable of.

Wrapping our heads around what we know, and have yet to learn, about mushrooms is a monumental task. Dr. Simmons has written a guide so thorough that it can turn a person with no background in the study of mushrooms into a responsible and informed consumer. I believe *Mushroom Pharmacy* will remain an essential reference for years to come.

Use this book as your most up-to-date guide to help you establish connectivity to not just mushrooms but also to the mystery of life itself as you explore the unique beauty of your own individuality inside the mycelial network of life on earth.

Will Van Derveer, M.D.
Integrative Psychiatry Institute
Boulder, Colorado
March 2024

INTRODUCTION

A RENAISSANCE IN the world of psychology and psychiatry is underway thanks to advances in mycology, the study of mushrooms and other fungi. New products from coffee to health supplements contain nonpsychedelic fungi like Lion's Mane (*Hericium erinaceus*), known for its anti-inflammatory and antioxidant properties, or *Cordyceps* (*Cordyceps sinensis* or *Cordyceps militaris*), which are sought after for enhancing physical and cognitive performance as well as their purported anti-aging properties. Everywhere you look these days, there's a fungus among us offering a new solution to an old or challenging health problem.

The possibility of psychedelic fungi as a treatment for mental health challenges is revolutionary. For decades, the pharmaceuticals prescribed by psychiatrists have been accepted as blunt instruments. Most condemn patients to debilitating and often demoralizing reactions. Weight gain, flattened emotions, and loss of libido are all well-known side effects of accepted psychopharmaceutical treatments. Many of these medications are worth their side effects only when the situation is dire: when grief is overwhelming, when someone is suffering a psychotic episode, when depression keeps someone in bed for months, or when someone believes suicide is a better option than waking up tomorrow.

The first modern discussion of psychedelics began with the discovery of lysergic acid diethylamide

(LSD) by Swiss chemist Albert Hofmann. Hofmann was in the process of testing numerous substances, looking for potential drugs as part of his work at Sandoz Laboratories. He synthesized the compound from part of the ergot plant, combining it with an acid. He marked the compound LSD-25, the last in a long list of attempted compounds using the LSD base. In testing the compound on animals, the response was not what Hofmann was looking for. The animals became agitated, but otherwise there was no change in the animals' heart rate, respiration, or circulatory systems, the areas of research that Hofmann was investigating. His research focused on finding a drug that could aid in circulation during labor and childbirth. In 1943 Hofmann tested the compound on himself with what he thought was a small dose, 0.25 mg. We now know his experimental dose to be more than 100 times what is considered an effective dose of LSD. Hofmann reported disturbing, distorted imagery at first, followed hours later by feelings of oneness and joyful acceptance.[1]

Several years after this discovery, amateur mycologist Robert Gordon Wasson and his

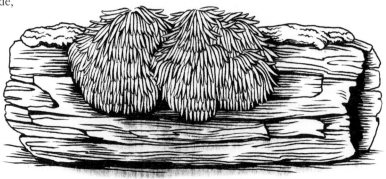

wife, Valentina Pavlovna Wasson, had begun researching mushrooms. After a weekend foraging trip, the couple became curious about culinary cultures that had developed around mushrooms. They engaged in research organizing fungi by cultures that were either mycophilic (liking mushrooms) or mycophobic (mushroom-averse). The Wassons began a study of different varieties of mushrooms they encountered, eventually authoring a compendium with hand-painted watercolor images titled *Mushrooms, Russia, and History* in 1957.[2]

But it was Wasson's interest in the mind-altering effect of some mushroom varieties that eventually led him to Mexico and the Mazatec people's use of native mushrooms in healing rituals. This encounter is now enshrined in the stories of how "magic mushrooms" became popularized in the United States. Wasson was introduced to Maria Sabina Magdalena Garcia, a Mazatec curandera (traditional healer) in the town of Huautla de Jiménez in the state of Oaxaca. The town lies about six hours from Mexico City by car. Sabina shared her healing ceremony, called a valada, with Wasson. She probably served him *Psilocybe mexicana*, a strain sometimes called Pajaritos (little birds) during an overnight valada. This is the experience he described in his incredible 15-page photo essay for *Life* magazine titled "Seeking the Magic Mushroom" in 1957.

This essay opened the door for a cultural revolution with psychedelics at the center. The counterculture learned of the power of Sabina's "sacred children," as she referred to the tiny fungi. Within ten years, seekers, hippies, CIA agents, and doctors descended on Oaxaca, seeking the mind-altering experience associated with mushrooms. Wasson eventually shared samples of the mushrooms he had taken with Albert Hofmann, the chemist who discovered LSD-25. Hofmann synthesized psilocybin from the mushrooms and created a pill that he shared with Sabina on a trip to Huautla de Jiménez in 1962.

More than 60 years later, it is easy to mythologize Sabina's and Wasson's roles in sharing *Psilocybe* mushrooms with the world. The story of how these mushrooms first found their way into the modern Western consciousness is one of mystery, intrigue, and scientific discovery. But the exposure of psilocybin mushrooms to the world of Western science, psychedelic tourism, drug manufacturing, and New Age consciousness includes a cautionary tale of colonialism and a debt that has yet to be paid to the Mazatec people, and Maria Sabina in particular. Sabina suffered greatly from sharing her "sacred children" with the Americans who visited her. She was accused of trafficking drugs by Mexican authorities. She was blamed for bringing ruin to her hometown. Her house was burned down, and her son was murdered. She died in poverty in 1985 at the age of 91.[3]

Though Sabina's initiation of R. Gordon Wasson into the world of psychedelic mushrooms in the 1950s marked the first modern introduction of naturally occurring mind-altering substances, "magic" mushrooms have been known for millennia across cultures for their healing and psychotropic properties. Indigenous peoples from the Americas to

Asia have used mushrooms for shamanic and healing purposes.

As of this writing, there are more than 180 varieties of *Psilocybe* mushrooms known to mycologists. Not all the species in this genus of mushrooms produce enough psilocybin to be effective as a psychedelic. We know about them because of the determination and dedication of mycologists across the world like Paul Stamets, R. Gordon Wasson, Valentina Pavlovna Wasson, Michael Beug, Jonathan Ott, and many more. Even outside the realm of mushrooms with psychotropic effects, mushrooms are rich with healing properties. It is only in the last decade that we have begun to scratch the surface of the range of medicinal capacities that mushrooms offer humans. Psilocybin is one of the most potent of these compounds.

In the last 15 years, some of the world's leading research institutions have conducted original research and groundbreaking experiments into the healing properties of psilocybin mushrooms. Prestigious research institutions like Johns Hopkins University Medical School's Center for Psychedelic and Consciousness Research have found that psilocybin offers unprecedented relief to people suffering from grave disorders like treatment-resistant depression, obsessive-compulsive disorder, eating disorders, and debilitating anxiety, to name just a few—giving new hope for patients who suffer from severe mental health disorders. As the US Food and Drug Administration examines the results of the last decade of research, those of us in the psychedelic community expect to see new pharmaceuticals, laws, and practices emerge. In my own practice we have several therapists certified in psychedelic therapy. We work with leading physicians and nurse practitioners and are developing new protocols based on the latest research. As the laws and practices change, psychotherapists and psychiatrists will need to update their training. Psychedelic therapy is a unique practice that calls on multiple disciplines, including depth psychology, psychopharmacology, somatic psychology, and trauma research. In the next eight chapters we will discuss the history of these powerful fungi, the resurgence in research that is underway, and the hopes for a future that is made magical by the promise of mushrooms.

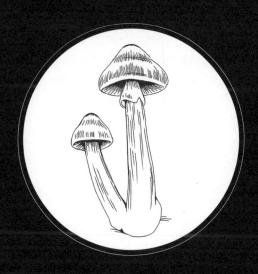

B+

Nature doesn't hurry, and yet everything is accomplished.

—LAO TZU

CHAPTER 1

A Brief History of Mushrooms and Psychedelics

Most of us think of using psychedelics as a modern phenomenon. We think of posh retreat centers like in the book *Nine Perfect Strangers*, or the story of NFL quarterback Aaron Rodgers taking ayahuasca and regaining his love of football. Culturally, the first exposure most Americans have in learning about psychedelics is in the history of the counterculture movements of the 1960s. But psychedelics have been part of our cultures since the beginning of recorded history. Their names haven't always survived, but whether we are discussing kykeon in Greece, San Pedro in parts of Central and South America, ayahuasca in Peru, peyote in the Rio Grande Valley of the United States, soma in India, iboga in Africa, or pituri in Australia, almost all cultures have had access to substances that induce a psychedelic state or form of altered consciousness.

Ethnobotanist and self-proclaimed mystic Terence McKenna proposed his hypothesis of the "stoned ape" based on the idea that psychedelics are responsible for humans developing into our current form. In his book *Food of the Gods*, McKenna challenged readers to consider the stark change in hominid brain development from our closest ancestors to anatomically modern humans. Hominid brains increased in size and volume very quickly by evolutionary standards around 10,000 BCE. McKenna proposed that eating psychedelic mushrooms changed our early hominid ancestors' brains by a gain of almost a third in volume, with most of the development happening in the frontal cortex. This part, found behind the eyes, is responsible for our larger brain volume and is the reason that humans are capable of complex thought and extensive memories. Most serious scientists don't consider McKenna's hypothesis to be based on science. However, recent laboratory studies on lab animals injected with psychedelic substances have shown immediate neurogenesis, the generation of new neurons, in the presence of these substances, at the very least raising an eyebrow toward McKenna's hypothesis.[1]

In the Louvre Museum in Paris there is a funerary stele titled *The Exaltation of the Flower.* The stele was excavated in what is modern Greece but was created more than 2,000 years ago in the city-state of Thessaly. The stele is dated to the fifth century BCE and depicts two women holding up either flowers or mushrooms, as though examining them. Scholars over the last 100 years have offered very different ideas of what the two women are holding and why the funerary stele was carved with their likenesses. Some scholars believe that the two women represented the goddesses Demeter and Persephone. Later scholars pointed out that this type of stele was primarily created as a tribute to a person who had died. The ancient Greeks didn't often think of women as worthy of permanent remembrance, so this created some stir. Would the Greeks have honored two women with a funeral carving?

Contemporary theories point to a culture in Thessaly that existed prior to Athenian colonization and suggest that the stele depicts women who worked as healers or midwives. The reigning theory of the stele is that the women are holding pomegranate flowers. But there are several, including English classicist Robert Graves and Italian ethnobotanist Giorgio Samorini, who argue that the flora in the hands of the ancient women are mushrooms.[2] Their hypothesis purports that people in Thessaly used mushrooms for healing and ritual purposes. Samorini adds that the site where the stele was discovered is part of an area along the route to the temple of Eleusis, home of the famed Eleusinian Mysteries. Anthropologists and scholars know that the participants in these secret ceremonies,

sometimes numbering in the thousands, drank a magical concoction called *kykeon*. While we do not know the ingredients used in the creation of kykeon (some speculate ergot; others, psychedelic mushrooms), we know that it was a powerful intoxicant that aided in the life-changing rituals at Eleusis. People of the period extolled the rituals as changing their lives, with a passion similar to that expressed by modern psychedelic enthusiasts.

After decades of academic exile renewed interest in the transformative powers of compounds like psilocybin, ayahuasca, dimethyltryptamine (DMT), and other psychoactive substances has fueled a renaissance in research in these substances. Sometimes referred to as entheogens, meaning "god or divine within" in Greek, these substances are widely accepted to produce a non-ordinary state of consciousness by ingesting them. The temple at Eleusis was destroyed by the Gothic invasion in 395 CE. Its relationship to Athens and its demise are perhaps instructive regarding contemporary considerations of psychedelic experiences. Greece had entered its "classical" period, focused on logic, cynicism, skepticism, and stoicism—all philosophies that denied the mystical and unconscious aspects of human endeavors. Hellenistic Greece became more rigid, and it finally ended with the death of Alexander the Great in 323 BCE. Unified Greece soon fell apart; wars and skirmishes plagued the Greek city-states until they were eventually conquered by the Roman Empire.

Across the world, from Greece to Asia and South and Central America, all ancient peoples have used non-ordinary states of consciousness to increase spiritual, psychological, or physical knowledge. Usually this is accomplished using a substance like psilocybin. Cultures like the Tsatan in Mongolia do this through practices like trance, and the Lakota, indigenous to North America, do so through multiple means, from inflicting pain during a ritual Sun Dance to sweat lodges.

Our hyperrational "modern" cultures in the West have long overlooked the value of altered states of consciousness and the importance of traditional practices in healing. In the United States and Europe, scientists banish anything smacking of mystical experience to the realms of religion, folklore, and psychosis. The scientific method demands reproducibility. The Cartesian ethos of *cogito ergo sum* (I think therefore I am) has for almost 500 years promoted the idea of the conscious mind being the seat of the individual psyche. While some psychologists and theologians have challenged this over the centuries, they have frequently been overruled. Science requires objective observation. When a transformation is happening at a subjective, individual level, observation isn't possible. In research, zero reproducibility equals zero effect.

Contemporary research into these states is proving that the transformative power of psychedelic experiences is partly responsible for psychological healing (the other parts are neurological or neurochemical). This is true whether the recipients are cancer patients facing their mortality or patients suffering from multiple years of treatment-resistant depression. Research into the effects of entheogens is opening doors for healing experiences that our ancestors across every continent once knew, and that Indigenous cultures in colonized areas have often shared to their detriment.

The Beginning of Psychedelic Science

In the United States it was the work of R. Gordon Wasson that opened the door to psychedelics in the 1960s. Wasson and his wife were amateur mycologists fascinated by mushrooms. Wasson was hardly a counterculture type. He was a respected executive at J. P. Morgan & Co. His research interests eventually led him to seek out "magic" mushrooms that were part of healing ceremonies in the Oaxaca region of Mexico. With typical colonial naïveté, he sought to understand and proselytize his "discovery." His 1957 photo essay, "Seeking the Magic Mushroom," in *Life* magazine shifted psilocybin mushrooms from their role in Indigenous healing to a postwar counterculture symbol in a world starving for meaning.

It didn't take long for Maria Sabina, the Indigenous shaman who first served Wasson psilocybin in her healing ritual or valada, to become a sought-after guru for seekers who ventured to her Oaxacan village of Huautla de Jiménez. Timothy Leary made a journey there, which began his research into the combination of psychology and psychedelics and led him to instruct an entire generation to "Turn on, tune in, drop out." The Beatles made the trek. Bob Dylan and Keith Richards are also reported to have made their way to her door. In the decades since these events took place writers, researchers, anthropologists, and Indigenous rights activists have all weighed in on the events that followed the publication of Wasson's essay. Sabina and Wasson are responsible for the reintroduction of psychedelics in the modern era. Their naïveté is also responsible for the watering down of the fungi's original sacredness. First, psychedelics became valued as a counterculture door to alternative spirituality, and more recently they've been studied for their potential as a powerful drug to treat intractable psychiatric problems.

In the 1950s and '60s Sandoz Laboratories provided LSD-25 (under the name Delysid) and psilocybin to researchers around the world who were experimenting with novel treatments for a myriad of problems. From alcohol dependence to schizophrenia, psychedelics were employed to treat suffering patients, and many experienced positive and profound changes in behavior. Starting in the 1950s British psychiatrist Humphry Osmond had successfully used LSD to treat alcoholism.[3] Osmond reported that a single dose had produced significant results. His patients continued to be alcohol-free 12 months after treatment. In medical research treatments, the outcomes that last more than 12 months are considered durable, and conditions are found to be in remission when there are no more symptoms. Osmond's first patients suffering from alcoholism reported 100% remission after 12 months following just a single dose of LSD.

Osmond pioneered the use of LSD in hospitals, marrying it with traditional psychotherapy, art therapy, and movement therapies. While these are common practices now, they were considered novel and edgy when he introduced them. Osmond and his colleague John Smythies administered LSD to more than 2,000 patients for alcohol dependence by the end of the 1960s and reported that 40% of their patients experienced durable effects, with remission of alcoholism present one year

after treatment.[4] The pair also experimented with mescaline derived from the San Pedro cactus. Osmond and Smythies noted that patients who had been administered mescaline demonstrated behaviors like those of patients with schizophrenia. This led the duo to conclude that schizophrenia was a malady of brain chemistry. Their hypothesis was widely derided and dismissed, though today managing schizophrenia is achieved through altering the brain chemistry of those suffering from this disease.

Timothy Leary and Richard Alpert (later known as Ram Dass) began their Harvard Psilocybin Project after Leary's visit to Mexico to visit Maria Sabina in 1960.[5] The staid Harvard psychology department proved somewhat skeptical, but it was not immediately dismissive. At the time, LSD-25 and psilocybin were not illegal substances, and the research potential was being pursued by other well-respected psychiatrists and psychologists. But in 1962, a Harvard Divinity School student named Walter Pahnke undertook an experiment under the ostensible supervision of Leary and Alpert. The double-blind study took place on Good Friday in the Marsh Chapel on the campus of Boston University.[6] Pahnke was curious whether divinity students who were obviously already inclined toward religion would have a religious or mystically laden experience under the influence of psilocybin. Twenty divinity students participated. Ten received niacin as an active placebo, meaning that they felt some physical effect (niacin makes one feel flushed) but didn't receive any psychoactive substance. The other ten received psilocybin. The students who had received the psilocybin reported experiences that Pahnke determined were indistinguishable from other mystical experiences that happen organically. This opened a door even wider into both the possible positive effects of psilocybin and the dangers of doing sloppy research in controversial areas.[7]

However, Pahnke failed to report the occurrence of some adverse effects in the psilocybin group. And in another experiment Leary was accused of administering psilocybin to an undergraduate student off campus, a violation of a previous rule that had been set by the Harvard psychology department. Their sloppy, cavalier attitude toward research—with accusations of sharing psilocybin more as a recreational drug than a research endeavor—got the pair into hot water. After much hand-wringing and attempts to corral their research protocols, Leary and Alpert were dismissed from Harvard.[8] The dismissal made them famous—or infamous, depending on your point of view—and it cemented their status as outcasts not just from Harvard, but from the academy more broadly. As psilocybin became popularized through the countercultural narrative in the 1960s and '70s, a backlash against psychedelics arose.

Leary was a polarizing figure. He reported that his trip to Mexico in 1960 was the most important experience of his life,[9] and he dedicated his efforts to popularizing, studying, and assisting others in their psychedelic pursuits. After being dismissed from Harvard in 1963, Leary found himself at times writing books on spirituality, leading antiwar protests, going to prison, being a fugitive from the law, living in exile in Algeria, and engaging in public debates with his onetime nemesis G. Gordon Liddy, who would later go on to Watergate fame. Leary was once called "the most dangerous man in America" by President Richard

Nixon. His greatest contribution was as an outspoken evangelist, extolling the benefits of psychedelics as gateways to enlightenment, an alternative to the buttoned-down life he was raised to embrace.

Prior to Leary's popularization of psychedelics, hundreds of people had participated in clinical trials of LSD, psilocybin, mescaline, ibogaine, and other psychedelic substances. Enthusiastic and hopeful experimentation flourished from 1950 to 1965. Some 40,000 people were treated with LSD or psilocybin, and more than 1,000 research papers were published in scientific journals. Like many early research projects, many of those studies were exploratory, with small numbers of participants and no control groups. The results were encouraging. The direction for more robust studies was set.

But in 1965 Sandoz Laboratories stopped producing psychedelics after public concern increased pressure on the company. Toward the end of the 1960s the countercultural revolution was in full swing, the Vietnam War was dividing the country, and highly charged desegregation efforts were contributing to a sense of Americans' feeling unmoored. Music, drugs, and the attending counterculture were blamed as the catalyst for all of society's ills at the end of the 1960s. To constrain these movements, President Richard Nixon signed the Controlled Substances Act into law in 1970. This law segregated substances into five "schedules" or classes of drugs that needed to be regulated based on the danger of abuse, addiction, or health risk. One of the positive aspects of the law was that it created a "cradle-to-grave" system for substances, so that manufacturers would be responsible for tracking the creation and distribution of their medicines.

This ensured that medications weren't tainted and that substances' purity, potency, and safety could be tracked across domains from synthesis to administration.

Schedule I includes drugs that are considered to have no known medical use, are easily abused, and have no safe means of administration. According to the official definition Schedule I drugs have a high potential for abuse or dependence, and include heroin, marijuana, and cocaine. Schedule II drugs have a known medical application and can be prescribed, dispensed by pharmacies, or administered in hospitals; they include morphine, codeine, oxycodone, and fentanyl. Schedule III drugs have moderate potential for abuse and include aspirin, ibuprofen, ketamine, and acetaminophen. Schedule IV drugs have even less potential for abuse, but still have some—they include benzodiazepines like diazepam (Valium) and alprazolam (Xanax). Schedule V drugs are considered to have the least likelihood of abuse among controlled substances; these include medicines like the cough medicine Robitussin and drugs used for allergy symptoms.

In the system created to support the 1970 Controlled Substances Act, the drugs considered most dangerous are the Schedule I drugs. Included on the list (in addition to those listed in the previous paragraph) are psilocybin, LSD, MDMA, peyote, and several others. The inclusion of some drugs in certain schedules was somewhat arbitrary and, according to some activists, racist, as at the time of the passage of the law substances like marijuana were more likely to be used in communities of color. The current research into the medical use of cannabis, and more recently psychedelics, aims to change the classification of these substances by demonstrating that they can be safely administered and that they have been proven effective as medications with positive treatment outcomes.

Resurrected after Decades of the War on Drugs

In the 1980s Rick Doblin formed the foundation of what is now called the Multidisciplinary Association for Psychedelic Studies (MAPS). The group didn't garner much attention even as Doblin made plans to create substantive research agendas and gathered a group of well-respected researchers, policymakers, and socially prominent people at the Esalen Institute to discuss the future of psychedelics. In the last 30 years MAPS has focused on developing rigorous protocols for large cohort studies of psychedelics, the most notable being its multiyear studies on using MDMA in the treatment of post-traumatic stress disorder (PTSD).[10]

Research opportunities became possible again thanks to the pioneering work of Rick Doblin and other brave leaders in the field. In 1996 medical researcher Rick Strassman at the University of New Mexico reported on the experience of research participants administered N,N-dimethyltryptamine, also known simply as DMT. Strassman and his research team observed that subjects experienced elevated blood pressure, heart rate, and elevated blood concentrations of growth hormone, beta-endorphin, corticotropin, cortisol, and prolactin. They found DMT to be short acting (approximately 30 minutes in duration) compared to other serotonergic psychedelics like LSD and psilocybin, whose effects can last hours. Subjects reported similar strong, vivid, and comforting psychedelic experiences despite their short duration.[11]

In 1998 Franz Vollenweider[12] at the University of Zurich's Medical School demonstrated that psychedelics like psilocybin activate serotonin 5-HT2A receptors in the brain. This neurological pathway is important, as the 5-HT2A receptors are widely distributed throughout the central nervous system and play an outsize role in learning and cognition. When there is disruption in the system of neurotransmitters in the 5-HT2A system, it is common to find dramatic changes in behavior and function. Depending on which systems are affected, psychologists and psychiatrists may diagnose someone with obsessive-compulsive disorder (OCD), schizophrenia, addiction, depression, or other conditions.

Prior to investigating psychedelics, Roland Griffiths studied the effects on brain chemistry of substances such as caffeine, nicotine, and cocaine, and the likelihood of their abuse. In 2019 the Center for Psychedelic and Consciousness Research launched at Johns Hopkins University. Griffiths published a paper in 2016 examining the effects of psilocybin on a group of patients with terminal cancer.[13] It showed that patients who had been administered a psychedelic had durable decreases in depression and anxiety. Then after completing a separate study of patients who were administered psilocybin to help them quit smoking,[14] Griffiths noted that both the cancer patients and the smokers had

reported mystical experiences and both groups had decreased activity in the default mode network (DMN) in the brain.[15]

The DMN is a connected set of neural structures that are responsible for our everyday processing. Parts of the DMN include the amygdala, the hippocampus, and the temporal lobe. In disorders like OCD, anxiety, and depression, imaging studies have demonstrated that the DMN is overly active. The possibility that a medicine could deactivate the DMN while preserving function is revolutionary. Up to this point, most psychiatric medications have focused on blunting symptoms. Traditional antidepressant medications work by reducing feeling and access to emotion overall. Common psychopharmaceuticals and antipsychotic medications blunt libido and create a flat, anhedonic mood, and many cause weight gain, not to mention other side effects that must be monitored. This often discourages patients who want to experience a range of emotions in life, especially those who have been on psychotropic medications before.

As of this writing there are more than 100 active studies listed at clinicaltrials.gov using psilocybin to treat various conditions. That list doesn't include past studies or privately funded research, but it shows that the humble mushroom could change psychiatry as we know it. A new tool that improves clinical outcomes without daily dosing is a revolution that doctors and patients are more than ready for.

and into the forest I go, to lose my mind, and find my soul.

—JOHN MUIR

CHAPTER 2

Mushrooms as Medicine

Neuroanatomy, Neurochemistry, and Psilocybin

The study of neuroscience has had a boom in the last two decades because of new research, some of it from investigations into psychedelics and other substances at the molecular level. If, like me, you find yourself getting curious about neuroscience as a result, I highly recommend deeper study on the topic. There's not a moment I don't find myself fascinated. To keep us focused, I'm going to direct my work here to the areas that are relevant to psilocybin and psychedelic therapy and experiences. But please know that this topic is vast, and the research that's going on now is opening pathways for the next hundred years of neuroscience, in which psychedelics are poised to play a significant role.

The neuronal architecture of our nervous system is complex. Neurons and their expansive structures permeate the whole body. Every system of the body is innervated, with neurons (nerves) connected to the structures that make the systems function together as a whole. When a neuron or nerve is in the brain or spinal cord, it is called a neuron, but when it is elsewhere in the body, connected to muscle

or organs, it is called a nerve. Signals travel along nerve fibers from every part of the body to the spinal cord, which carries those signals to the brain. The brain acts as both a conductor and respondent to millions of signals in a day. Signals travel from the brain and back through the spinal cord in microseconds. The system of neurons within the human body and its communication structure is incredibly complex and efficient. Everything from hunger and heart rate to pain and pleasure are generated, accelerated, and decelerated by the nervous system.

But how does all of this work? And why does it matter for the study of psychedelics? Psychedelics are interesting in relation to neuroscience and evolutionary biology for similar reasons. The molecules in psychedelics act structurally and functionally like neurotransmitters in the body. This is because both the neurotransmitters in the body and the compounds in mushrooms are forms of chemicals called tryptamines. These molecules are derived from the amino acid tryptophan, and they are used throughout nature. In the human body, serotonin is a particularly important tryptamine; it is not produced in great amounts in the brain, but it is pervasive in systems from the brain to the digestive system.

Thinking about these compounds from a functional perspective leads to both a better understanding of our bodies and the world around us, as well as to fascinating philosophical problems. Why would a compound in a mushroom growing on the detritus of a dead tree have a similar structure to a critical chemical in the mammalian brain? Is it because all things that communicate via networks use similar types of compounds? (Nerve fibers and mycelia do look surprisingly similar, implying similar function.) Is there a biological connection between people and fungi? What does evolution say about commonalities between organisms that aren't just different species but are categorized into wholly different kingdoms of living beings?

Researchers have known since the 1950s that neurotransmitters play a critical role in how the nervous system functions. There are many neurotransmitters that work in the body. The most important ones are glutamate, GABA, adrenaline/epinephrine, norepinephrine, acetylcholine, dopamine, and serotonin. These seven neurotransmitters have more than 100 variations that act on specific receptors inside our nervous systems. In psychedelic studies, you'll often see researchers refer to "classic psychedelics"; when they use this term they are describing serotonergic psychedelics, or substances that work on the serotonin pathways of the nervous system. The reason traditional psychedelics—lysergic acid diethylamide (LSD), psilocybin, N,N-dimethyltryptamine (DMT) and mescaline—are so powerful is because they act on the same pathways as serotonin, hence the term *serotonergic*.

To dive into these questions and why they are important, a little basic neuroscience knowledge is useful. In this chapter we'll get a little nerdy with the science, and we'll discuss ways of thinking about psilocybin and other psychedelic compounds in order to help you understand what's happening to your brain in the presence of these powerful substances.

What Is a Neuron and How Does It Work?

For hundreds of years scientists have created an artificial separation between the body and the brain. In some texts you'll see this described as the mind/body problem. Philosophically, you'll hear this idea resonating in Rene Descartes's famous dictum, *cogito ergo sum*: "I think therefore I am." Descartes was trying to make a point that it is the capacity for abstract thought that makes human beings different from animals, plants, and, dare we say, fungi. But while we can point to variations in brain structure between ourselves and other animals, we really have no idea whether or not those beings are "thinking" in the same way that we are. However, based on our brain structures, we can presume that there is a fundamental difference.

What we do know is that since the time of Descartes, we have separated ourselves from the other living things on our planet. What's more critical, though, is that we have separated ourselves from ourselves. The basic biology of the nervous system should remind us that we are not a brain simply directing a meat suit that's walking around. The same types of neurons that accumulate in the brain populate our entire body. It's just that the

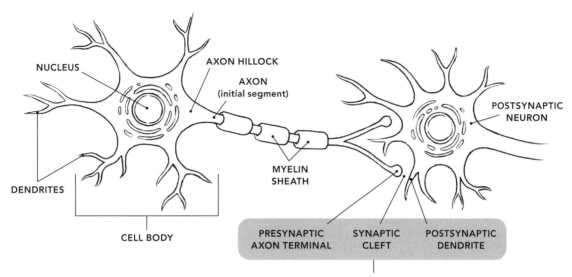

NUCLEUS

AXON HILLOCK

AXON
(initial segment)

POSTSYNAPTIC
NEURON

DENDRITES

MYELIN
SHEATH

CELL BODY

PRESYNAPTIC
AXON TERMINAL

SYNAPTIC
CLEFT

POSTSYNAPTIC
DENDRITE

SYNAPSE—the region where an axon terminal
communicates with its postsynaptic target cell

neurons in the brain are more densely congregated and organized for more efficient and complex communication. That density and complexity organizes itself around structures with simultaneously specific and diffuse functions.

A neuron is a complex cell. It has a nucleus, a cell body, an axon, dendrites, and a complex microcellular structure. For our purposes, the most important area to understand is the synaptic cleft. This part of the neuron sits at the outer edge of the structure, making it the chemical gateway of the neuron. It is the boundary between the synapse—or the area between neurons and the neuron itself. This chemical doorway between neurons is the place where they spill their neurotransmitters and other chemical compounds. The action in the synaptic cleft determines what a neuron does and, in turn, how we experience our own consciousness.

Science loves metaphors for helping to explain complex phenomena. If you were thinking of the structure of the synaptic cleft on a macro level, the best metaphor would be a shipping port. We understand that the different commercial ships in a port are run by different companies with varying specialties. Some ships might sail regionally, moving cargo around the country and into rail yards; other ships might focus on private commercial travel, like fancy cruises. Cargo ships deliver shipping containers across the ocean. We are familiar with different sizes of ships, and we understand that some are meant for traveling short distances, while others are meant for taking longer trips. In thinking about docking a boat or a ship, we inherently understand that the whole reason for a dock is to secure a vessel so that it can be loaded and unloaded. There is water in between the boat and land, and the dock is there to help secure the boat so that people can move their cargo wherever it needs to go.

Each boat or ship has a brand, and because of their different purposes, their presence

THE SYNAPTIC CLEFT

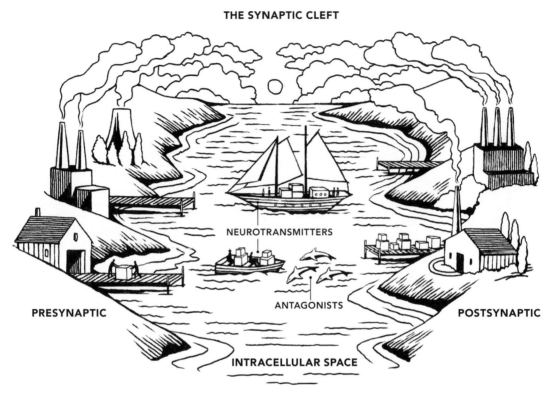

NEUROTRANSMITTERS

ANTAGONISTS

PRESYNAPTIC

POSTSYNAPTIC

INTRACELLULAR SPACE

requires different groups, activities, and functions to take place. An international voyage will need to gather more people and resources around it relative to a shorter domestic trip, which might consist of a quick sail between two cities located along the same coast. Water is also useful for our understanding of this concept, because between the neurons in the synaptic cleft the intercellular space is filled with liquid into which different compounds and molecules are released. The substances then facilitate what happens in the neuron—that is, the sending and receiving of signals from your brain.

You might have learned in high school or college biology that the activities of the neuron begin with the creation of action potentials through the work of potassium and sodium ions in the brain. It's kind of like priming a pump in a boat's engine room. Once these actions begin in the neuronal structure, the action potential is there, revving the engine and waiting to release the boat. Once the boat is ready to go, a cascade of neurochemicals is released into the waters of the intercellular space. Neurons are limited in what kinds of neurotransmitters they can produce, but they are more diverse in the types of neurotransmitters that they receive. A neuron might produce one neurotransmitter, like glutamate, (the most widely produced neurotransmitter), but it might have receptors for several others, like glutamate, serotonin, and GABA.

Once the neurotransmitters are released by the neurons that produced them, the action potential releases the boat from the dock, energizing it so that it can make its journey. The boat is branded and filled with whatever unique cargo has been produced by the neuron—that is, glutamate, serotonin, GABA, etc. It then sails across the intercellular space, or the space between cells, on the other side of which are specific docks that have the right crews waiting to manage the boat's neurotransmitter cargo when it comes into port. Importantly, this system is integrated. When one side gets enough serotonin (or other type of neurotransmitter) it tells the other neurons to hold back production. This helps maintain a delicate balance in the neuronal channels, and this signaling system becomes critically important when using some kinds of medicines that affect serotonin, because the body will respond to artificial levels of serotonin or serotonin-like compounds (like psilocybin) by slowing down production of naturally occurring serotonin. This effect can be mild or, in some cases like serotonin syndrome, dangerous.

Most neurons can produce only one type of neurotransmitter, like a factory that sits at the edge of a dock in our metaphorical shipping port. As we know, a neuron might only be able to create one type of neurotransmitter, but its receptors are able to receive many different types of neurotransmitters. However, too much of a particular neurotransmitter can be dangerous; too little and the system doesn't work efficiently, which can lead to negative consequences. To help manage this balance, when the skipper of the neuronal boat realizes that there is too much of a particular chemical in the waters, they'll send up a flare that tells the other workers on the docks that they need to send an inhibitor or antagonist. Like a school of dolphins, these inhibitory

neurotransmitters make their way to the docks on the other side and block them. This system of docks is quite specific on the production side of things and more generalized on the receptor side of the equation. Specific neurotransmitters can fit into a few different docks. How a neurotransmitter binds to its dock then determines what actions come next. Blocking those docks means that some neurotransmitters just sit in the water, and eventually they will be recycled. This recycling process is called reuptake.

Complexity and flexibility are built into this system. If your brain finds there isn't enough serotonin in the boats, the system can block other neurotransmitters to make more room for more serotonin (or GABA, adrenaline, etc.). Sometimes the way to make sure more neurotransmitters are available is to leave them in the water for a longer period of time before recycling. This is how drugs called reuptake inhibitors work. Another way to get more of a particular kind of neurotransmitter is simply to activate more serotonin release, which is a little more difficult to do, since less of it is produced. The system is flexible and provides multiple ways to achieve the goal of increasing any particular neurotransmitter concentration when needed.

For our purposes in this book, we will focus on serotonergic substances like psilocybin and their activities. In pharmacology-speak, psilocybin is what is called a prodrug. This means that the body takes the form it's given—psilocybin—and transforms it into a compound that can actually be used by the body: psilocin. This secondary compound is not unique to the human body. Psilocin is found in psychedelic mushrooms and a handful of other organic materials. As a molecule it is relatively unstable and short lived. Psilocybin is more stable. When psilocybin is digested, the body sends it to the liver to have one of its phosphate groups removed, thereby transforming it into psilocin. This process takes about 20–30 minutes, which is approximately the amount of time after which most people will start to feel the effects associated with psychedelics. Sometimes in a clinical environment, psilocybin is administered intravenously, in which case the effects are almost immediate. Psilocin and psilocybin are very similar in structure to serotonin. As such they can fit into the receptors/ports that on most days make room for, and process, serotonin.

While neurons that *produce* serotonin are not very prolific in the brain (about one per 1 million), receptors that can recognize and use serotonin are found across all the different brain structures and in other parts of the nervous system as well. From a behavioral viewpoint, serotonin is involved in almost everything that we consider psychological. Mood, perception, anger, aggressive behavior, reward, appetite, sexuality, memory, attention, and many others all are mediated by the presence of this one neurotransmitter.

Serotonin is also implicated in a number of mental health challenges. Studies have shown that people with treatment-resistant depression have fewer active serotonin receptors in strategic areas of the brain. People who suffer from schizophrenia show damage in a critical portion of the brain where a substantial portion of serotonin is created and used (the raphe nuclei). In addition, some people with a genetic predisposition toward low serotonin efficiency may experience problems in their moods that may look like, or actually be diagnosed as, a form of bipolar disorder.

In recent years the *Diagnostic and Statistical Manual of Mental Disorders*[1] has collapsed all of the forms of bipolar disorder into one diagnosis. Currently bipolar disorder is diagnosed simply as either bipolar I, which is characterized by more episodes of mania and fewer episodes of depression, and bipolar II, which you would correctly suspect is characterized by less-intense and fewer instances of mania and more instances of depression. Previous diagnosis standards included a milder form of bipolar disorder called cyclothymic disorder, which proved useful because it made room for subclinical presentations that may not be detectable by most patients and therefore not cause serious problems. These helped psychologists and psychiatrists make better recommendations for patients. Today, cyclothymia doesn't appear as a diagnosis in the *DSM*. This is an important distinction because someone who has subclinical tendencies toward a serotonin disorder should be cautious when using any serotonergic substance like psilocybin. A person with cyclothymia might be more sensitive to psilocybin than someone else. Maybe the *DSM* will reconsider this in the next edition.

An interesting fact about serotonin is that it is more widely distributed outside of the brain than within, with the largest concentrations circulating in the bloodstream and found in the digestive system. Receptors for serotonin populate multiple nerve systems, including the concentrations around the heart and the gut. This proliferation implies that serotonin has a much larger role in biology than previously thought, one that researchers in medicine and neuroscience are actively working to understand. The implication for a person taking psychedelics is that depending on your own personal neurobiology and the types of mushrooms or psychedelics that you may choose to work with, the sensations could ripple in a complex combination of places, including your intestines, heart, or head. Anywhere your body or brain can use serotonin, it can also use psilocin/psilocybin, though the effects of the drug will mostly be experienced at the level of consciousness, meaning in the brain and central nervous system.

The Brain's Key Structures

The brain has a complex architecture that we are only beginning to understand. Since the beginning of the study of medicine, understanding the brain has been seen as a critical endeavor. We have used whatever metaphors were available to discuss the way the brain works. When we didn't have language to describe electricity or machinery, the brain's workings were explained using the imagery of liquids via the form of the four humors (blood, black bile, yellow bile, and phlegm). When we began to develop pneumatic machinery, the brain was likened to a hydraulic engine. With the discovery of electricity, we began to think of the brain as receiving impulses across nerves that were themselves conceived of as wires, with the spark of life being likened to an electrical current. In the age of computers, we think of the brain as a central computer. While each of these metaphors has allowed scientists to make sense of the brain and its various functions, none of them is capable of encapsulating exactly what the brain is and how it works. The brain is more significant and meaningful than any metaphor we have to describe it.

For decades researchers have debated whether the functionality of the brain can be mapped onto its structure, or if the connections and networks that exist within the brain are redundant and flexible enough to allow certain functions to move to different areas. The process by which this happens is called neuroplasticity. The merging of functionality with a topographical understanding of the brain has changed how we understand the brain's capacity over the course of the last century. We now know that the brain is dynamic. It changes and can grow or atrophy throughout the course of a person's lifespan. The first scientific progress into understanding the brain began with associating particular regions of the brain with discrete functions. The research into topology and function began as a result of examining patients who had survived severe traumas and for whom critical functions were either lost or enhanced.

There is ongoing interest into how functions migrate across the cortex or outer structure to other areas of the brain. There is ample research to show that after injury or stroke, the brain will often heal by migrating a function (or functions) to a new area of the brain. We now know that the structure and substructures of the brain are not exclusive, independent areas. We have learned that neuronal hubs and pathways organize themselves following the principle that form follows function. When there's injury or a specific need, the brain is complex enough to allow for some aggregation and healing, which means that neuronal structures may diversify to support more complex function.

In the last 70 years neuroscience research has exploded as people have begun to explore ways that neurons interconnect into proximal

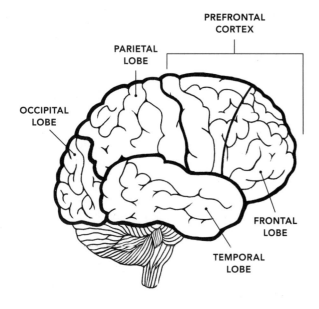

PREFRONTAL CORTEX

PARIETAL LOBE

OCCIPITAL LOBE

FRONTAL LOBE

TEMPORAL LOBE

(close) and distal (distant) networks in the cerebral cortex. The latest research shows that the brain organizes itself around network hubs that interconnect and function in complex synchronies. These networks first share information between themselves and then to the rest of the central and peripheral nervous systems. Of these, the default mode network (DMN) is one of the most critical to our well-being, and one of the most recently researched. Investigations into the DMN have changed our understanding of the brain's structure and function. We will spend a little time discussing the basic neuroscience so that when we discuss the effects of related tryptamines like psilocin and psilocybin you will have a working understanding of how your brain interacts with these compounds, and how the structures of your brain respond to outside stimuli.

THE PREFRONTAL CORTEX

For decades we have considered the prefrontal cortex (PFC) to be the seat of memory, logic, and critical thinking. This is based on studies of patients who have suffered lesions or injury to this part of the brain. The PFC extends from the middle of the skull forward to the face and forehead. Research indicates that the function of the PFC centers on memory, but perhaps not in the static ways that earlier models implied. The latest research shows that the PFC receives inputs from multiple network hubs within the cerebral cortex. In addition, the PFC also sends signals to hubs inside the brain and to various areas in the peripheral and autonomic nervous systems.

The most interesting data in the current research on the prefrontal cortex is the interdependence between regions. If either the PFC or an area with which it is in regular communication—for example the hippocampus—is injured, then both areas may degenerate or atrophy over time.[2] In other words, an injury to an area that is connected to another area may eventually create impairment or cellular death in the connected area as well.

The function of the PFC was first defined by examining cases of people who had survived devastating injuries. Phineas Gage is probably the most famous of these examples. His was the first case that showed how a severe injury to the brain might impact the behavior, demeanor, and personality of a human being. In 1848, Gage was a railroad foreman. While setting explosives on a patch of land in Vermont that was meant for a new railroad line, Gage suffered a destructive injury when an accidental detonation launched a tamping spike through his face and brain like a javelin.

Miraculously, he survived, though the spike cut through his face beneath the jawbone and exited out of the top of his skull. A huge portion of the left lobe of Gage's PFC was destroyed, and connections to the temporal lobe and its structures were severed.

Gage lost the use of his left eye and reportedly became unable to regulate his emotions after his injury. Contemporaries reported that Gage went from being a well-mannered young man to someone who was ill-tempered, used the most obscene profanity, and became quickly angry and agitated. Neuroscientists are still interested in Gage's story. He survived for 12 years after his injury, working jobs like driving a long-distance stagecoach, which required planning and logic, therefore implying migration and/or preserved function of the PFC. Gage died in 1860 from an epileptic seizure that was certainly a result of his injury 12 years earlier.[3]

Damage to the PFC often impacts the ability to learn and perform tasks like reading and spatial organization; it can also affect one's ability to connect thoughts with feelings. Current research into the functions of this area of the brain reveals that the prefrontal cortex integrates data about context, memory, complexity, history, and future forecasting from multiple areas in the brain, including the amygdala, the hippocampus, and other cortical structures. In this context, the PFC appears to be a complexity engine. This section of the brain conducts ideas, context, and future planning into an elegant symphony that defines higher-order thinking.[4] This part of the brain also appears to be filled with 5-HT2A receptors, which implicates the PFC in psychedelic experiences and neuroplasticity,

as will be discussed a little later in this chapter. In the last two decades researchers have discovered that the brain engages in communication of hierarchal layers across hubs and nodes of neurons. Depending on where the brain's attention is directed, different networks in the cortex activate or deactivate in response. A particular network is activated, depending on whether the stimuli is coming from an internal or external source.[5]

THE TEMPORAL LOBES

The temporal lobes are often associated with emotion and memory. This may be because of the proximity of the neurons in this area to the hippocampus and the amygdala. Many of the critical structures of the brain appear underneath the blobby mass of the cortex and are situated toward the spinal cord. Those that inhabit the deepest part of the cortex have connections and protrusions into other areas of the brain, like the temporal lobes. The temporal lobes are found on either side of the brain behind the "temples" of the forehead and extend just past the ears. Parts and connections of the hippocampus and amygdalae extend into the temporal lobes. The temporal lobe includes functional anatomy that supports olfactory (smell), visual, language, auditory, and semantic memory. We will go into a little more detail later with regard to the specific areas of the temporal lobes that are relevant to the default mode network, but know that there are many areas in the temporal lobes that are serotonergic, implying that psilocybin and other tryptamines will have a deeper effect on areas within the temporal lobes and therefore a deeper impact on emotion, memory, and olfactory and auditory stimuli.

THE DEFAULT MODE NETWORK AND ITS PARTS

The default mode network (DMN) was first described in 2001 by Marcus Raichle and his team at Washington University in St. Louis, Missouri.[6] The work of this research team built on previous work by Gordon Shulman, also at Washington University in St. Louis.[7] That earlier research had detailed what appeared to be synchronization between different areas of the brain while it was at rest. Raichle's team conducted imaging studies that specifically looked at what was happening inside the brain when it was not given a specific task. Their discovery completely changed how neuroscientists and psychologists think about the brain.

The researchers observed that when subjects participating in the study were asked to do nothing but either close their eyes or look at a small crosshair image on a blank screen, their brains lit up in similar ways. Specifically, there were areas of the brain that were "on" when the subject was not engaged in a task. The original research identified that the brain rested in a "default mode" when not given a specific task to complete. Researchers noticed that when a subject was resting, this network was active, and this name stuck after their original paper describing the DMN was published.

When the same subject in the study was asked to think of something specific and to engage in a task like identifying a color on a screen or studying a list of words, the DMN would deactivate, and other areas of the brain would increase their activity. Researchers were

able to observe these changes in a functional magnetic resonance imaging machine. When subjects were at rest, the areas associated with the DMN lit up, and when the same subjects were asked to engage in a given task, the DMN would deactivate, and other brain networks would light up. This has led to more than two decades of research into the DMN. We now know that the DMN is implicated in several areas that are associated with over-thinking, ruminating, anxiety, and depression. The following areas of the brain are the most significant for understanding the DMN, relative to our purposes in this book:

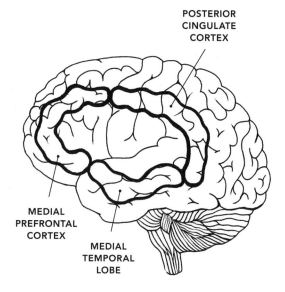

POSTERIOR CINGULATE CORTEX

MEDIAL PREFRONTAL CORTEX

MEDIAL TEMPORAL LOBE

THE MEDIAL PREFRONTAL CORTEX

The medial prefrontal cortex (mPFC) is located in the front middle part of the brain. It is sometimes described as the central switchboard of the nervous system because it takes in data from disparate parts of the brain and sends messages to update various systems in response. Research has demonstrated that the mPFC assists in regulating consciousness, self-awareness, motivation, emotions, and social behavior and understanding. It is the central place for self-referential thinking, meaning that when you are imagining yourself in any activity, you are engaging the mPFC. Dysregulation or injury to the mPFC has been implicated in several diseases like Parkinson's and Alzheimer's. Lack of development in or damage to this area has been implicated in depression, anxiety disorders, schizophrenia, and autism spectrum disorders.

THE POSTERIOR CINGULATE CORTEX

We know less about the posterior cingulate cortex (PCC) than any other area of the brain that has been identified to date.[8] Before the advent of complex imaging techniques, the majority of studies on structure and function were based on examining cases of people who suffered from invasive tumors or injuries in a specific area of the brain. The PCC occupies a place in the brain that hasn't been the subject of many studies based on malfunction or injury. Instead, this area of the brain has only recently been isolated from surrounding structures in functional imaging studies. The PCC benefits from the greatest density of blood vessels in the brain structure, giving it ample access to oxygenated blood. This is important for multiple reasons, including risk for stroke, but more important, the ready access to oxygen-rich blood implies that this part of the brain performs a critical function. The most consistent theme across research of the PCC is its role with regard to episodic memory. The PCC is often activated in retrieving memory, but it shows less activation in creating memory. Further, the PCC is activated more

profoundly during tasks where research subjects are asked to focus on subjective memory and the details of those memories. So, when you're thinking about that time that you went on a waterslide in Idaho wearing a purple bathing suit with your cousin Timmy, you're definitely engaging the PCC. This has led researchers to think of the PCC as a contextualization engine. It works in concert with the mPFC and other structures to make sure that the experience being reflected on is in the proper context.[9]

THE MEDIAL TEMPORAL LOBE AND LATERAL TEMPORAL CORTEX

As mentioned, the temporal lobes are associated with emotion and memory. There are many complex structures in these areas of the brain. Their functions are manifold, including everything from emotional awareness to language centers. To keep things simple, we'll focus on the amygdala and the hippocampus, two structures located in the medial temporal lobe (MTL) and lateral temporal cortex (LTC) that activate during emotional situations and help us create memories that make sense of our experiences. The amygdala is actually not one structure but two (plural: amygdalae), one on either side of the corpus callosum that gives the brain its well-known appearance of two halves divided by a center line. The amygdala's name comes from the Latin word for almond, because each of the halves shares that same shape. Though the role of the amygdala is still an active area of scientific research, the historical view has been that this structure regulates the brain's responses to threat, aggression, and our sense of safety.[10] This structure can activate and process a threat before you are even aware of it. A signal will come from the eyes, ears, nose, or peripheral nervous system, and the amygdala will respond in milliseconds. Immediately glucose elevation signals energize the muscles, telling them to run, and signals are sent to the adrenal glands, which then release adrenaline to help prepare to either make a quick getaway or engage in a fight. How many of us have noticed our own reactions—like hitting the brakes or deflecting a tennis ball to the head—only *after* we've already safely avoided a threat? That's the amygdala at work. Though historically we've associated this small structure as wholly focused on threat, new research is proving more intriguing. Contemporary studies reveal the amygdala's capacity to discern and make meaning of incoming sensory data in more nuanced ways. We still see the amygdala as a threat detector, but soon we may learn that there is much more to this small, critical structure.[11]

The hippocampus is necessary for the formation of memory. Its name derives from the fact that structurally its shape resembles a seahorse. The word for seahorse in Greek is *hippocampus*. The Greeks could be very literal: *hippo* = horse, and *kampos* = sea monster. Patients with damage to the hippocampus struggle with forming and retrieving memory, especially when it comes to new tasks learned after a hippocampal injury. Research into the function and connectivity of the hippocampus is ongoing, with new details emerging about how this component of the brain integrates spatial information and new data into memory.[12] These two structures, the amygdala and hippocampus, work together to transform experience into useful data. Other functions associated with structures that reside within the MTL and LTC include emotional

processing, olfactory processing (smell), as well as auditory (hearing) and motor (muscle action) connectivity.[13] They connect to the hubs of the mPFC and PCC via the amygdala and hippocampus in an elegant design that allows the brain to function with or without conscious awareness.

The DMN and Psilocybin

Robin Carhart-Harris of the University of California, San Francisco, and Imperial College London has developed a revolutionary theory of neurodynamics.[14] He calls it entropic brain theory. Carhart-Harris's background in both neuroscience and psychoanalysis guided him and his team to make connections between the types of altered consciousness experienced when using psychedelics and states of consciousness that might have existed before the evolutionary development of the DMN and its characteristic synchronization of brain activity. Over multiple studies Carhart-Harris and his research collaborators explain that the brain on psychedelics appears to lose its synchronization abilities, a state Carhart-Harris aligns with the principle in Newtonian physics called entropy.[15]

If you took a physics class in high school or college, you might recall that entropy is an active state of falling out of organization. Some people liken it to decay, but that term sometimes gives the wrong impression of how entropy works. The second law of thermodynamics in physics states that while all systems move toward entropy or disorganization, the overall entropy in a system remains constant. It's kind of like what happens to an old Chevy left sitting in a driveway. Even if the car is old, if you maintain it and keep it in good working order, it will still be able to run. But if the car sits and you never touch it, it will degrade, rust, and fall apart. The gaskets will dry out, mechanisms of the engine will seize up, the brakes will fade. The act of ongoing disintegration of the car is a *form* of entropy, not the result of entropy. The system of the car moves toward further and further states of disorganization over time as nature reclaims the car molecule by molecule, returning its structures to particles of rust and steel.

The entropic brain theory proposes that when the brain is exposed to psilocybin and other classic psychedelics, its state of entropy will increase, becoming more disorganized as its synchronization efforts are interrupted by the psychedelic experience. The implication of this theory is that a "normal" brain state requires the brain have a dynamic relationship with its internal structures. According to Carhart-Harris, this dynamic state generates a form of consciousness that identifies with a person's internal ego for stability. From a psychoanalytic perspective, without this internal ego, the brain is more likely to fall into a state of increased entropy. The experience of the personal ego consciousness is the psychic structure that corresponds to the feeling of being "whole" or the experience of "I am." Carhart-Harris argues that this capacity for the internal ego to provide a sense of psychic stability allows adolescent and adult humans to experience their consciousness differently from babies or animals.[16]

Babies, for example, identify with other babies and with their mothers for the first two years of their lives, more or less. They are unaware of their individual differentiation, which is why when one baby starts to cry

pretty soon any other babies nearby will cry as well. The ability to create a reference to the self in its current state alongside an abstraction of the self from which a person can plan for the future or imagine alternative options is the result of the synchronization of hubs in the brain. The self becomes a self *because* of the limiting container of the ego, not in spite of it. Based on this theory, the experience of the ego or the "I" is wholly dependent on the self-reference that exists as a result of the DMN and its related brain structures.

In one of the studies that informed this theory, Carhart-Harris and his team performed a meta-analysis of studies looking for neural correlates of the psychedelic state. Carhart-Harris and his team found that in modern studies using imaging techniques there was significant decoupling of critical areas like the PCC of the DMN from other areas like the hippocampus while using psychedelics.[17]

The state of normal waking consciousness is defined by structural hierarchies. Without them, the brain can't prioritize information from the environment or from a person's internal homeostatic functions. The higher entropy state experienced while under the influence of psychedelics (i.e., more disorganized) is likened to what researchers call a "primary" state of consciousness. This state is hypothesized to be more in line with what infants and animals experience of themselves. Evolutionary psychology proposes that our primate ancestors would have experienced consciousness in a similar fashion, and that the development of the DMN serves the purpose of enabling ego development and higher-order thinking that includes the abstraction of self that's associated with the kinds of thought (self-awareness) and future-casting that are enabled by the structures in the DMN.[18]

Subjects experiencing psychedelic states often report not feeling constrained by the ego. Sometimes psychonauts, those who explore the depths of the psyche, report that they can feel their own rigid ego transforming into something more permeable and abstract while in a psychedelic state. Sometimes this experience is blissful, and other times it can be felt as a frightening kind of "ego death." When examined in a functional MRI machine, the mechanics of these experiences reflect the decoupling of the central connective hubs of the brain from one another, resulting in a reduction in brain synchronization between nodes and structures. This creates a diffuse, conscious, and simultaneous experience of multiple brain systems at once, resulting in a loosening of our rigid concept of the ego. In the absence of sensory prioritization, which is typically handled by the central connective hubs of the brain, hierarchies associated with the DMN and other self-referential thought processes alter the experience of conscious awareness.

The term *synesthesia* can be described as a blending or unusual coupling of sensations. Psychonauts commonly report feeling mixed sensations during psychedelic and mystical experiences. Participants report having difficulty in distinguishing between sensations, or connecting sensations that don't align in a normal state, like tasting music or hearing colors. This is a result of the decoupling of cortical hierarchies associated with psychedelics.

Another study led by Richard Daws, part of the Carhart-Harris team, followed research subjects who were clinically depressed after psilocybin administration and found that there were two sequential activities that occurred in the brain. First, a decrease in DMN activity took place, and this was associated with the first administration of psilocybin. Later, there was an increase in activity in the DMN. This correlated with findings that the research subjects participating in this study experienced improvements in their mood over time. Daws and the research team proposed that what may happen in the DMN with regard to psilocybin is that the brain actually produces a reset for the DMN as a result of the complex cascades of different neurotransmitters that occur over days and weeks following the use of psilocybin.[19]

Research into the DMN has shown that it is overactive in disorders like depression, obsessive-compulsive disorder (OCD), and anxiety. The higher activation of the DMN during normal consciousness in people who suffer from these disorders means that these folks are overfocused on their experience of self. This does not mean that they are self-serving or narcissistic; it means that they are self-referential. These people are worried more about their performance or the ways that they can or should behave. As a result of Carhart-Harris's discoveries, researchers have begun to consider psychedelics as possible treatments for these disorders, as well as others where the DMN figures prominently. Following the discovery of the DMN, researchers have begun to look for other flexible networks in the brain. These networks and their effects could revolutionize our understanding of what the brain is and what creates consciousness. It is an incredible time to be engaged in the examination of psychedelics and how these remarkable substances may interact with the higher-order networks within our bodies that make us conscious.

Psilocybin's Mechanisms of Action

If you aren't interested in the nitty-gritty of neuroscience, feel free to jump ahead, but bear with me, because understanding even a little of the complexity of how your brain responds to psilocybin will be very useful as you consider your own experience. As I've written, psilocybin is a serotonin agonist. This means that psilocybin facilitates connections within the brain and increases activity at the receptors that work with serotonergic neurotransmitters.

Serotonin is critical for many pathways throughout the central and peripheral nervous systems. While your body can use serotonin in a number of ways, there are very few neurons that actually produce serotonin in the brain. Despite this imbalance between production and use, serotonin is critical for a healthy nervous system and brain. Serotonin regulates mood, emotional capacity, and some aspects of memory, and it is necessary for the proper functioning of several neural structures like the hippocampus and amygdala.

Serotonin itself is a tryptamine; its chemical name is 5-hydroxytryptamine (5-HT). It is a monoamine that has specific sites within a neuron where it can work. There are more than seven discrete forms of serotonin receptors within the brain, and as many as 14 different subtypes. Serotonin is derived from tryptophan, a naturally occurring amino acid. It is then manufactured in the body by translating tryptophan, which we get from the foods that we eat, into serotonin. The body does this in two phases. First, two hydrogen and three oxygen molecules are added to the tryptophan molecule. Then, one hydrogen molecule and two oxygen molecules are removed from the resulting metabolite (5-hydroxytryptophan) and transformed into water. This turns, or translates, the original molecule into serotonin.

Another critical substance for neuronal health is a key protein called brain-derived neurotropic factor (BDNF). This protein assists in regulating neurotransmitter connection and binding, and it also plays a critical role in neuronal health and regeneration. Some studies also find that BDNF is important in reducing inflammation. Without sufficient BDNF the brain struggles to modulate, heal, and grow. This protein is critical for neuroplasticity. If there isn't sufficient BDNF, the brain has difficulty creating new pathways or generating new neurons. High levels of BDNF have been found in the hippocampus, amygdala, cerebellum, and cerebral cortex, indicating that these parts of the brain require higher levels of BDNF to engage in their normal functions.

Because psilocybin is an agonist for the 5-HT2A receptor, this receptor site garners the most attention in research. Agonism means that the cell's adoption and binding of a compound is promoted. The 5-HT2A receptor is a serotonin receptor and as such it plays a significant role in mood, emotional regulation, and memory. Psilocybin has also been shown to work on the 5-HT1A receptor, which is the main inhibitory pathway for serotonin.

Researchers have learned this by blocking the 5-HT2A and activating the 5-HT1A receptors experimentally. When the 5-HT2A receptor is chemically blocked or inhibited after psilocybin administration, any psychedelic effect is prevented.

When psilocybin is administered to someone, a series of activations occurs in the central nervous system. The 5-HT2A receptors are activated, binding psilocin (which has been translated from psilocybin in the liver) to the neural pathways and causing many different experiences to occur based on where the 5-HT2A receptors are located. Some of these are located in the PFC, hippocampus, PCC, and amygdala. Remember that the default mode network keeps us in a self-referential mode. Because the DMN is deactivated in the presence of psilocybin, there is less personal investment in memories that may come forward during your journey. The context of these memories is readily available, but it comes without the personal identification associated with ego states. Depending on the dose administered, the DMN's desynchronization may be mild or intense, thereby increasing the likelihood of a reduction in a person's overall sense of rigidity and ego-centrality.

Depending on the dose you've taken and your personal neurochemistry, activation of the 5-HT2A receptors in the visual cortex may create visual disturbances or the appearance of shapes or forms. Activation in the auditory and emotional areas that are associated with the temporal lobes may make any music you're listening to seem more engaging and meaningful. You may find yourself remembering music from important periods in your life, or you might feel a connection to sounds that you hear during the psychedelic experience.

Mood disorders, especially depression, are often associated with mild to severe inflammation in the brain.[20] There are several neurochemical indicators associated with brain inflammation, like the presence of interleukin. In contrast, the presence and availability of the protein BDNF is one of the most significant neurochemicals for addressing and reducing inflammation in the cortex. Elevated BDNF implies greater neuroplasticity and is positively correlated with increases in functional connectivity between hubs in the brain. Psilocybin increases the release of BDNF in the brain. This release promotes a reduction in inflammation and an increase in neuroplasticity. The reduction in inflammation may partially explain why patients who have been administered psilocybin may experience relief from depression. In addition, the increase in neuroplasticity may also make it easier for these patients to find new routes of thought to assist them in problem solving or simply helping to break patterns of rumination by providing alternative pathways out of depression or rigid thought patterns.

An increase in neuroplasticity correlates to a decrease in psychological rigidity. When a person has more available neurological pathways, they have a greater capacity for problem solving, acceptance of negative affect, and depth of processing. This may also help to explain why the use of psilocybin appears to help people who suffer from depression, OCD, and other disorders where cognitive rigidity plays a significant role.

Science hasn't teased out all the biochemical effects of neurotransmitters like serotonin, despite engaging in research on the subject for more than 60 years. Meanwhile, research into psilocybin's effects on the nervous system is in its infancy. The discovery that psilo-cybin works on the serotonergic system in such profound ways opens up a host of new possibilities for treatment, drug research, and novel approaches to solving often intractable psychological problems like treatment-resistant depression (TRD) and obsessive-compulsive disorder (OCD). The effect of substances like psilocybin on the central nervous system also opens up areas of new research into disorders like schizophrenia, where science has often struggled to make significant improvements in the lives of patients.

Psilocybin and Depression: The Research

Depression in all its forms is a major public health problem. In the United States, depression is the primary cause of disability for people between the ages of 15 and 44. The economy loses over $200 billion annually due to mental illness, the most common of which is depression. According to the National Institutes of Health, in 2020 approximately 21 million people over the age of 18 experienced at least one episode that would qualify as major depressive disorder. That equates to approximately 8% of all adults in the United States. What's even more compelling is that the statistics describing depression among the adolescent population was double that number. Approximately 4.1 million adolescents aged 12–17 years reported having had at least one depressive episode in 2020. The number for female adolescents was much higher than the reported number of male adolescents, 25.2% versus 9.2%.[21]

Major depressive disorder (MDD) and treatment-resistant depression (TRD) are challenging problems to say the least. They impair cognitive and social function, and they can lead to suicidal ideation and behavior. Over the last decade there have been few new treatment options for these disorders. In order to be diagnosed with TRD a patient has to have tried and failed at least two separate courses of different antidepressant medications.[22] There are multiple reasons that someone might suffer from TRD. There are biological factors, trauma history, and genetic possibilities that all coalesce to make TRD problematic. If a person has a deficiency in neurological processing caused by an injury or a structural problem in the brain, it can be very difficult to get them the help that they need. Research has shown that most people with TRD have structural limitations because parts of their brains struggle to produce enough serotonin, usually as a result of damage to the cortex.[23]

There have been only a few clinical trials that examine the effects of psilocybin on depression. There are even fewer studies that compare psilocybin to the current medicines used to treat depression. A class of medication called selective serotonin reuptake inhibitors (SSRIs) is the first response for a patient who is struggling with depression; these medications are also sometimes used for people struggling with anxiety. You may recall, from our discussion of the synaptic cleft and our metaphor of the shipping docks earlier in this chapter, that sometimes the brain needs more of one particular neurotransmitter. This SSRI class of medications has been developed to help keep more serotonin molecules floating in the "waters" between neurons, and thereby preventing it from being recycled or reabsorbed by the body (the recycling process is called reuptake). For decades, one of the ways that doctors tried to help people with depression was to make sure that they could get more serotonin into their neural pathways when needed. The SSRI class of drugs has been developed over decades with increasing precision. The goal has always been to keep serotonin in the waters long enough for the right kinds of receptors to be able to use it.

This class of drug has proved to be a useful but blunt tool. It can take weeks or months to get the right dosage that fits a particular patient's unique neurochemistry. SSRIs also cause problematic side effects, and the science isn't absolutely clear on how this class of drugs interacts with other systems, like the dopamine reward system, or with other organs where serotonin is used differently, like the heart. We know that the serotonin that exists in the gut tends to behave more like a hormone than a neurotransmitter, and historically SSRIs can interfere with some individuals' metabolisms, causing them to gain weight. In other people, taking SSRIs affects the reward system in the brain as it pertains to sex, making sexual behavior uninteresting or undesirable.

For these reasons and others, many people resist taking SSRIs. Though a person who is struggling with anxiety and depression should always consult their physician about the best course of treatment, SSRIs may not be great for everyone. Indeed, there are some classes of SSRIs that are dangerous for people with serotonin sensitivities. People who have any genetic predisposition to bipolar disorder, even a subclinical presentation, will also find that the increased availability of serotonin and the subsequent natural downregulation

that the body engages in as a result will negatively affect the delicate balance of their central nervous system. The body has a natural set point for neurotransmitters. When too much is in the system—for example, after taking a serotonergic substance like psilocybin—the brain will downshift and return to its set point, making less natural serotonin. When a person is taking SSRIs regularly, the brain will adjust to that set point and slow the production of neurotransmitters; this is why it is dangerous to go off of SSRIs too quickly. The brain needs time to adapt.

Because psilocybin works on serotonergic pathways, researchers have begun investigating the efficacy of treating ailments like major depressive disorder with psilocybin as an alternative to SSRIs. In multiple studies over the last decade, researchers have administered psilocybin to patients to see if psilocybin is a viable alternative to the current protocol of SSRIs for treatment of depression and generalized anxiety. The results have been surprising. In most cases the studies have shown great promise. Some have shocked the medical, psychiatric, and pharmaceutical communities. Others have come and gone with little fanfare.

In these trials researchers ask participants to fill out usually multiple standardized questionnaires that measure for depression or changes in mood throughout the trial. The most frequently used questionnaires are the Hamilton Depression Rating Scale (GRID HAMD, an updated version), the Beck Depression Inventory (BDI), the Quick Inventory of Depressive Symptomatology (QIDS-SR-16), the Montgomery-Asberg Depression Rating Scale (MADRS), and the Laukes Emotional Intensity Scale (LEIS). Each of these questionnaires measures slightly different aspects of depression, well-being, and ability to cope with psychological or emotional pain.

Before any drug or therapy is administered, the participant must fill out one or more of these standardized tests. This gives the researchers a baseline score against which to determine if there is a therapeutic effect from the treatment protocol (drug, psychotherapy, or a combination). Participants repeat the questionnaires after the intervention has been made (i.e., after they have been administered a dose of psilocybin), and researchers examine the scores and assess if there is any significant difference between the baseline and post-intervention scores. A significant change is one that can't be explained by normal healing or random chance; in statistics this is given a numeric comparison called a *p*-value (*p* is for *probability*).

A Sample of the Research

Several convincing studies have been performed whose results have been published in the last several years. At the moment there are also currently more than 100 trials underway around the world. A section in chapter 7 of this book looks at some of the new research that is underway using psilocybin for the treatment of different disorders. The research that has had the longest and most consistent body of work has been in treating depression.

In a 2022 phase 2 double-blind study, Guy Goodwin of Oxford University's medical school worked with an extensive research team to test the efficacy of a single dose of psilocybin for patients suffering from treatment-resistant depression (TRD). The findings,

published in the *New England Journal of Medicine*, were intriguing. The researchers administered different doses of psilocybin to three groups of participants. Participants received either a 1 mg dose, a 10 mg dose, or a 25 mg dose, depending on which group they were randomly assigned to. There were more than 200 participants in the study across multiple countries in Europe.[24]

The study provided initial preparation with a psychotherapist prior to the administration of the medication, and two integration sessions immediately following administration. Each individual participant was assigned a therapist, who worked with that participant throughout the study to maintain therapeutic trust and consistency. The researchers conducted follow-ups after the initial administration of psilocybin, and at several points (3, 6, and 12 weeks) after administration. This research was sponsored by Compass Pathways, a pharmaceutical company developing medications based on psychedelic research. They provided the experimental medications for the study.

At baseline, all of the participants reported moderate to severe TRD with corresponding scores on the MADRS depression scale. The highest experimental dose of psilocybin given, 25 mg, produced a significant improvement in participants' scores. The 10 mg dose didn't produce a significant improvement and was relatively consistent with the 1 mg dose. The study was designed to measure effects at three weeks after administration. The maximum possible MADRS score is 60. A higher score indicates more serious depression. A treatment effect (meaning that the experiment caused some kind of measurable change that can be attributed to the intervention) was considered a 50% reduction from the participants' original baseline score. Researchers defined remission (meaning no more depression) as testing at less than or equal to a score of 10 on the MADRS assessment post treatment.

The average MADRS score at baseline was 31.9 in the 25 mg group, 33.0 in the 10 mg group, and 32.7 in the 1 mg group. Between the first measurement at 3 weeks and the last at 12 weeks, 37% of the participants in the 25 mg group reported a treatment effect compared to 19% in the 10 mg group and 18% in the 1 mg group. The remission scores, meaning a score of 10 or less on the MADRS, were 29% in the 25 mg group, 9% in the 10 mg group, and 8% in the 1 mg group. Effects were durable when measured again at 12 weeks, for 20% of the 25 mg group, 5% for members of the 10 mg group, and 10% for members of the 1 mg group. These scores indicate that 29% of the members in the 25 mg group reported a change and an average drop of more than 21 points in their MADRS scores.[25]

Goodwin and his team reported that more research is required to better understand the mechanisms and potency of these medicines with regard to this particular population of people who suffer from TRD. They acknowledged that more trials are needed, especially trials that specifically look at even broader populations and for longer experimental durations. Despite the limitations of this study, the results are very encouraging.

Natalie Gukasyan at the Johns Hopkins University School of Medicine recently ran a study with several other leading authors at the Center for Psychedelic and Consciousness Research that demonstrated that psilocybin could provide durable results for patients suffering from depression. Their paper was published in the *Journal of Psychopharmacology*

in 2022. In this study the researchers administered two doses of psilocybin over eight weeks. Participants received a dose of psilocybin early in the trial, and then a second dose two weeks later. All of the participants were provided with supportive psychotherapy to help prepare them for treatment and to help them integrate the psychedelic experience after the medicine sessions. The team of researchers followed up with the participants one year after their treatment and found that there was a significant improvement for all members of the cohort even 12 months later.[26]

Robin Carhart-Harris was the principal investigator in a study that compared the effects of psilocybin against the effects of escitalopram (Lexapro), which is a common SSRI. Carhart-Harris, who founded the Centre for Psychedelic Research at Imperial College London and is now the director of the psychedelics division of Neuroscape at the University of California, San Francisco, published results that seemed to contradict earlier findings. In this study, which was published in the *New England Journal of Medicine*, researchers found that while the respondents' scores were encouraging, the difference in effects between the group taking psilocybin and the group taking escitalopram was so small as to be statistically insignificant.[27] The psilocybin group reported an 8-point improvement in their symptoms, while the escitalopram group reported a 6-point improvement. Both groups had a margin of error of 1 point, and a high p-value (probability value) of 0.17. This combination reflects a statistical environment where there is sufficient unknown data in the system as to confound the results. A p-value of 0.17 means that there is a 17% chance that the hypothesis the researchers were trying to disprove is true. In other words, the experiments could not prove that psilocybin is a more effective treatment than escitalopram in treating depression. By statistical standards, there is too much random chance in the system to explain the results in any definitive way.

In addition, the researchers proposed that the six weeks over which their subjects were administered escitalopram was an insufficient span of time to measure the comparative effects. The dosing window is significantly different between escitalopram and psilocybin. Psilocybin's anti-anxiety and antidepressive effects are immediate, while escitalopram can take weeks to measure, presuming it is effective at all.[28]

Despite the researchers' conservative interpretation of the primary data, their secondary data (effects that are meaningful but not the goal of the study) showed major differences in the reports from the psilocybin group versus the escitalopram group. According to the study, 57% of the psilocybin group showed remission of symptoms as reported on the QIDS-SR-16, while the escitalopram group reported a remission rate of 28%. That is a significant improvement, with the psilocybin group having more than twice the remission of the escitalopram group. The researchers said that these secondary results were not controlled for and so should not be considered conclusive.[29] While this is a somewhat frustrating finding, it is important to note that scientists report their results as accurately as possible in clinical research. However, even if we do not consider the results of this study definitive, they are still informative. Psilocybin has greater potential than SSRIs to help people in immediate need of relief.

Research conducted by Matthew Wall and his team at Imperial College London revisited this question about the effects of escitalopram versus psilocybin by examining brain images of research participants engaged in an emotional task. This study was published in *MedRxiv* in 2023.[30] Since the development of neuroimaging techniques, neuroscientists have engaged in research that uses advanced imaging to see how the brain responds to different stimuli. It's a little nerdy, but researchers have figured out how to cancel out the noise in the brain to look for increases in activity based on blood oxygen density. The more resources the brain is using, the higher the blood flow will be to a specific area of the brain. So, by examining the blood oxygen level density signal, researchers can tell what parts of the brain are the most active. Researchers can thus use functional MRI imaging techniques to learn what areas of the brain are activated when engaged in a certain task or behavior.

Wall's research team examined the effects of escitalopram and psilocybin on the brain while participants were engaged in the emotional task of viewing facial expressions. Researchers recruited participants and asked them to submit to a functional MRI that would examine what parts of the brain were active while participants were looking at faces that reflected expressions of fear, happiness, and neutrality. The participants were also asked to provide baseline and follow-up measures of several standardized tests for mood, well-being, and depression. Their scores were measured at baseline, at three weeks, and again at six weeks after beginning either psilocybin or escitalopram treatment.

Tests from this experiment provided physical evidence of something that patients who have taken SSRIs have often complained about over the last several decades. The participants who took escitalopram showed reduced activation across multiple areas of the brain when compared to the psilocybin group. One of the most remarkable findings, however, was that the participants in the psilocybin group had a greater capacity for feeling while the escitalopram group had blunted emotions, but it appeared that after the six-week evaluation, the psilocybin group's functional MRIs showed continued or improved internetwork connectivity, meaning that different parts of the participants' brains improved in how much one part of the brain talked to another. The psilocybin group also had higher emotional responses in the Lauks Emotional Intensity Scale, which was one of the first objective measures used to capture emotional blunting associated with the use of SSRIs in clinical research.[31]

These and other clinical research trials point to psilocybin as a powerful alternative in the treatment of depression. Psilocybin appears to improve emotional awareness and tolerance of varying emotional states. It also increases the network connectivity in the brain, and while there are sometimes unpleasant side effects that come along with this, like headaches and nausea, the overall tolerance of psilocybin is often preferred to the long-term effects that patients taking SSRIs have reported. It is important to note that while SSRIs are often prescribed along with therapy as a recommendation, the use of these medicines is not dependent on having a skilled therapist at the ready. In all of the trials involving psilocybin, therapy has been instrumental in helping support patients as they make sense of their experiences. Only time will tell if there is a way for the molecular properties of psilocybin and other classic psychedelics to be used in the same way as more recognizable medications like SSRIs. For now, it is safe to say that we have not come close to that threshold. Psychedelics stimulate the psyche in ways that require conscious integration of unconscious material. Working with the imagery and experience is a minimum requirement. Ideally, anyone doing psychedelic work for healing would work with a skilled guide or therapist trained in psychedelics and/or depth psychology.

Psychedelic research is opening up neuroscience in new ways. Neuroscientific and psychedelic research are still in their early stages. Working with psychedelics to help neuroscientists uncover the mysteries of the mind is particularly intriguing. Neuroscientists don't completely understand how the brain works or how its different systems, neurotransmitters, and receptor systems work or interact with one another. The field is a vast undiscovered dimension, and new medicines and psychotherapeutic techniques are still emerging. If we continue to encourage research in this domain, we will certainly benefit from new scientific and clinical discoveries that could emerge as early as this decade.

Neurogenesis

For decades doctors and scientists believed that nerves didn't regenerate. Early biology textbooks told students that people are born with a given number of neurons, and that's all we get. But this is not at all the case. The discovery of stem cells in adult bodies showed scientists that some neurons do regenerate. This led to the belief that there are limited places within the body where neurogenesis is possible.[32] For a time, the research seemed to indicate that the only place in the brain where neurogenesis occurred was in the hippocampus. However, more contemporary research has shown us that there is more to neurogenesis than just birthing new neurons from stem cells, and that the hippocampus is not the only place where neurogenesis occurs.[33]

Translational research seeks to take findings from laboratory results and make them useful for treating patients. It can unite many seemingly disparate areas of research from psychopharmacology to genetics. In the last decade, translational research has demonstrated that there are changes that occur at the gene, RNA, cellular, and morphological levels that activate different types of neuronal growth. In some instances, this can lead to the development of whole neurons. Depending on the gene expression and the conditions in the cell, the neuron may experience dendritic growth, which is growth of the spiny lengths of the dendrite alone. Or the cell could undergo increases in the capacity, length, surface, and volume of the axon, called axonic growth. In some instances, there is an expansion of the synaptic area and, with it, opportunities for new connections in the neuronal structure.[34]

Neuroplasticity is a term used in neuroscience to describe the capacity of the brain and nervous system to reorganize and adapt. For the longest time dynamic adaptations were thought to be the result of stress, injury, structural changes, or invasive tumors.[35] New research has demonstrated that neuroplasticity is also the result of therapy, learning,

and, as more recent research has shown, the introduction of psychedelics. Laboratory and clinical studies have demonstrated that neurons do amazing things in the presence of psychedelics, literally accelerating growth and improving neuroplasticity by encouraging the creation of new neural pathways and the growth of new neuronal structures. Psilocybin and other classic psychedelics have demonstrated that they have the power to catalyze different types of neurogenesis. This astounding result opens incredible new potential in how we consider medicating all kinds of neurological conditions.[36]

The current research implies that psychedelic related neurogenesis is concentrated in areas that have high densities of 5-HT1A and 5-HT2A receptors. In animal models several psychedelics have demonstrated the ability to create a higher density of presynaptic neurons in the PFC and hippocampus.[37] In human beings imaging tests have demonstrated increased signaling between glutamate receptors in the PFC.[38] Since glutamate is the most prolific neurotransmitter in the human brain, this implies that there is increased production and reception of glutamate. Efficient or improved use of neurotransmitters in the brain is a key aspect of neuroplasticity.

The timing of neuroplastic changes in the nervous system may provide insight into why there is a clear difference in the efficacy of escitalopram and psilocybin. In animal models, psilocybin affected the genes necessary for neuroplastic changes within 1.5 hours of exposure, and in some animals these changes continued for more than 24 hours after administration. In some instances, neuronal growth continued for 72 hours after exposure.[39] These numbers are based on studies done with animals, so translating the results to human populations isn't advised. However, the fact that there are these kinds of changes occurring in animals supports many of the working theories of how psychedelics work in the brain and nervous system of humans. Solving the mysteries of neurogenesis in the presence of these substances could help create new medications for diseases ranging from Parkinson's disease to Alzheimer's disease. Several studies are currently in the planning stages to test the efficacy of psilocybin on these disorders. Some of these research plans are discussed later in this book.

While the technical explanation of the genetic and translational effects of psilocybin are outside the scope of this book, the data that exist support the idea that almost all psychedelics support neurogenesis in one way or another. There is not yet enough research to inform us of the optimal doses for these changes, or at what doses these substances either lose their efficacy or possibly become toxic. We know that while psilocybin toxicity is rare, it is possible. More research is required to help scientists better understand the positive and negative effects of psilocybin on the central nervous system.

Experiential Avoidance

The idea of experiential avoidance first became part of the psychotherapeutic toolbox with the development of acceptance and commitment therapy (ACT), which began with Steven C. Hayes at the University of Nevada in the 1980s.[40] This form of psychotherapy was one of the first to integrate mindfulness techniques into the practice of therapy. In the last

two decades there has been a growing interest in helping patients increase their capacity for emotion and feeling. While this may seem like an obvious goal of psychology and psychotherapy, it has only recently been introduced as a discrete experience of healing. At its core, the goal of this approach to therapy is to stress the idea that feelings and emotions, regardless of whether they are positive or negative, must be accepted. In ACT this is called "radical acceptance." The term *radical acceptance* is not meant to describe a passive acquiescence. It is not the promotion of suffering or the idea that we should welcome suffering or seek out pain. Rather, radical acceptance means that we must accept that there *is* pain in life. That less-than-ideal conditions should and do exist proves to be a difficult idea for many people to accept, especially at the beginning of therapy.

Experiential avoidance is the opposite of radical acceptance. Experiential avoidance (EA) is distinguished by holding negative opinions of painful emotions, feelings, psychological states, memories, and sensations, and actively engaging in behaviors that are meant to dissuade, avoid, or negate the experiences associated with these negative emotions coming to the fore.[41] EA is a necessary behavior; after all, avoiding pain is a key to survival. But when the avoidance goes to an extreme, it can become pathological. Psychologists and psychiatrists often use EA as one of the hallmarks of some disorders. These include eating disorders, obsessive-compulsive behaviors, addiction, alcohol use or dependence, and many other milder conditions.

In day-to-day life, everyone engages in a little EA. In certain circumstances, like a student who is focusing on an important exam or a doctor in the middle of performing surgery, people are able to focus on the task at hand by setting troubling thoughts and memories to the side of their awareness. In these cases, a person's ability to focus on a single task is a form of EA that is actually useful. While EA may be adaptively helpful in some circumstances, it has become a widespread form of coping that is often at the root of deeper problems. If we fear feeling sad and push that pain away with shopping, that is a form of EA. If we judge ourselves for being unhappy, and then immediately reach for a funny movie to avoid that feeling, that is another example of EA. If we tell ourselves that we don't have anything to be depressed about, even when our lives are filled with sadness, that is a form of EA. When EA is overused in a person's life, it is maladaptive. To put it simply: habitually avoiding negative feelings and experiences is a direct route to depression and possibly to other destructive behaviors.

Acceptance and commitment therapy is one of the core foundations in my own practice. Regardless of what my client and I are working on, or what modality or intervention we are using, routing out EA is one of the core concepts of our sessions. I often explain to my clients that the quickest way to understand the emotions that they're struggling to process is to look at the places where they are experiencing the two R's: resistance and rigidity. What do you resist feeling? What is the forbidden terrain in your own mind? Where, or under what circumstances, are you not allowed to be sad, angry, frightened, or quiet?

In psychology we know that the integration of difficult feelings is actually the key to happiness. It sounds crazy, but making room for and accepting challenging experiences and feelings is the only way to truly find mental health. Western culture is primarily built on EA. Just think of some of our expressions: "Keep a stiff upper lip," meaning don't let yourself cry. "Don't worry, be happy," which is self-explanatory. "Just do it," which is usually interpreted to mean "Do it no matter what." I could list a dozen more examples of how EA permeates our cultural mores. In the United States in particular, we promote the ideal and the goal of "being happy" as the ultimate version of success. Social media has also promoted the idea that shiny happy people are supposed to be the norm of the human experience. Accepting challenging emotions is a lot more difficult in practice than it is in theory.

Addressing experiential avoidance requires a person to first find the places where they are avoiding feeling. As we've already discussed in this chapter, SSRIs are usually the first medicines prescribed for people who are struggling with either depression or anxiety (both disorders tend to engage the same systems in the brain). The mechanism of SSRIs appears to work by blunting emotion, thereby making it difficult for people to feel as deeply, regardless of whether they're feeling sadness or joy. Psilocybin, on the other hand, tends to enhance feeling. While SSRIs seem to make feelings less painful by dulling the whole emotional spectrum, psilocybin appears to enhance feeling and to help people tolerate sensations by engaging them via a novel approach.

Richard Zeifman and his colleagues at the Toronto Metropolitan University and the Langone Center for Psychedelic Medicine at New York University's School of Medicine led a small team that reexamined the data from Robin Carhart-Harris's study that compared the use of psilocybin and escitalopram, discussed earlier. In this new study researchers did a complex analysis of participants' responses to several measures that examined EA and some of the known experiences associated with psychedelic experiences and therapy.[42]

Specifically, the study examined the order of how participants arrived at an improved mood and whether or not the two different medications made a difference in the sequence of therapeutic interventions. The study, which was published in the *Journal of Affective Disorders*, demonstrated that reductions in experiential avoidance predicted increases in well-being and decreases in depression and anxiety. These results are not surprising given the ongoing research into the effectiveness of ACT and EA. However, what was very interesting was that the use of psilocybin was much more effective than escitalopram in helping clients living with treatment-resistant depression reduce their incidences of EA. Researchers discovered that psilocybin reduced EA by improving participants' sense of connectedness to life, other people, religion, the earth—whatever gave their lives meaning. Ego dissolution was the best predictor of improved mood and well-being via the experience of connectedness. The test group that was administered the SSRI did not experience the same gains. They did not report improved connectedness or ego dissolution.[43]

The researchers who performed the study concluded that psilocybin can help reduce EA, and therefore it can also help increase a person's capacity for feeling. This state change makes it easier for patients to experience a range of emotions. Researchers reported that based on their own study and other related findings, it is likely that psilocybin assists patients by increasing the capacity for active coping where SSRIs facilitate passive coping, meaning that by amplifying a patient's capacity to feel emotion, psilocybin effectively resets their window of tolerance rather than dulling their emotions overall.[44]

If we put all these pieces together—dosing with psilocybin and learning to cope with our emotions—we start to form a picture that shows an entirely new way of thinking about mental health, psychological and emotional well-being, and the mechanisms of healing. For the last 100 years psychiatrists and psychologists have sought to understand mental health by understanding the structure and function of the brain, almost thinking of the brain as if it was an isolated bowl of jelly. The last 70 years of neuroscience have shown us that the brain is a great deal more complex than the hydraulic pumps of a machine, the wires of an engine, or the circuits of a computer. The brain and nervous systems comprise a labyrinthine architecture whose structures are influenced and altered by a dynamic dance of neurochemicals and proteins.

Psilocybin appears to reset that neural and psychological architecture without causing loss to the memory, structure, or core personality of the person who is taking it. It appears to do this by first deactivating the default mode network, which allows a person to step outside of the self-referential world of their ego. Next, research seems to suggest that the experience of the DMN going offline creates a sense of ego dissolution that helps a psychonaut feel less alone and more connected to other people and the living world. Psilocybin also contributes to neuroplasticity. The release of BDNF and glutamate affords the sojourner greater insight via increased intracortical connections. The presence of psilocybin may also increase neurogenesis by providing more structure to help make these changes in the brain long-lasting. If the findings produced in the studies we've discussed here continue to be reproduced by neuroscientists and psychopharmacologists, they will completely change the practices of psychiatry and psychology. We must continue to advocate for responsible research and administration of psilocybin in order to offer the next generation better medications and tools for mental health and improved wellness.

Healing and Mystical Experiences

It is a common stereotype that it is mostly yoga-loving New Age folks and tie-dye-wearing hippies who are enthusiastic about psychedelic experiences. This image has changed in the last two decades as increased research into the efficacy of psilocybin and other psychedelics has started to become more widely distributed and discussed. But researchers have noticed that a greater sense of healing is reported by people when they have a more spiritual and/or more ritualized experience while taking psilocybin.

This is a controversial idea. Most scientists are loath to endorse any kind of spirituality, even though research shows us that people who have an active spiritual belief system often experience greater meaning in life. Before the advent of modern research into psilocybin, it was easy to say that the spiritual dimension reported by people who were enthusiastic psychedelic users was occurring because they were self-selected. The people

who took these drugs were interested in spiritual topics before they took an interest in psychedelics, so it was natural that their experiences would take on a spiritual hue.

Contemporary research into altered states of consciousness has changed the focus of that argument. Research into awe and mystical and psychedelic experiences shows that these states can change the brain's physiology. Awe, mystical experiences, and psychedelics all reduce the activation of the DMN. They also promote the release of oxytocin, a critical neuropeptide that aids in helping a person feel connected and loving. Psychedelic experiences, regardless of whether they are spontaneous or induced by a psychoactive substance like psilocybin, also promote reduced inflammation, increase BDNF, and reduce interleukin 6, a key marker of inflammation in the body.[45]

Those who engage in even a single psychedelic experience often report powerful encounters with something greater than themselves or other spiritually oriented experiences. These often include the sensation of ego dissolution, awe in the presence of feelings of profound connectedness, and powerful encounters with cultural symbols like God or important symbols from the personal unconscious. While most often positive in nature, these types of encounters can be dysregulating.[46] As such, having a touchstone that has been worked out in a preparation session (or sessions) with a psychedelic guide or therapist is recommended (see "Journeying" in chapter 5). A psychonaut in the depths of their psychedelic experience is in a vulnerable, suggestible state. Ritual-like elements can help create a setting and anchor an experience not only in place, but also in time. A sense of ritual can also help ground the participant, making it safe to open themself to the types of meaning that arise during a psychedelic experience.

In the West, there is a decrease in religious affiliation but an increase in nonreligious spiritual identification. In other words, fewer people are going to church. Not as many people belong to a specific religious group, but most still believe in *something*, and they can be easily moved by spiritual ideas and experiences. In population research that has investigated religious life in the United States, these individuals are often referred to as Nones, people who report no religious affiliation. Research on spirituality's influence in psychology has pointed out that though Nones often have no official connections to a religious institution,[47] they often exhibit a "religious residue." This is demonstrated by religious feelings, attitudes, and behaviors in Nones that are historically associated with adherents of a particular faith. Nones experience awe, mysticism, and ethical concerns without the orthopraxy or orthodoxy associated with being a member of a religious community.

A study by Keri Mans and her team at the Centre for Psychedelic Research at Imperial College London found that individuals who sought out psychedelic experiences with the hope of improved well-being typically achieved their goal.[48] This group reported increased spirituality scores as well as improved well-being that was durable at a 24-month follow-up. In other research, scientists studied the effects of psilocybin on patients who were diagnosed with terminal cancer.[49] The results demonstrated that these patients found it much easier to let go of their fear of and resistance to dying. They were able to place their lives in a more meaningful

context, and this led to an overall reduction in anxiety.

Many areas of psychology have become more friendly to spirituality in the last several decades. People who find it easier to ascribe meaning to events in life and who aren't haunted by nihilism often find life easier and tend to have better mental and physical health outcomes. While psychologists have been hesitant to promote religious or spiritual beliefs as a means of healing, we have learned that people who participate in a religious practice or who hold a set of spiritual beliefs are often happier and tend to find life more meaningful. After psychedelic experiences occur, individuals often find that the experience of even mild ego dissolution, and the resulting feelings of connectedness, lends itself to more interest in spiritual ideas and beliefs. Roland Griffiths and his team at the Johns Hopkins University Center for Psychedelic and Consciousness Research have authored several papers that describe these outcomes.

In one study, Sandeep Nayak and Roland Griffiths examined participants who had a single psychedelic experience, and they found that these individuals reported a greater attribution of consciousness to animals, plants, fungi, and even inanimate objects.[50] In another study Griffiths and his team examined the correlation of experiences reported by those who had a mystical experience without any substance against those who had a psychedelic experience. They found that there were striking similarities in the descriptions given by participants from both groups. In this study, more than two-thirds of participants who identified as atheists before their medicine session no longer identified as atheists after their session was complete.[51]

All the Things That Heal

Spirituality, neurotransmitters, brain-derived neurotropic factor—all of these things interconnect in the experience of psychological and emotional healing when discussing psilocybin. *What* someone believes is less important than the simple fact that they believe in anything at all. When it comes to working with psilocybin it would be foolish for me to tell you what you will see, hear, or feel during your trip, but I can offer that you are likely to encounter the depths of whatever matters to you most. Whether that is love, God, Goddess, family, ultimate reality, or the web of all that breathes—you are likely to encounter significant emotions during your psychedelic experience. To honor that encounter, it is best to go into the experience with respect and an appreciation for awe. Healing comes easiest and deepest when we allow ourselves to be open to all the different ways that our psyche can make sense of our experience.

The difference between animals and fungi is simple: animals put food in their bodies, whereas fungi put their bodies in the food.

—MERLIN SHELDRAKE

CHAPTER 3

Mushroom Anatomy

Mushrooms have been used as medicine or food for thousands of years. Every culture on the planet has a relationship with mushrooms. Some are mushroom averse, or mycophobic, and therefore they avoid them, perhaps due to a proliferation of poisonous mushrooms in the local environment. Other cultures are mycophilic, meaning that they love mushrooms and are attracted to mushrooms for food or healing purposes. Likely this is due to a host of inverse reasons from mychophobic cultures, such has having a longer history of positive mushroom associations in the culture. In traditional Chinese medicine, the medicinal effects of certain species of mushrooms have been known for thousands of years.

A mushroom or, in mycology terms, a fruiting body, is the result of reproduction, much like the fruit of a tree. Spores from the gills of the fruiting body are classified as haploid, meaning that they have half of the genes needed for sexual reproduction. In animals, reproduction also requires haploid cells—eggs and sperm individually have half of the genetic material of their contributing parent. When an egg and a sperm meet, if the conditions are right, the two will form a zygote, which can then become a fetus. In mushrooms, the equivalent of the sperm and egg are called hyphae. Hyphae are usually denoted as positive and negative, only because there's no male/female distinction in fungi. The hyphae extend from the spores, looking for the right connection to a suitable counterpart. When one positive and one negative (or masculine and feminine, if you prefer) hyphae meet, the two connect and unite. The hyphae's haploid cells combine, and a mushroom will eventually result.

A mushroom is not a plant. The fruiting body is one part in a larger fungal organism. If you continue thinking of a mushroom like the fruit of a tree, then think of a pear tree: the pear that grows on the tree would be a mushroom. Fungi are an entire kingdom unto themselves in the living world. Animals as a kingdom are defined by their ability to move about independently, by their unique methods of reproduction, and by a need to feed themselves from external sources. Plants as a kingdom are defined by their ability to feed themselves from sunlight through a process called photosynthesis and by their lack of mobility—they maintain a stable footprint throughout the entirety of their lives. The majority of a plant's movement consists of turning slowly toward sunlight, growing upward and outward to create more leaves and fruit, and growing downward to deepen a root system. Like animals, fungi need to seek out nutrients, but they are also stationary like plants. Fungi in general are fascinating life forms. They are neither animal nor plant, but their presence is essential to preserving the ecosystems of both.

Mushrooms are an active subject of scientific and medical research. The biochemicals within mushrooms and other fungi produce antioxidant, anticancer, antibiotic, and anti-inflammatory effects in humans and animals. There are more than 200 mushroom species that have demonstrated immunotherapeutic properties. We know from the explosion of available antibiotics in the last century that fungi can assist in many ways that we now take for granted. It was just over 100 years ago that an infected wound could kill a person. Today a simple round of antibiotics produced from a fungal culture like penicillin is taken easily and with little thought about how magnificent a medical achievement it is to be able to assist the body as it heals using its own natural immune system.

Just as a plant has a system of roots used for gathering nutrients, a fungus has a mycelial structure that accomplishes a similar purpose. An animal feeds itself by consuming nutrients, and a mushroom does the same. Plants reproduce by producing flowers and seeds, usually clothed in fleshy fruits that sustain the seeds when they fall. One of the ways fungi reproduce includes producing spores that travel on the wind or on the legs of animals. The other way is a complex form of sexual reproduction whose elements are reminiscent of both animal and plant reproduction.

Basic Mushroom Anatomy

Most people recognize the familiar shape of mushrooms. At first glance it's easy to see how a mushroom could be confused with a plant. They have what appears to be a stem, but it's something called a stipe, which grows up from the ground. When you pick one, you'll find little threads hanging from the ends—slender fibers that resemble roots but are part of the structure of the mycelium connecting the various parts of the larger fungal structure together.

As a whole, the fungus is not just the mushroom, which is essentially the reproductive product. A fungal organism includes its fruiting body, what we call the mushroom, and its mycelia, which connect the networks of the fungi to its substrates, which provide nourishment. The mushroom is the easiest way to identify the organism. It's not easy or practical to try to identify species by examining their mycelia. We instead rely on the appearance, morphology, and structure of the fruiting bodies to help identify the species that we encounter.

The mushrooms you come across in your daily life will have similar features. Whether you are foraging for them, growing them, or find yourself suspicious about some you were gifted, understanding the morphology and anatomy of mushrooms will help you make better decisions about what to do with the mushrooms that cross your path. All the mushrooms you encounter will have similar features.

BASIC MUSHROOM ANATOMY

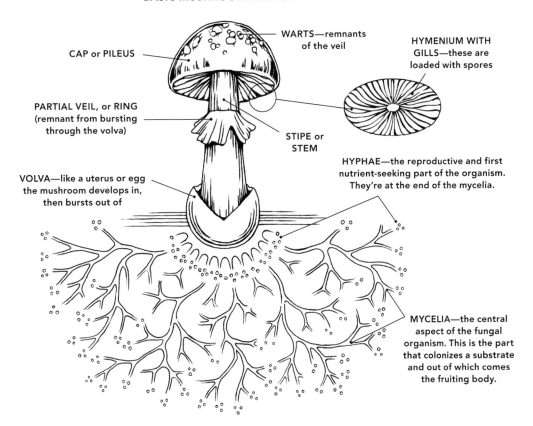

CAP or PILEUS

WARTS—remnants of the veil

HYMENIUM WITH GILLS—these are loaded with spores

PARTIAL VEIL, or RING (remnant from bursting through the volva)

STIPE or STEM

HYPHAE—the reproductive and first nutrient-seeking part of the organism. They're at the end of the mycelia.

VOLVA—like a uterus or egg the mushroom develops in, then bursts out of

MYCELIA—the central aspect of the fungal organism. This is the part that colonizes a substrate and out of which comes the fruiting body.

But because there is such diversity within the world of mushrooms, it is beneficial to have a broader understanding of the different parts of the mushroom because this will help you identify which specimens could be useful and which could be harmful. Learning to examine and compare specimens is a skill that takes time to cultivate.

If you are foraging, it will be critical for you to have a lot of exposure to different mushrooms in order to understand what you're looking at and in order to safely distinguish them from what you are looking *for*. This is the first time in this book that you will read the words *BEWARE THE LITTLE BROWN MUSHROOM*. It cannot be overstated that there are different species of mushrooms that look almost identical. Some mushrooms may appear identical, but it is common to find very different individual specimens living in close proximity to one another. They produce wildly different experiences when ingested and can have profoundly different properties from one to the next. A psychedelic mushroom can grow immediately next to a poisonous one, and without testing each individual mushroom, you'll be hard pressed to tell the difference between them. In the next chapter, it will become more clear what to look for when examining a mushroom. For now, let's discuss the anatomy of a mushroom specimen from the Basidiomycota phylum, one of the most diverse and prolific groups in the kingdom of fungi.

THE CAP OR PILEUS

When looking for mushrooms, it is critical to learn how to describe each individual mushroom in detail. Let's start with the cap, the most recognizable part of the mushroom. Sometimes this is referred to by the Latin term *pileus*. The word *cap* is also an abbreviation for the Latin word meaning head: *caput* or *capita*. If you were to watch the development of the mushroom through its life cycle, the name would start to take on a more complex meaning. The fruiting body grows in a closed, egglike structure called a volva. The mushroom cap breaks through the volva and stands on its own.

A particular species will be identified first by the cap's shape, color, and features. Some have "warts," which aren't warts at all but remnants of the veil and volva after the mushroom emerged from it. The edge of the cap is called the margin, and at its bottom is where the cap and hymenium meet (more on this in a little bit). Mushrooms will have different shapes of cap, depending on what species you are describing. A conical or convex cap will be long and narrow. A bell-shaped or campanulate cap will look like the traditional shape of a church bell. Flat caps will look like pancakes lying atop the mushroom's stipe or stem. An umbonate cap will have an umbo, which is a reference to the raised center section of a Roman shield from antiquity. Another type of cap is a papillary, where the cap has a much smaller button at the apex. While an umbo resembles an outie belly button, one that is

papillate suggests a nipple. Ovoid shapes, of which there are a few, look egglike. Because a mushroom cap doesn't open as easily with ovoid shapes, their spores don't spread as easily or as far. As mushrooms age, the cap may change color or split.

The pellicle is another feature of the cap that's worth noting. The term *pellicle* comes from the Latin, meaning "film." The pellicle is a thin membrane that covers the cap of the mushroom. In some mushrooms it is visible; in others it is difficult to identify. In field guides, you'll often read that a pellicle is "separable" or not. This means that you can

COMMON MUSHROOM CAP SHAPES

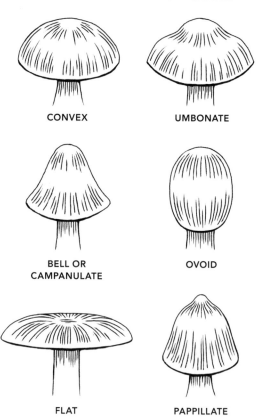

CONVEX UMBONATE

BELL OR CAMPANULATE OVOID

FLAT PAPPILLATE

identify the pellicle and peel it back from the surface of the cap.

When you look at field guides or read books to help you identify species, you'll see words and descriptions of the cap like these. Becoming familiar with the shapes and how they appear in living specimens will be helpful in foraging for any specific mushrooms. Identifying the shapes of the caps will also help you avoid some species that you don't want to bring home by accident.

THE VEIL OR RING

Prior to emerging from the egglike volva that protected it, the spores were covered by a protective layer called a veil while they developed. The veil protected the spores in the hymenium, the area under the cap where you will find the gills. Once the mushroom is mature, the spores are safe to release. Sometimes you'll see a mushroom and notice that it has a torn circle around the stem, or stipe. This is the veil, ring, or annulus. The presence of a partial veil or ring is one of the ways mushrooms are identified in the wild. The ring remains around the stipe and looks like a torn collar. Some mushrooms have a veil that remains, while others lose their veil early on.

HYMENIUM

The hymenium holds the spores of the mushroom before releasing them out into the world. Mycologists examine how the spores are arranged to help them narrow down the species. There are several types of spore arrangements. Gills, teeth, pores, and veins all release spores from the underside of the hymenium, which is located on the inside of the cap. In most mushrooms you will see gills, which are little ridges that expand from the center of the

stipe toward the edge of the cap. Inside these ridges there are millions of haploid spores.

Recognizing the different forms that the hymenium can take is quite useful. In some species there aren't prominent gills or teeth, but rather ridges that look like veins located underneath the hymenium surface.

SPORES

Most people who want to learn about mushrooms aren't terribly interested in the microscopic differences between the species. But mushroom spores are unique to each species, and because there can be millions of spores within a single mushroom, a microscope can be very useful. A spore is to a mushroom what a seed is to a fruit. They hold the genetic material necessary for the reproduction of the species. Spores travel on the wind, on the legs of animals, through the digestive systems of animals that eat mushrooms, or through the grass where those animals have pooped. When identifying a mushroom, a spore print is one of the most reliable ways to tell what type of mushroom you're examining. I'll discuss making a spore print in the next chapter.

Mycologists use the spore size, color, and shape to help distinguish one species from another. A microscope comes in very handy— if you are looking for a reason to buy one, examining mushroom spores is a very good reason! Most serious field guides will provide a little information on the microscopic features of the spores, and you'll find that the spores are typically described as part of the identifying marks. You'll also find a description of their color. Their shape may also be described, usually as either ellipsoid or round. A description of the spore may also list its size in micrometers, as measured by examination through a microscope.

The rest of the typical mushroom description that you'll find in a field guide may not be very useful to you. You'll find words like *lageniform*, *cavitate*, and *central germ pore*. While this additional information is useful in studying mushrooms from a mycologist's perspective, it may not be terribly useful for the kinds of personal research that you're interested in undertaking as you read this book. For our purposes it's important to know that there are differences in spore shape, structure, and color. If you are identifying mushrooms that you have picked in nature or that you are growing (or maybe you're even developing your own strain), you'll want to get familiar with looking at spores under a microscope.

STIPE OR STEM

A mushroom has a stalk or a stem; in mycology this is referred to as a stipe. This structure makes a mushroom similar to a plant, but the stipe doesn't perform the same function as the stem of a plant. The stipe's primary job is to support the cap of the mushroom (though it does also conduct moisture), whereas the stem is part of the nutritional system of a plant. One of the ways that mushrooms are identified is by examining the stipe. As you'll see when we start describing mushrooms and the different strains that exist within a species, the type of stipe is often an important identifier. For instance, the strains of *Psilocybe cubensis*, which is the most prolific species of psychedelic mushroom, often have descriptive names, and some of those names reflect the shape of the stipe. In Penis Envy, for example, the stipe is obviously a central feature in identifying that strain.

The stipe's job is to hold the mushroom above the ground layer so that the spores can leave the hymenium and be distributed as widely as possible. The taller the stipe, the more distribution the spores can achieve. The dangerous little brown mushrooms that we discussed earlier, which include many *Psilocybe* species, typically have very thin stipes. Sometimes people avoid eating the stipe of edible mushrooms. Typically, the stipe is just as edible as the cap, so this is a matter of aesthetics rather than nutrition. With psychedelic mushrooms there is some debate as to whether the stipe has as much psilocybin or other psychedelic compounds as the cap.

STIPE TYPES

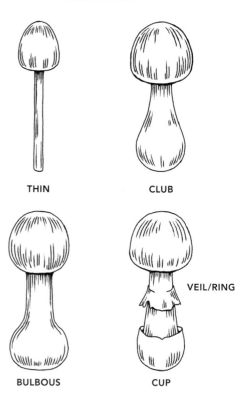

THIN

CLUB

BULBOUS

CUP

VEIL/RING

While it depends on the species, the stipe may have ample psilocybin and can be used in the same way that you would use the cap.

VOLVA

The volva can be likened to an egg. It is from this structure that the mushroom will emerge. I have more to say about the reproduction of mushrooms in a little bit. It's important to know that not all mushrooms will have a visible volva. However, if you see a volva, it will be important to note this, since some poisonous mushrooms are identified by the presence of a robust volva at the base of the stipe.

MYCELIA

The mycelia are the most important part of the organism we call a mushroom. They form a network beneath the mushroom that seeks out nutrition that will sustain the whole organism. They colonize substrates to get that nutrition. Once the substrate is colonized and has maximized the feeding potential, it will begin the reproductive cycle by creating a mushroom that will release spores, and thus the whole process begins again.

Mycelia make up the largest part of a mushroom's anatomy. They look like nerve fibers, and they act like an external digestive system. They colonize substrates like wood, and then often eat the nutrients from the inside out. It is the mycelia that provide the critical functions of the organism. They reach out, grow into new areas, and find themselves making connections with similar species and creating new fruiting bodies (mushrooms) as a result. Our entire ecosystem is dependent on the mycelia that exist within fungal colonies. Fungi consume plants and animals; the process we call decay is comprised of fungi

that consume whatever has lost its "aliveness," whether it is a tree, a piece of pizza, or the body of an animal.

In nature, mycelia function as a network beneath the floor of forests and grasslands. They communicate with the other mycelial branches and plants around them, and work with—and sometimes against—other species. Because mycelia are responsive to environmental changes, some researchers, like Paul Stamets, consider them to be sentient. While that is an intriguing proposition, we have no idea whether the kinds of communication going on between fungi and redwood trees in Yosemite National Park is a conversation or merely a set of biological signals. Researchers have placed mycelia in all kinds of situations to test their capacity for communication. My favorite test is one Stamets quotes in his book *Mycelium Running: How Mushrooms Can Help Save the World.*[1] In it he describes biologist Toshiyuki Nakagaki, who placed a mycelial fiber at the start of a maze. At the other end of the maze, he placed a nutrient that the mycelium would normally seek out. In every experiment the mycelium chose the shortest route possible to get to the nutrient.

We have also learned through both neuroscience and network science (which is just what it sounds like: the study of complex networks) that systems that work on redundant connections are some of the most robust systems that exist in nature. Brains, computer networks, and mycelia all work on very similar structures. Without mycelia, there would be no life on earth. The work of mycelia in the fungi kingdom is to break down everything and recycle it for use by other species. Fungi are all around us, digesting and returning nutrients back to the earth. They are also carrying important messages between trees and other plants. Their presence ensures that the nutrients from a decaying stump are recycled into beneficial molecules like nitrogen and carbon, which can then be used by living trees and saplings in the forest. We need them much more than they need us.

A Crash Course in Mycology

I remember being a kid and having an instant aversion to mushrooms. Anything that was described as a fungus was automatically gross, disgusting, inedible. Mushrooms looked slimy and unappealing. But fungi are more than just mushrooms, and we depend on them for more than simply their use in our cuisine. Fungi are responsible for some of the biggest breakthroughs in medicine over the last 100 years. We use different compounds developed from fungi in antibiotics and cancer treatment, but fungi can also do damage: blighting crops or spreading parasitically through forests and killing trees and decimating habitats. Despite this, humans collaborate with fungi fairly easily. Spending more time befriending and studying them may ultimately help us save ourselves from some of the devastation in our world like famine, cancer, and global warming. The world needs more professional mycologists, so if you're fascinated by this subject and are looking for a new career, consider mycology. You'll be fascinated forever, and while most of the animals and plants of the world have been discovered, only 10% of fungi have been discovered and described by scientists.[2]

When was the last time you had a grilled cheese sandwich? Did you have a beer the last time you watched a football game? What about that fancy dinner party where you had wine and cheese? None of these culinary events would be possible without fungi. The yeast that helps the bread to rise and the beer to ferment is a fungus. Vintners use fungi that grow naturally on grapes or sometimes selective ones to initiate the fermentation process and transform grapes into wine—some of these are penicillium strains. The cheeses you enjoy all use different fungi, including mold, to take on age and flavor. Generally speaking, our food sources would be fundamentally different without fungi.

MAKING MUSHROOMS

Mushrooms are only one form of fungi. We'll focus on these given that mushrooms are the focus of this book. There are other fungi that are incredibly interesting. As we've discussed, the part of the mushroom that reproduces is called a spore. When a fungal spore leaves the comfort of its mushroom cap, it goes in search of a new home and a connection to another spore. The spore will land in an appropriate substrate, like moist soil or rotting wood. When it arrives it will form long, cylindrical filaments called hyphae (singular: hypha). These hyphae grow through the substrate, and as they colonize, they act like an externalized digestive system. They excrete enzymatic proteins that help break down the surface of the substrate so that the hyphae can use its nutrients. The hyphae will find the sugars in the substrate that it has broken down, and they will use those sugars to continue to grow and infiltrate the substrate. As this process unfolds, the hyphae develop mycelium, which are a more organized and robust system that can colonize the substrate more efficiently.

The science of organizing living things in the world is called taxonomy. It was developed by the Swedish scientist Carolus Linnaeus. He created the organizational system we still use to this day when we organize specimens or describe new ones. When you read about a particular species of living thing, you are usually reading its last position in a phylogenetic tree. My dog is categorized as a member of the genus *Canis*, and the species *lupus familiaris*. We don't usually go to the trouble of saying, "This is my dog, Pepper; she is from the kingdom Animalia, from the phylum Chordata, of the class Mammal, of the order Carnivora, from the family Canidae, of the genus *Canis*, and the species *lupus familiaris*."

> **KINGDOM:** Animalia
> **PHYLUM:** Chordata (having a spinal cord)
> **CLASS:** Mammalia (mammal)
> **ORDER:** Carnivora (omnivorous plant and meat, or just meat-eating)
> **FAMILY:** Canidae (dog family: wolves, coyotes, foxes, jackals, dogs)
> **GENUS:** *Canis* (dog genus, includes lots of doglike creatures: wolves, coyotes, wild dogs, dingos)
> **SPECIES:** *Canis lupus famialaris* (when writing the species we always include the genus as part of the name.)

When you write the genus and species in a scientific description the genus is capitalized and the species is not. So now let's try for a psilocybin mushroom: *Psilocybe cubensis*.

> **KINGDOM:** Fungi
> **PHYLUM:** Basidiomycota (can create sexual spores, called basidia)
> **CLASS:** Agaricomycetes (create fruiting bodies, have hyphae, and create a positive and negative haploid reproductive structure)
> **ORDER:** Agaricales (have veils or partial veils, gills, pores, or other distribution types)
> **FAMILY:** Hymenogastraceae
> **GENUS:** *Psilocybe* (produces psilocybin)
> **SPECIES:** *Psilocybe cubensis*

The fungal kingdom is broad, consisting of eight groups or phyla. The phyla are distinguished by how they reproduce, the structure of their hyphae, their spore production and distribution, and microscopic features like DNA and cell wall structure. Within the fungi kingdom only the phyla Basidiomycota and Ascomycota create fruiting bodies.

Taxonomic classification is a description based on different types of observations. Some of these observations are macro (sometimes called gross) features, meaning that they are based on observing a specimen from the outside and describing its features based on what can be observed without a microscope. Thus, micro features are those that can only be observed with the aid of a microscope. Taxonomies were created before the invention of the microscope or the discovery of DNA. As such, taxonomies in the fungal world are actively shifting. There are regular discussions and debates in mycology about the reclassification of species based on new data emerging from microscopic differences or DNA analysis.

FRUITING BODIES

Agaricomycetes are a class of fungi that create fruiting bodies that take on the familiar mushroom shape. These are usually referred to more simply as agarics. They are easily recognized by the gills beneath the cap of the mushroom. When examining the gills, you may notice different types of attachments among the different species of agarics. Some will be free, meaning that they do not touch the stipe, while others will be attached. Gills take on the color of the spores.

VEILS

Universal and partial veils are not unique to the agarics, but they are common features in the *Psilocybe* species. A partial veil protects the spores during development and connects the stem to the cap's edge via a thin membrane. As the mushroom matures, the film of the membrane ruptures. In some species a universal veil covers the entire mushroom as part of the volva when it is in its primordial stage. Recognizing the veil and distinguishing it from other parts like the pellicle will help in identifying certain species of mushrooms and differentiating them from other species. While you may not understand how to apply these details right away, it will become easier with practice. So, spend some time examining all kinds of mushrooms. You can even practice by looking at everyday grocery store mushrooms!

MUSHROOM REPRODUCTION

By now you're hopefully starting to feel comfortable with all the parts of the mushroom. You know that mushrooms have fruiting bodies—the actual mushroom itself—and that they reproduce using spores. You know that the spores travel and eventually germinate

and colonize a substrate. Now let's dig a little deeper. First, let's discuss the general way that mushrooms develop, and then we'll focus specifically on *Psilocybe* mushrooms. This will come in handy in later chapters when we discuss how mushrooms are grown.

The mushroom's life cycle is similar to that of both plants and animals. While there is no such thing as male and female in the mushroom world, there are haploid spores that are frequently described as simply positive and negative. Each haploid spore carries half of the genetic material that makes up a mushroom. In animals, haploids are found in spermatozoa and oocytes (sperm and eggs). Haploids aren't just a random count of half the genetic materials, but rather they carry half of the DNA structure that can be recombined as part of sexual reproduction. Humans have a set of 23 chromosomal pairs. When humans reproduce, one set of those 23 chromosome pairs is found in the gametes of each parent. So far, we are early in mapping the genome of psilocybin mushrooms. Recent unpublished research has identified 13 chromosomal pairs in *Psilocybe cubensis*.[3] So, in each of the haploid spores, you'll find 13 chromosomes. When two hyphae carrying their unique positive or negative haploids find each other, they fuse. The new cells carry the full complement of 13 pairs.

The biology is important because scientists aren't sure yet if all psilocybin-producing mushrooms use the same genes and mechanisms to create psilocybin, or if the variation in the different species is actually a result of different genetic actions. We are very early in the process of understanding how mushrooms produce psilocybin and other compounds in nature.

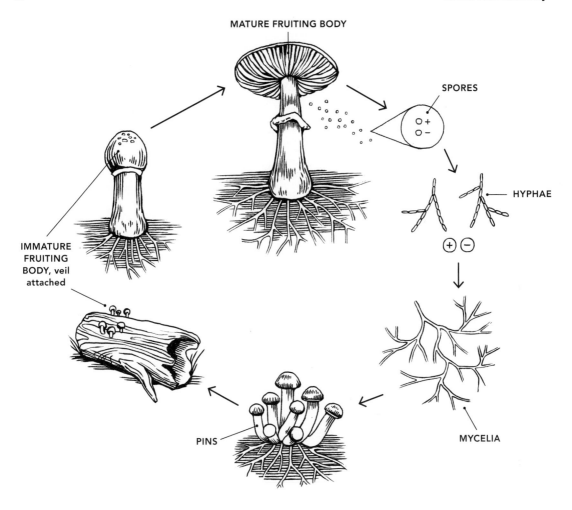

MATURE FRUITING BODY

SPORES

○ +
○ −

HYPHAE

⊕ ⊖

IMMATURE
FRUITING
BODY, veil
attached

MYCELIA

PINS

Haploid reproduction is an evolutionary means of increasing diversity that allows for greater combination of genetic information. Almost all the world's diverse species use a combination of haploid and diploid reproduction to ensure individual diversity within a species. Haploids are found in the separate gametes as a reproductive set, and without haploid reproduction each individual would just be a clone of its parent. In biology this is dangerous, since a lack of diversity means there is an inability to generate stronger traits that can respond to evolutionary or environmental pressures.

The spores of the mushroom carry its haploid cells. Spores are particularly well suited to be carried long distances without being noticed. While they are delicate, they are also robust enough to survive traveling great distances even in harsh environments. When a spore finds its way into a friendly substrate, like soil, a rotting tree, or animal dung, it will start to divide and extend its structure into a hypha, which is a precursor to mycelium that is uniquely designed to seek and digest the contents of the substrate. The hyphae do this by excreting enzymes that break down the complex structure of the substrate.

Many mushrooms are specific to the types of substrates that they "like." To that end, many psychedelic mushrooms prefer decomposing trees or woody substrates. The enzymes in their hyphae are particularly talented at breaking down very hard materials like the cell walls found in wood. When a hypha of one haploid meets its positive or negative complement, they fuse and begin to form a complex network called mycelium. The mycelium, as described earlier, is the most complex and critical part of the fungal structure because it colonizes the substrate. This process is complete when the mycelium has completely subsumed the substrate or when the mycelium "decides" that it has enough nourishment to reproduce. Sometimes these cues come from the environment, as when there is a change in temperature or in the density of light.

As the mycelium colonizes the substrate, it forms something called a hyphal knot, which begins the primordial reproduction phase. The hyphal knot is created when a subset of the hyphae organizes into a structure that will become a fruiting body. In some species this happens inside the volva, and in others it begins later, with the pin stage. Some of the most dangerous mushrooms in the world—the deadly *Amanitas*—have a prominent volva; however, most of the psilocybin-producing mushrooms do not generate a volva. Instead, their fruiting bodies appear via the formation of "buttons" or "pins" that emerge from the substrate.

This happens during the primordial phase of development. When the mushroom is in this phase, it is gathering all of the nutrients it can via the mycelium, and the nourishment that's coming from the mycelium is going directly to create the fruiting body. The additional nutrients help the fruiting body develop all of the various structures that are necessary to complete the structure of the mushroom: stipe, cap, gills, and spores. Once the primordial fruiting body emerges, the stipe will grow and push the fruiting body upward so that as it reaches maturity it can shed its spores. Once a mushroom has reached maturity and shed its spores, the process begins all over again as new spores take root in new substrates.

Understanding the mushroom's unique anatomy will help you understand which mushrooms you're looking at, and this knowledge will also help you recognize mushrooms that you should avoid. Whether you are foraging, growing, or just shopping, knowing which characteristics denote a particular species or strain is a necessity in the world of mushrooms. Understanding the anatomy and reproductive cycle of mushrooms generally and of psilocybin mushrooms specifically will make you a more informed consumer of these magical species. We'll get into the specifics of identifying psilocybin mushrooms in the next chapter.

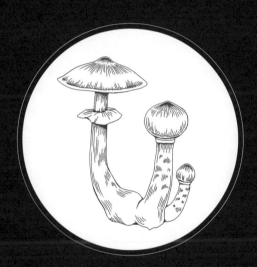

ALACABENZI

Through the genius of evolution, the Earth has selected fungal networks as a governing force managing ecosystems.

—PAUL STAMETS

CHAPTER 4

Mushroom Environments

Fungi are everywhere. Without them life would not be possible. They're in your garden and on the produce you picked up from the farmers market. They're in your cheese, beer, wine, and bread. Mushrooms sometimes appear suddenly in your yard or along a familiar walkway. They show up in rings, apparently fully formed, in places you'd least expect. This penchant for quick growth is one of the reasons that mushrooms of all kinds have been considered magical throughout history. When you add the trippy effects of psychedelic mushrooms or the healing power of medicinal and nutritional mushrooms, it is easy to see why these fungi have been held in such mystical esteem for so long. So far in this book we've covered some of the critical points for understanding what a mushroom is. In this chapter I'll go into ways to identify mushrooms that produce psilocybin and how to tell them apart from those that produce more dangerous toxins. Remember: beware the little brown mushroom! This directive is my primary warning throughout the remainder of this book.

Identifying Psilocybin-Producing Mushrooms

There are multiple habitats where psilocybin-producing mushrooms grow, from the mountains of Mexico to the Pacific Northwest in the United States to New Zealand. One of the most interesting consequences of human activity is the way that mushrooms have accompanied us on our journey. As humans have expanded the ways we travel and the places we travel to, it is not at all uncommon to discover that a species of mushroom once found only in a small mountain village in Germany has somehow made its way to Mongolia on the trousers of an international student heading off on a hiking trip. The student would likely have no idea that they spread the spores of the mushroom. Air travel would have played a part in that transmission, but another way that we are finding psilocybin mushrooms spreading is in wood chips that are used as landscape materials like mulch or fertilizer. In the case of mulch or decorative wood chips, the wood is being sourced from places where there are existing spores or mycelia. When the spores in the wood chips find a complement, they start the mycelial process, and soon there are little pinheads sprouting up in the roses you planted in your garden.

In his book *Psilocybin Mushrooms of the World*, Paul Stamets offers a very simple way to identify mushrooms that produce psilocybin. Ask the following questions:

- If you handle the mushroom, does its skin turn blue? If the answer is yes, that is a good indicator that the mushroom you're handling contains psilocybin.
- On what kind of substrate did you find the mushroom? If you found it on decaying logs or near or on manure, that is another good indicator that your specimen contains psilocybin.
- What color are the mushroom's spores? If they're purplish-black, then the mushroom likely contains psilocybin.

Even if you get all the positive indicators that you have found a psilocybin mushroom *DON'T EAT IT!* You still have more to do to make sure that this mushroom isn't a poisonous imposter.

While I'd love to say that you can just toss this book into a backpack and go find some shrooms, that would be dangerous advice on my part. Reading one book will not make you an expert mushroom hunter. Indeed, the best thing you can do is join a local mycological society and participate in organized gatherings called forays, where whole teams of people go foraging in the woods together. But more on that a little later.

If you want to recognize psilocybin-producing mushrooms, your first step is to study everything you can on what they look like and where you are likely to find them. In the United States the most likely places to find them are wooded areas, preferably those with at least a little bit of old-growth forest available to serve as food for the mushrooms. Most psilocybin species prefer wood substrates or grassy substrates with loads of fertilizer, usually in the form of animal dung. So, a field where cows or horses graze that happens to sit next to a wooded area would be an ideal environment. However, it would be good to know how long the pasture has been a pasture. If it was recently cut back, then there's no telling what kinds of mushrooms you'll find. It's always best to use the utmost caution when foraging.

Areas where old wood growth has been newly exposed are also excellent places to find psilocybin mushrooms. Areas where a river might have recently flooded and or receded or locations where construction has exposed long-fallen trees would be likely places where you'd find psilocybin mushrooms. However, be mindful that a dangerous habitat doesn't make for a pleasant foray. So be careful that you don't decide to go hunting in a newly exposed landslide, or trespass onto a construction site in hopes of getting lucky with the mushrooms.

Any land area that doesn't experience sustained extreme temperatures and that gets sufficient rainfall can host psilocybin mushroom growth. However, the plain reality is that there are far more nonpsychedelic species of mushrooms than there are psychedelic species. It is critical that you do your homework and make sure that you can distinguish poisonous mushrooms from the other mushrooms you might come across. Get a good field guide and join a local mycological society or club. Besides finding like-minded people with more experience in identifying species, you'll also have a new group of friends who won't think it's weird that you want to talk about mushrooms all the time.

Foraging

If you are planning to forage for mushrooms, you'll need some tools. First and foremost, get at least one good field guide (you'll benefit from having more at home). A handful of excellent ones are available. When in doubt, stick to the classics: those produced by the National Audubon Society or almost any book by Paul Stamets. Sometimes you can also find great options in your local used bookstore. I've found dozens of guides over the years; many of them are hand-typed treasures written by local enthusiasts. They can be invaluable. Don't throw out one that was printed on purple mimeograph paper just because it's a few decades old! While the scientific data might not be up to date, you're likely to find some local specialist knowledge that you can't get from a bigger, more encyclopedic treatment.

You will also need a good bag or basket, some gloves, a pencil or pen, a knife, a dusting brush (like archaeologists use), some specimen bags (try to avoid plastic as it speeds the decomposition process), and a small field notebook for noting the location where you found your specimen, the date, temperature, etc. If it's not clear that you'll be doing a slow hike as you forage, I will point it out now. If the foray you're going on is in a wooded area (most are), you'll want to wear appropriate clothing such as hiking boots, light trousers, and a hat. And you'll want to be sure to bring sunscreen and insect repellant. In my bag I also like to pack some white tissue

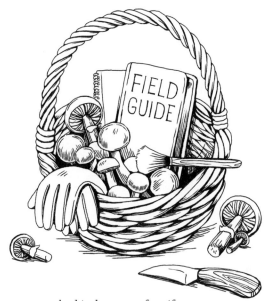

paper—the kind you use for gifts, not the kind in the bathroom. The tissue paper is excellent for wrapping delicate specimens. To avoid confusion when I'm unpacking them later, I typically make a note somewhere on the paper that corresponds to a description in my field notebook. For example, my first specimen might have this written on the paper: "9-12-22, Sp 1A." This is my own nomenclature that includes the date and the specimen number. For me, the A denotes the first place I found any mushrooms, and the number is the order in which I collected them. This is especially important because many little brown mushrooms look alike *and* flush (fruit or grow) together, even though they are completely different species! Be sure to wrap each individual specimen separately, even if you found them together. Remember that different types of little brown mushrooms can grow right next to each other and be dramatically different in their properties.

It is best to go into a foray with a goal in mind. If you have the patience for it, go in the first few times with the goal of finding something—anything—and identifying it correctly. The journey to being able to identify psilocybin-producing mushrooms requires a lifetime of education. Many enthusiasts share humbling stories about going out for years, only to find a rare specimen on their 100th foray. Other folks tell stories about finding a huge flush of some rare mushroom on their first or second outing, only to never find the flush again, even after looking in the same place year after year. Have patience and treat the mushroom spirits respectfully.

When you do find a specimen, take a quick photo of it in situ (where it lives) before collecting it. Wear gloves to protect yourself from toxins and to protect specimens from contaminants. Be sure to be gentle with the mushroom. Use the knife to separate the stipe from the substrate. If you can, dig a little bit underneath to preserve the base of the stipe. Next, use the brush to remove any dirt or debris. Lay the specimen on white tissue paper if you have it. Some people like to take specimen photos right away (the in situ photos are not the same as the specimen photos). There are good reasons for both methods. Some people find it easier to identify the species when they have all the photos taken close to the same time. I usually wait until later. I find it helpful to compare the in situ photos with the specimens at home, and then take the photos. Decide for yourself which works better for you.

Mark the paper with the date and specimen number and note the location where you found it. If you're on a foray with others, you may not have a lot of time to write field notes. In this case, make a quick note in your notebook so that you can retrace your steps.

> **5-15-24:** Woods near Montecito hiking trail.
>
> **SP 1A:** Little white mushroom, with mycelial threads, small, no immediate bluing. Found on base of rotting stump.

You can write a more detailed description later. At the end of most forays there will be time to look at one another's specimens. This is also a great moment to make notes, like "Bob says specimen is likely *Psilocybe caerulescens*; will check against key or field guide," or what have you.

A word of caution. Please don't rely on a photo app to help you identify mushrooms. There is far too much subtlety from mushroom to mushroom, and the apps are not always able to discern the differences between species. Don't bet your health or well-being on an application created by someone who is great at visual recognition software alone. Apps can be useful, but they shouldn't be relied upon as your sole source of information. If you use a photo app and a field guide, and they provide different information, then you need to find another source. Ask someone more experienced than you for their advice, or look to a different field guide for more information.

Which brings us to keys. These are handy checklists that have been created by experienced foragers and mycologists to help you discern what species you are examining. Some keys can be quite long, but they are invaluable tools. They ask you questions that help you identify what species you have found. Keys have always reminded me of a schematic or an engineer's flow chart; they're basically asking yes/no questions, and each answer will send you in a new direction depending on your response.

I'll show you how it works by creating a key for animals that you're very familiar with—a cat and a dog—to help you understand how keys work. In this exercise you're trying to identify a cat.

1. Is it (or should it be) covered in fur?
   A. Yes (continue)
   B. No (stop: Sphinx cat)

2. Does it appear to be more than 25 pounds in weight?
   A. Yes (stop: unless a wild cat or extremely overweight, dog)
   B. No (continue)

3. Does it have retractable claws?
   A. Yes (stop: cat)
   B. No (continue) (a cat whose claws have been removed would garner a no)

4. Does it make barking sounds when alarmed?
   A. Yes (dog)
   B. No (cat)

This is a silly example, but you get the idea. A foraging key is similar in concept, but it may be several pages long. One of the best I've ever seen was in a small field guide called *Poisonous and Hallucinogenic Mushrooms* (1977 edition) by Richard and Karen Haard.[1] It also had amazing illustrations. If you can find a copy in print, I highly recommend it! Their key to discerning poisonous species of mushrooms has more than 30 points in the checklist. At several points in the list the authors tell you which species you're examining based on how many questions you've answered so far.

If you're joining a foray, keys and guides might be shared by the group's organizers. If you receive useful keys, I highly recommend saving them for ongoing research and field trips. Some of these will remain useful for many years. Keys are very helpful after a foray or when you have been out gathering specimens on your own. If you haven't been given a key or can't get one from your local foray group, then I recommend you start your own.

Separate your specimens and write down in excruciating detail everything that you can observe. Your notes should look something like this.

5-15-24: Woods near Montecito hiking trail.

SP 1A: Little white mushroom, with mycelial threads, small, no immediate bluing. Found on base of rotting stump.

Bob says specimen is likely *Psilocybe caerulescens*; will check against key or field guide.

White mushroom approximately 2 inches tall found on rotting oak tree stump near running stream.

Stipe is bulbous with mycelial fibers at the bottom. Fibers are blue in color.

Cap is white at margins, but caramel colored on top.

Cap margin curls downward and colors blue.

> There are some remnants of the veil at the margin.
> There is a clear pellicle that isn't separable.
> At the base of the stipe and on the cap there is bluing from handling.
> The stipe has some fibers and a partial veil.
> The gills appear grayish, nearing black, looking like soot or ash.

✖

The Spore Print

Looking at these field notes, it seems likely you have found yourself a *Psilocybe* mushroom, but we need more data for the identification to be conclusive. It's time to make a spore print from your specimen. Get some white paper, some black paper, and some aluminum foil. Aluminum foil can be useful if you want to germinate mushrooms from the samples you discover, and it is easy to sterilize with alcohol. To begin making your spore print, gently remove the cap from the stem.

If you notice that the gills appear to be white, then you'll want to use either black paper or aluminum foil to get the spore print. The white spores will be easier to see this way. Based on the sample notes we created in the last section for the hypothetical specimen we found in Montecito, we would use white paper or aluminum foil to make our print because the gills were dark in color. Next, place the cap of the mushroom from the specimen gently on either the white paper or the aluminum foil with the gills facing the paper. Use a drop of water at the top of the mushroom to encourage it to drop its spores onto the

paper. Next, cover the cap and the paper with a drinking glass (ideally, its circumference should be similar to that of the cap). It will take the mushroom a little time to release its spores, usually a few hours.

Once you have the spore print, you'll be able to make a more educated guess about the color of the spores. A purple color in your print denotes the presence of psilocybin. Once you've narrowed your options down by making a spore print, you're in a much better position to offer an educated guess about the sample you've collected. The spore print we made using our hypothetical sample from Montecito yielded purple spores that had a slight brown hue. This result, along with our description of when and where we found it, indicates that we have a psilocybin mushroom. It looks like Bob might have been right about the specimen being *Psilocybe caerulescens*! Since this is your first time examining a mushroom, it's best to check with someone who has more experience before you make your final identification.

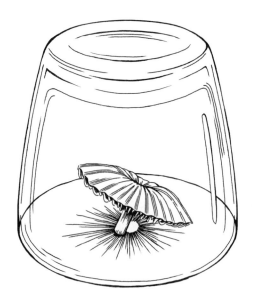

Foraging for psilocybin mushrooms can be great fun, but remember, it is also much easier to find something poisonous than it is to find something magical. So, it's best to learn with more experienced foragers and develop your mycology skills over time. A word of warning about other foraging risks. Mushrooms are excellent at recycling heavy metals from substrates. Depending on where you are foraging, you may find wild mushrooms that have begun to do some cleanup of their environment by leaching heavy metals and toxins from the earth or wood. You won't have any way of knowing whether this is the case, so I will repeat my recommendation that you forage with more experienced people and that you use significant discernment in deciding whether or not to ingest what you've found.

Another quick warning: there is a condition called wood lover's paralysis that can occur after ingesting wood substrate–loving mushrooms. The effects don't last long (roughly 24–48 hours), but they are very frightening. As the name implies, the patient often experiences partial or full paralysis of the body or limbs. Sometimes this extends to the larynx, so the person may struggle or be completely unable to talk. When in doubt, don't eat the mushrooms you find. You can always use your spore prints to safely germinate your own mushrooms later if you found something magical. (Wood lover's paralysis tends to come from the substrate, not the spore prints.)

Growing Your Own Mushrooms

Now we're getting into tricky territory. Consuming mushrooms you find in the forest comes with risks, but there are different kinds of risks that come with growing your own mushrooms. Later in the book we will discuss places where mushrooms are being decriminalized and what the changes in the law will mean for those of us interested in the powerful potential of psychedelics as tools for healing. Until there is an actual reduction in the scheduling of psilocybin, it is still an illegal drug in the United States and in many other places. Bear that in mind as you consider whether you want to grow mushrooms for either scientific or personal purposes.

With the risks made abundantly clear, from here on out everything I'm going to share with you is theoretical and for scientific purposes only. I am not endorsing these methods, nor am I recommending that you engage in any illegal activity. As such, the methods described in this section are abbreviated. Should you want to read an authoritative guidebook on all the ways that you can grow mushrooms, try *The Psilocybin Mushroom Bible: The Definitive Guide to Growing and Using Magic Mushrooms* by Haze and Mandrake[2] or *Growing Gourmet and Medicinal Mushrooms* by Paul Stamets.[3]

We are going to focus on the PF Tek method. Please note that this is one of the most well-established methods for growing mushrooms, and there are companies that specialize in providing PF Tek kits to help get you started. This method is great for growing any kind of fungi, and you can use it to germinate Lion's Mane or other nutritious mushrooms; it's not only for psychedelics. The person who is famous for this technique is a man named Robert McPherson. He went by the pseudonym Psilocybe Fanaticus (PF) to protect his identity.

Here are the basics of what you'll need to get started:

- A clean place to work where there's not a lot of circulating air
- Vermiculite (substrate much like a fertilizer)
- Brown rice flour or rye seeds
- Big mixing bowl
- Hammer
- Nail
- Wide-mouth 16-ounce mason jars (make sure the mouth is wide; traditional ones are narrower at the top, which can make it difficult to get the resulting mycelium cake out of the jar)
- Alcohol swabs, or rubbing alcohol and cotton balls
- Aluminum foil
- Permanent marker
- Big pot with a tight-fitting lid, or a pressure cooker (to sterilize)
- Wire rack or trivet (for cooling)
- Lighter or long matches
- Syringes (for inoculating the substrate with spores)
- Spore solution
- Transparent tape or masking tape
- Larger clear grow box with a lid (like the kind you use to store holiday decor)
- Gloves
- Mask
- Shallow pan
- Distilled water, cold
- Sponge
- Thermometer

This technique has been used repeatedly by people who want to grow all kinds of mushrooms. It is very reliable when followed closely,

it makes it easy to see contaminants, and it is excellent if you are growing for yourself. If you're planning on sharing your mushrooms, you might need more than one mason jar. Enthusiasts say creating four small PF Tek cakes should be perfect for your own personal use. The whole procedure takes three to five weeks, depending on the species or strain of mushrooms being cultivated. If you are growing psilocybin-containing mushrooms and decide to dry them, their potency will last about a month. Of course, they're excellent fresh, but if you want to keep them for any length of time you should consider drying them to preserve their potency.

STEP 1: PREPARE THE SUBSTRATE

Set aside about ⅓ cup of vermiculite for each 16-ounce jar so that you can cover the substrate in each of the jars at the end of this preparation phase. For every 16-ounce mason jar that you'll use, mix ⅔ cup of vermiculite and ⅔ cup brown rice flour in a large bowl and stir in enough water so that the mixture is wet but not soupy. It should look a bit like oatmeal, or like cereal that doesn't have enough milk. Make sure that the vermiculite pieces are thoroughly covered in flour. The flour is going to be the food that the mycelium seeks out. The vermiculite is a helpful addition that holds water to keep moisture in the jar.

STEP 2: PREPARE THE JARS

You'll be injecting the spores into the jar using a needle, and the needle won't go through the hard metal top of the mason jar, so you'll need to make a few holes in the lid. Using a hammer and nail on a safe surface, make a few holes in the metal top. Three or four should be sufficient. Once you've made the holes, wipe both sides of the lid with an alcohol swab, being careful not to cut your finger on the metal lid. Next, cover the top of the lid with a piece of aluminum foil on both the top and the bottom. Mark the location of the holes with a permanent marker so you know where they are.

STEP 3: FILL AND PREP FOR INOCULATION

Fill the jars almost to the top with the substrate mixture. You don't want to pack the jars, so don't tap them for the substrate to settle and don't force it down. Add the plain dry vermiculite you had set aside to the top of the substrate. Leave a half inch to 1 inch of room at the top, so that the mycelium can expand. Next, wipe the area around the lid with a fresh alcohol swab, making sure that there are no bits of substrate lingering around. Any contaminants could use bits of substrate to colonize and compete with the mycelium, so be sure to wipe down those areas. Also, make sure that the jars are covered by the aluminum foil and that the lid is tightly screwed on before proceeding to sterilize the jars.

STEP 4: STERILIZE THE JARS

Place the jars on a steamer tray inside a large pot, or you can use a pressure cooker. Add a couple of inches of water to the bottom of the pot. Cover the pot and slowly warm the jars and water together as you bring the water to a boil. Let the jars steam for 1 hour, checking the water level occasionally so the pot doesn't boil dry. You will need at least 1 hour for four 16-ounce jars, and you should add 15 minutes for each additional jar. If you have more than six jars, you should work in batches. Don't try to sterilize more than six jars at a time. If you

have a pressure cooker, you can save a little time in this process. You can use the pressure cooker for 45 minutes at approximately 15 psi for up to six jars. Be sure to read the instructions on your pressure cooker to find out how much water you need to use to make preservatives or canned fruit, as this is basically the same procedure.

STEP 5: COOL

The substrate must be 100% cooled before you introduce the spores. Place a wire rack or raised trivet in a clean area that is out of the way. Remove the jars from the heat and set them on the rack so there is air flow around the bottom of the jars while they're cooling. Be careful when handling the hot jars and *DO NOT OPEN THEM!!* It will take at least 2 to 3 hours for the substrate to cool to room temperature. Most cultivators wait 12 hours or more to be 100% sure that the jars are ready to go. Be mindful that even a little warmth is not okay. Heat will kill the spores, and warmth will encourage bacteria growth. The jars must be *completely* cooled before you can perform the next, critical step.

STEP 6: INOCULATE

When the jars are completely cooled, inoculate the substrate with the spores. Wipe the needle of the syringe with an alcohol swab, then use the flame of a lighter or match to heat it until you see the needle change color to red or orange. Allow the needle to cool (don't touch it to test). Once it's cool, inject the spore solution into the jar through one of the marked spots where you made a hole in the foil-covered lid. You should be able to see the needle through the glass jar. Repeat this injection process with each of the holes, covering each hole with tape immediately after you're done. Aim the needle toward the glass wall of the substrate as you inject the spore solution. This will help you watch the process unfold more clearly. You'll be able to see where the spores start the germination process.

STEP 7: INCUBATE

This is when the magic happens! Place the jars somewhere dark and warm, like a closet, wardrobe, or cabinet. The mycelium is going to begin the process of colonizing the substrate inside the jar. The incubation time will depend on the species. As long as the dark storage location doesn't experience extreme variations in temperature, it should be fine to just leave the jars alone and check on them every couple of days. When you can see the mycelium has completely taken over the jar, you'll have what's referred to as a cake. Be sure to check the bottom of the jars to make certain that the mycelium has completely taken over the substrate. If you're in doubt about its progress, it's best to wait a few more days. A note on contamination: if the jars smell weird, like spoiled fruit or mold, or if there are different-colored blobs showing up in the substrate or on the glass, you can be pretty sure that your jars are contaminated. Toss that sample and start over.

STEP 8: PREPARE THE GROW BOX

Get the grow box/fruiting chamber ready. Use an inexpensive clear plastic storage box like those typically used to store holiday supplies so that it's easy to see into and move around. Wipe down the inside, outside, and the cover of your box with alcohol swabs, wearing gloves and a mask. It is important to stay cautious about contamination. Once you've wiped

down the grow box, cover the bottom of the box in vermiculite and prepare a separate pan with vermiculite before moving on to the next step.

STEP 9: RELEASE THE CAKES

Wear a pair of sterile gloves for these next steps, and I recommend wearing a mask. Some people believe that the need for a sterile environment is much lower at this stage, but I recommend continuing to be careful. Once the mycelium has completely colonized the substrate it should be relatively easy to remove from the jar. As mentioned earlier, the mycelial substrate in this state is called a cake. Remove the cake from each of the jars and rinse it off with distilled water. Place each cake in a bowl with cold distilled water and cover it with foil, wax paper, or parchment paper. Leave the bowl filled with the cake and cold water in the fridge for between 6 and 12 hours—the longer you do this, the better your results will be, but don't go past 18 hours. If you live in a dry climate, do your best to really dunk the cakes in the water. The cold water stimulates the fruiting process and will provide some much-needed moisture. Roll the cakes in the dry vermiculite that you set aside in the pan earlier.

STEP 10: PUT CAKES IN THE GROW BOX

Place the cakes into the grow box. They shouldn't be too close to one another; you want the fruiting bodies to have plenty of room to grow. Home growers often grow four at a time, because you can have one grow box at a time, and it's not a challenge to manage. If you live in a cold environment, make sure that the grow box won't get too

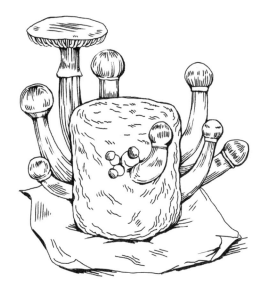

the stipe and the margin of the cap will be torn. That tells you the mushrooms have matured. Once you've harvested the mushrooms, you can use the same cakes again. The critical part of the mushroom is the mycelium. So long as the mycelium has nutrients, it will continue fruiting. When the cakes start to collapse, you'll know it's time to start the process over, but don't throw the cakes away! Use them as part of your substrate in the next batch. They typically yield even better fruiting bodies this way.

Acquiring Mushrooms

A handful of states have decriminalized possession of psilocybin-producing mushrooms, and a few states have introduced legislation to allow mushrooms to be shared in either a ceremonial or psychotherapeutic setting. The restriction in those instances is against the *sale* of the mushrooms, not their use. There are some places where even though it is not legal to buy or possess mushrooms, you can still buy them in a cannabis dispensary. It's all very confusing. Be sure to know the laws of your jurisdiction to protect yourself.

The most important thing I can say about getting mushrooms from someone else is caveat emptor: buyer beware! If you are buying or being gifted mushrooms, don't be afraid to ask where they came from and how they were grown. My hope is that by reading this book you will have gained some valuable knowledge into the species and strains of mushroom that you might encounter. In the same way that the cannabis industry has invested time and resources into adding higher concentrations of THC and CBD in their products, so too

cold. If you live in a dry environment, make sure that the grow box won't get too dry. Place a sterilized sponge soaked with distilled water in the bottom of the grow box. That is enough to keep the contents in the covered box moist. Some people get super fancy and use equipment that measures humidity inside the box; if that is too much work for you, the sponge method should work fine. The distilled water is to avoid introducing any pathogens using the water. Placing a thermometer in the room where the box resides is a good idea, especially if it's winter, or if you live in a cold place. The temperature shouldn't swing too much in the room, and the box should stay relatively temperate—between 68°F and 74°F is ideal.

STEP 11: HARVEST

Once you see the mushrooms starting to form pins, you're just days away from having a wonderful mushroom flush (a fancy name for a crop) that's ready for harvest. When you have mostly mature mushrooms, harvest *all* of them, not just the ones that look grown. You'll know they're ready because the veil between are cultivators of magic mushrooms working diligently to increase the tryptamine concentrations in their mushrooms.

Because *Psilocybe cubensis* is the most prolifically cultivated psychedelic mushroom in the world, it is the one you are most likely to encounter. You may hear references to the name of its strain, and indeed many of those strains have been developed for higher psychedelic effects. The strain names could be anything from Penis Envy to Snow White. So be sure to ask about whether or not the mushroom you have is a "cube," meaning a *P. cubensis*. Don't be afraid to ask what the expected tryptamine concentration is for that particular strain. Depending on the kind of experience you're looking for, you'll want to be sure you're aligning your desires and goals with the kinds of mushrooms that are available to you. The varieties section in this book will give you a place to begin. Bear in mind that strains wax and wane in popularity with each passing day. What was popular a month ago may have been replaced with some new strain developed by a new cultivator. The most important thing is to know what questions to ask, and you should be well prepared by the time you finish reading this book.

Storing Mushrooms

Most people find that dried mushrooms tend to last the longest, while fresh ones will have the most potency. If you acquire fresh mushrooms and can't use them right away, you should dry them. If you grow them, you'll most certainly want to dehydrate them so you can keep them longer. Dried mushrooms are also much easier to microdose, as you can

pulverize them and measure out the dried powder more easily.

Most cultivators use a dehydrator because it's easy. Some people have complicated ways of drying, from placing specimens in an oven with no heat to setting them close to heating vents in their house. Before you can place a specimen in a dehydrator, you will need to air-dry it a bit. Set it on a clean towel or sheet that has been placed on a flat surface like a table or counter. If you're drying multiple specimens, separate them so that they're not touching each other. After a few hours, place the specimens into the dehydrator. Before you do this, check their sizes. If one is too big and maybe still a little moist, you'll want to cut it into two pieces. This isn't always a necessary step, but you want to at least give the mushroom a chance to dry out properly.

I had a colleague who swore by the oven method, but I've found that mushrooms lose their potency this way. In this method you place the mushrooms on a pan or baking sheet and set it in the oven. If you're using a gas oven with a pilot light, no heat is necessary; they'll warm and dry by the pilot light. If you have an electric oven or a pilotless gas stove, preheat it on the lowest possible temperature and turn the heat off before placing the mushrooms in the oven. Leave them in for a few hours. If you don't have a dehydrator, this is the next best method, but I haven't seen it perfected yet.

Once the mushrooms are dried, they are good for about four to six weeks before they lose their potency. Place them in a cool, dark place, like a cabinet or a coffee can. Please note that putting them in the freezer or fridge is usually a sure way to lose potency. There is something about really cold temperatures that makes psilocybin break down more quickly. Some people pulverize mushrooms or chop them into small pieces and mix them into chocolate truffles; they tend to last a little longer in the fridge this way.

You have now been introduced to several ways to identify, forage, grow, acquire, and store magic mushrooms. Where we go next is the fun part! How do we work with these powerful compounds? What is the best way to use them for healing and deepening the mind, body, and soul? You may be asking yourself, *What will happen to me? What should I do? How do I prepare for a psychedelic trip? Should I do this alone? Or with others? What is the best experience for me?* Well, buckle up, because we're about to go on a wild ride as we explore the ways you can work with psychedelic mushrooms.

Psychedelic therapy creates an interval of maximum plasticity in which, with proper guidance, new patterns of thought and behavior can be learned.

—MICHAEL POLLAN

CHAPTER 5

Working with Mushrooms

We are in the midst of what many researchers, psychotherapists, and doctors have come to refer as the psychedelic renaissance. In the last several years, research into the therapeutic uses of psychedelics has exploded. Drug companies are trying to isolate the compounds found in psychedelic mushrooms. The known compounds psilocybin, psilocin, baeocystin, norbaeocystin, and aeruginascin are found in varying degrees, depending on the species of mushroom being studied. There may be trace compounds yet to be discovered as well. The research that is currently underway is in its infancy. Understanding how these compounds best interact with each other to produce positive psychological or psychiatric effects is the holy grail of psychedelic research.

There are many ways to work with psychedelic mushrooms. In this book I'm not talking about different ways to prepare them for ingestion, though there are plenty of those. From magic limoncello to spring psilo salad, you can find plenty of ways to enjoy magic mushrooms. There are dozens of ways that people get the active components into the body, from making tea to making chocolates laced with psilocybin mushrooms. But when it comes to how people use psychedelic mushrooms, there are three well-known primary purposes that have well-known methodologies: microdosing, recreational use, and psychedelic therapy. It is important to note that because the use of psychedelics is still illegal in most places, conducting traditional research has been challenging. Up until 20 years ago it was nearly impossible to conduct clinical research on psychedelics. There was a tacit embargo on any research that used these substances. Before 1968 and the creation of the schedule system for drugs in the United States, there were more than 1,000 studies on classic psychedelics, from LSD to psilocybin. Findings were generally positive. Researchers discovered that psychedelics were very effective in helping treat patients with addiction, depression, and other "neurotic" disorders, as they were called at the time.

The association of the counterculture movement with psychedelics was a sociocultural quagmire, and the US political establishment used the Comprehensive Drug Abuse Prevention and Control Act of 1970 to crack down on these substances. One of the results was that public opinion on research into their clinical uses shifted from being hopeful to disgraceful. Manufacturers stopped making drugs that could be used by researchers, and as a result psychedelics went 100% underground for almost 40 years.

Roland Griffiths's research team at the Johns Hopkins University School of Medicine began to quietly experiment with psilocybin in 2000. The group was the first to get federal approval for psychedelic research in decades. In 2006, Francisco Moreno's lab at the University of Arizona started to engage in clinical research on DMT. To everyone's surprise, both groups reported successful results. The research environment has become better for groups like these, though there is still a long way to go. It is difficult to get regulatory approval to work with compounds that are considered illicit drugs. But the research at Johns Hopkins and the University of Arizona has continued. Many other universities and medical schools have taken up the cause as well, including groups at Yale, Harvard, UCLA, New York University, and more. Research focused on smokers, people at the end of life, and those suffering from addiction has proven that psychedelics can be powerful forces for good.

The gold standard for any medical treatment is durability of results. That usually means that the patient in the study has no symptoms for at least six months following treatment. When researchers started to show that smokers and alcoholics were still abstaining from smoking and drinking six months after being treated with psychedelics, the traditional biomedical establishment began to sit up and take notice. There are more than 100 studies of psychedelics underway worldwide as of this writing. Multiple high-profile research groups and centers have been established to pursue legitimate studies in psychedelic

medicine. The Center for Psychedelic and Consciousness Research at Johns Hopkins University Medical School was established in 2020 with a $17 million private grant.[1] The NYU Langone Center for Psychedelic Medicine is another that began in 2021.[2] Many institutions have been engaging in psychedelic research for more than a decade. The establishment of these research centers points to the durability of clinical results and the need to expand research in these domains.

More than two decades after Griffiths's work began there are protocols for psychedelic therapy, microdosing, and recreational tripping and trip sitting. While there haven't been many large-scale, double-blind studies to examine the efficacy of all of these protocols, more studies are being conducted each year. It is likely that once psilocybin is taken off Schedule I, it will open the door to the kinds of research that the world is waiting for. The schedule status of multiple psychedelics will likely be changed in the near future, moving these from illicit substances to ones that can be prescribed by a physician.

We are still relying primarily on anecdotal evidence for some of our guidelines, but medical research is widely available and shows promising results both in clinical findings and research designs. The lack of double-blind results doesn't mean that the available results aren't compelling. It means that people report benefits and that scientists can't control for all the variables in these experiences. Are the benefits because of a placebo effect? Are they from a prioritization of serotonergic 5-HT2A agonists in particular areas of the brain? Is the population who takes psychedelics self-selected based on personality traits? Or could it be a particular neurological profile that creates the likelihood of self-selection? We don't yet have the answers.

This is one of the most exciting times in history to be engaged at the forefront of research. Psychedelics open a whole new area of exploration that begins with pharmacology and neurobiology. There is a universe of possible outcomes because there is so much more that is unknown at this point in the state of psychedelic and neuroscience research. We could discover whole new actions of neurobiological agonists and antagonists in the research. We could discover neuro-regional hierarchal behavior in response to the presence of psychedelics. We also know that psychedelics are responsible for neurogenesis in research subjects. The idea that psychedelics can jump-start this process is revolutionary. In short, this space is dynamically changing each and every day! If you're curious about psychedelics and medicine, there is no better time to be learning. This subject can keep you fascinated (and busy) for the next 50 years.

In the next several pages we will go through some of the ways that people use psychedelic mushrooms. You'll find this list is comprehensive, but not exhaustive. If you are considering your own psychedelic journey, above all make sure that you are working with trusted people. If you are growing your own mushrooms, make sure you get spores from people you trust. If you are acquiring raw or dried mushrooms, make sure they are from someone who is experienced and knowledgeable. If you are using prefilled capsules, please don't get them from just anyone. Psilocybin production is still illegal as of this writing. Be incredibly careful and mindful of the fact that for most producers, this is a business. An illegal business will naturally have more risk,

and people who are willing to be on the cutting edge are also sometimes willing to take chances that you wouldn't be comfortable taking on your own. Though it is still illegal in much of the United States, the safest thing is to grow your own mushrooms from spores, which can be acquired legally for scientific purposes. It is a complicated process, but not as technically difficult as it may seem. Always use caution.

Understanding Dosing

There are loads of guidebooks, magazine articles, online forums, and personal advice available for people interested in using psychedelic mushrooms. Most psychonauts follow some rudimentary measures. The most available mushrooms come from the species *Psilocybe cubensis* (a comprehensive species list follows in chapter 6). Dozens of strains of this species are cultivated by professionals and amateurs. A strain is like a unique type within a species. For example, different strains of cannabis, like Indica or Sativa, have different properties based on their concentrations and balances of cannabinoids. Similarly, different strains of wine-producing grapes will have different flavors and properties. With psilocybin mushrooms, even within the same flush or crop an individual fruiting body may have a higher or lower concentration of psychedelic compounds than another. There are several reasons for this.

One is that a particular species itself aggregates the psychedelic or tryptamine compounds more than another based on its own genetic makeup. Certain *Psilocybe* species produce higher concentrations of psilocybin and psilocin than others. The species *P. azurescens* and *P. semilanceata* produce some of the highest known concentrations of tryptamines. Wild mushrooms tend to grow lower concentrations than cultivated ones. And the conditions of the substrate or growing environment also make a big difference in the concentration of tryptamines in the mushroom. Healthy substrates make for potent mushrooms.

A second reason why a mushroom might be higher in active compounds is because the specimen itself is young. The older the specimen, the more likely it is that the active components may have broken down. Paul Stamets has theorized that psilocin and psilocybin may be easily broken down by ultraviolet light. He noticed that mushrooms that grew in the shade tended to have more potency than those that grew in sunlight. So, a young mushroom that has grown in a shady place is likely to be more potent than an older specimen that has lived its life in the sun.

Another thing to consider is whether a mushroom is dried or fresh. And depending on the species, a mushroom that is picked and then quickly dried when young is more likely to have a higher concentration of tryptamines than an older mushroom.

In medical research, regardless of the medicine being tested, most scientific journals refer to very low dose (VLD), low dose (LD), moderate dose (MD), high dose (HD), and very high dose (VHD). For our purposes, we will include the language that is familiar in this domain, and we will refer to a VLD as a microdose. Psychonaut and ethnobotanist Terence McKenna coined the term *heroic dose*. This term usually applies to something between HD and VHD. Most people will

never need a heroic dose to have a meaningful experience with psychedelic mushrooms.

There are several ways to think about dosing. A microdose is considered a subperceptual or subtherapeutic dose. This means that the dose is so low as to not create any impairment, though there is debate on whether it creates minor alterations of perception. A microdose is usually 10% of the minimum therapeutic dose. A low dose of psilocybin is considered 1.0 to 1.2 g of dried mushrooms, usually of the species *P. cubensis*. This species of mushroom is a reliable producer of psilocybin, and its concentrations can typically be trusted. There is currently no reliable way to home test samples for psilocybin concentrations. Thus, it is important that you know your varieties and sources. When you read about mushrooms that have been tested, these are usually happening as part of scientific research, or perhaps as part of mycological research being done by enthusiasts or mycologists. Indeed, every measurement reported in this book has come from other researchers who have reported on the concentrations of psilocybin, psilocin, and other tryptamines— usually through mass spectrometry. One of the most well-known places for enthusiasts to get information on psilocybin concentrations by strain is the Hyphae (formerly the Psilocybin) Cup, a competition for cultivators to submit samples and test the concentration of active compounds. The goal is to breed the sample with the highest psilocybin content. The program is run by Oakland Hyphae and the related Hyphae Labs. The lab provides testing services, and winning the cup is a sought-after accolade for cultivators.

If you are new to psychedelics, please start at a low dosage. There are several important medical and psychological reasons to start out this way. First and foremost—and most obvious—is that you have no idea what your personal biochemistry is or how your own personal neurobiology will respond in the presence of psilocybin. If you've taken other psychedelics, like LSD, MDMA, or ketamine, you may have an idea how you *psychologically* respond. But ketamine and MDMA work on different neurotransmitters, and you may have a completely different experience with psilocybin. One of my favorite expressions is "slow is smooth, and smooth is fast." It's used a lot in sports. It basically means don't rush the basics. You'll do better if you go slow in the beginning so that you can go fast later.

Some people with certain psychological or psychiatric diagnoses may find psychedelic experiences unpleasant with these substances. Anyone who has a diagnosis that affects their neurotransmitter load should take extra time to research, discuss with their physician, and consider if taking mushrooms is the best course for them, and if they do decide to go ahead, they should take extra precautions. People who struggle with bipolar disorder in any form may not have good experiences due to the activation of serotonin receptors in the brain. Psychedelic mushrooms are a serotonin agonist, and as such they have an effect on the serotonin pathways in the brain and nervous system. In addition, there are certain medications that shouldn't be taken with mushrooms. Obviously, you should consult a physician about changing any medical treatment or protocol before considering a psychedelic trip. You'll find that many psychiatrists and nurse practitioners are interested in the research findings that are going on in the psychedelic world. If you trust your provider, please have

a discussion with them before discontinuing any medications or treatment. I'll cover contraindications later in the book, but as most people pick up a book like this and look at it piecemeal, it seems important to include it in more than one place.

HOW TO THINK ABOUT DOSING

The psychedelic experience reflects an altered state of consciousness, not a different place or dimension. This is sometimes referred to as a journey or trip. All cultures have some means of achieving an altered state of consciousness. When sacred plants are used, how fast and deep you go depends on the dose of medicine. The lowest doses are the microdose, very low dose (VLD), and low dose (LD). In psilocybin research the differences between a VLD and a microdose are negligible. Because this isn't a manual for a particular research study, we won't concern ourselves with the VLD descriptions. A microdose will be around 10% of the lowest effective dose. Since the lowest effective dose is usually around 1 g, that would mean that a microdose is 0.1 g. Because some varieties and strains have higher concentrations of tryptamines, be sure to check here or in another reliable guide before consuming any novel strains! An LD should almost always be your introduction to using psychedelic mushrooms. You may have a particular affinity for psilocybin, or you may have a potent strain. Always start low—don't rush your mush! Many times people are excited to have the kinds of experiences they've heard about from friends, seen in movies, or read about in books. But rushing might bring with it an unpleasant experience, so do your homework, prepare properly, and start slow. You'll be grateful you did.

The moderate dose (MD) for most of the mushrooms you will grow or procure will be about 1.5–2.5 g. This is an expected dose for most *Psilocybe cubensis* strains. At this dose you can expect to have a more psychedelic experience. You'll see some visual stimuli, likely fractal images, maybe colorful triangles or iridescent lines. They'll be there whether your eyes are open or closed. You may experience a "body high," depending on the strain or species you're working with. This may feel like a body that is energized and wants to move, or it could feel like a body that is heavy and wants to stay glued to the ground. Allow the experience to unfold; it won't last forever. You will probably feel some euphoria, though at this dosage it may not reach the level of oneness that some people report. You can also expect some mild synesthesia at this level, things like hearing colors and tasting sounds.

Some people who journey at this dose will have a challenging experience. This usually comes in the form of memories or feelings associated with trauma or shame. The important thing to note about this is that the psyche is serving this to you not as punishment but as clarity. If you have a challenging journey at this dose level, don't presume you have to immediately go higher next time to avoid it. Those images or feelings are being brought up for a psychological, spiritual, or emotional reason. Follow the inner healing intelligence of your deep self in that instance. You are being asked to (at least) acknowledge something that needs your attention. Most people who have challenging experiences at this level will vividly remember what they learned in their psychedelic voyage. Allow yourself to write in a journal, draw, paint, or talk into a recording app during or immediately after

your encounter. If you have a difficult journey, bring the images and lived experience to a trusted person trained in integration.

With a high dose (HD, anywhere from 2.5–5.0 g, depending on your biochemistry and the species or strain), you can expect the kinds of things you've read or heard about. This is the realm of full-blown psychedelia. There will likely be cognitive, visual, and auditory distortions. Your perception of time may change dramatically. You may feel far away from your body or struggle to find words. You may stare into or beyond the space you occupy, feeling yourself at one with the molecules in the air or in the walls. You might have the sensation of *being* music or art. People at this dose often report feeling the experience of ego dissolution. This is frightening to some people, as the loss of the ego can feel like death. The feeling that there is nothing without the ego is common, but untrue. Ego dissolution can be very unnerving, and this is one of the reasons to have a trusted person close by. If you find yourself going through ego dissolution, it is important to remember that whatever feels like it's dying is not real. The thing that is dying is a mask, a projection, a role. The connection in that moment is to the whole self, the deep self.

Preparing for your session includes knowing to reach for this profound self should you feel lost or afraid during the session. If you were raised in a religious tradition, you may find that there is a divine image at the center of this, and that's fine. Allow yourself to be pulled toward that image as comfort. A little later in this chapter we will discuss preparing for the journey, and there will be more about how to create a map for your encounter.

For most people, this is as far as one need ever go with psychedelic mushrooms. People frequently report that a journey at this dose is life changing. Sojourners who use this level of psychedelic find themselves understanding things that previously seemed out of their grasp. People who have experiences at this level often come away understanding messages of profound connection or spiritual enlightenment that bind people to one another and to nature in astounding ways. This dose can bring people to an entirely new experience of love and purpose in the world. It can also serve up the things that need to be addressed in order to find happiness in life. It is not uncommon for people who have a challenging experience at this dose level to follow up with another experience at the same dose that brings more clarity and peace. Don't presume that you must increase the dose to have a better or more enlightening experience.

The very high dose (VHD) or Terence McKenna's "heroic dose" shouldn't be on anyone's list of first experiences with mushrooms. This dose can bring about psychotic-like experiences. It is most likely the kind of dose that Gordon Wasson experienced in his first valada with Maria Sabina. He and his colleague found themselves sitting on the floor in total darkness having flashes of memory, insight, symbolism, all coupled with profound visions. If you undertake a VHD or heroic dose, you will likely experience some things that defy explanation and logic. Symbols might be intense. You may feel like you've been transported to another realm. When you return, you will likely lack the language to describe the experience. You will most likely have both positive and negative experiences in this state. Do not consider this dose if you aren't an experienced psychonaut, don't have a safe place with a safe person as a sitter, and can't be free for several days afterward without the intrusion of work, school, family, childcare, and the like. Most people I have worked with who have attempted a heroic dose early in their journey don't recommend it. It isn't fun, and sometimes the imagery or the feeling of disconnection is so overwhelming that the person comes back to themselves feeling worse or more disconnected.

DOSING BY WEIGHT

Most studies have dosed participants using a model of x g or mg per 70 kg of body weight (70 kg is a rough approximation of a fit adult, just under 155 lb). Researchers believed that, as with other substances, weight is what makes the difference in dosing. The belief has been that for scientific studies, researchers needed to control for the weight of participants to ensure a valid dose. This is true for most other drugs and substances. Someone at a low weight has a much more intense experience at a low dose of drugs like alcohol or opioids than someone at a higher weight.

Recent research suggests that blood serum concentrations of some psychedelics may not be affected by a person's weight or body mass index. These findings indicate that weight-based dosing is likely an unnecessary restriction, at least specific to the study of psilocybin. The concentration of psilocin in the blood is the most effective measure for drug efficacy, and recent research demonstrates that the body translates the prodrug form of psilocybin into usable psilocin at a constant rate regardless of weight. In investigating optimal doses of psilocybin for therapeutic benefit, researchers at the Johns Hopkins University Center for Psychedelic and Consciousness Research found that regardless of their body weight, there was no difference in the effects that participants experienced when given the same dosage of psilocybin.[3]

The researchers compared subjective experiences of two groups, a fixed dose group, and a weight-adjusted group. The researchers determined that there was no difference in subjective experience based on either weight or biological sex. They included a wide range of participants with vastly different body weights, from 49 kg (about 108 lb) to 113 kg (about 250 lb). The research team had a large sample population, more than 275 participants over 10 previous studies. They compared studies of weight-adjusted groups to those of absolute dosage groups. The researchers engaged in this systematic review of previous studies in an attempt to make sure that drug-to-weight ratios weren't the factor used to explain drug effects. Similar studies have upheld these findings, meaning that a microdose or a heroic dose for someone will likely be the same whether they're an elfin ballet dancer at 100 lb or a towering 300 lb football player.[4]

Microdosing

Microdosing is defined as using a subtherapeutic dose of a substance. To be considered a microdose, the amount of psilocybin should be small and the person should be able to function in their normal day-to-day manner. Most people who microdose psilocybin are doing so to improve wellness or mental health or to support cognitive abilities or creativity. An effective microdose is considered one that is below the perceptual threshold. The idea is that a microdose is meant to be consumed to unremarkable effect. For most people this is

around 1 g of fresh mushrooms, and significantly less if you're using dried mushrooms: around 0.1% of a gram, or 1 mg.

Though Indigenous shamans have been recommending microdosing throughout the ages of their cultures, it entered the public discourse in the West around 2011 with the work of James Fadiman and his seminal book called *The Psychedelic Explorer's Guide: Safe, Therapeutic, and Sacred Journeys.*[5] Fadiman collected stories from people who were independently experimenting with microdosing LSD and psilocybin. He collected their testimony and shared his research to report on the positive and negative effects of working with these substances, and also to create a blueprint for what is commonly called harm reduction with regard to psychedelics. People are going to use these substances whether they are legal or not. Harm reduction aims to educate people so that if they are going to move ahead with using psychedelics (or other illegal substances), they are empowered to use them from an educated perspective. In working with psychedelics, the typical harm-reduction approach is to educate users on what not to mix and how to understand dosing, and to help users understand what to expect from the experience.

Since the early 2010s many studies have examined the efficacy of microdosing psychedelics. Most of these have been surveys of current users or of those who are planning on beginning a course of microdosing. The majority of those surveyed report that their decision to microdose psilocybin was meant to improve wellness. But there is likely a subset of the microdosing population who are self-medicating to manage mental health. Whatever the reasoning, the practice of microdosing is expanding faster than the scientific community can study it.

Some researchers claim that due to the dearth of double-blind studies on microdosing psychedelics the data doesn't support a case for actual drug effects.[6] In some studies, the effects of microdosing and using a placebo are about the same.[7] This placebo effect doesn't take into account the possibility that there are longer-term effects beyond the immediate window, or that there are subclinical effects that are difficult to measure. It also doesn't concede that the hierarchy of the effects may be more robust for one person over another, depending on someone's own personal neurochemistry.[8]

Many recent studies that may not have made it into the public discourse as of yet show that regardless of whether we can measure the mechanism of action, there does appear to be an active medicine effect on the neurobiology of those microdosing psilocybin. One study reported that after microdosing psilocybin, study participants in the psilocybin group had a lower heart rate six hours after dosing compared to those in a placebo group.[9] Users sharing their experiences report positive results with microdosing ranging from improvements in energy and mood to better concentration and stress management.

In my own practice I have clients come in frequently who tell me that they have been microdosing. They report that this has given them improved access to both thought and feeling. One client in particular was embarrassed to tell me that she had been microdosing because she thought I would be offended. She thought I would take it personally that therapy wasn't "enough." But I was thrilled!

Microdosing greatly improved the efficacy of therapy for this client. She had more access to her feelings and was able to move through difficult emotions and old patterns faster. She saw her own motivations more clearly. This client, who had been in therapy with me for years, was soon in remission from depression and anxiety within a few months. When we held our last session, something therapists call a "termination" session, we shared some profound thoughts about her journey. I was happy to see her not feel crippled by her pain, and she was relieved to no longer feel broken.

MICRODOSING EFFECTS ON MOOD

Several studies and meta-analyses (examinations and comparisons of previous research) have found that people who microdose psychedelics report an improvement in overall mood,[10] including reductions in irritability, a greater overall sense of awareness, improvements in depression scores, and reductions in intrusive thoughts. There were mixed responses with regard to anxiety. Some respondents reported higher anxiety while microdosing. Others reported higher anxiety on days when taking psilocybin, but lower than baseline scores on days when they were not microdosing. This implies that psilocybin and its derivative psilocin may have an activating effect for some people, but that once the immediate drug action is over, there is a reduction in overall anxiety. This indicates that activation of neurons in some areas of the brain associated with anxiety may indicate a wavelike pattern. The short-term activation of neurons brings a longer decrease. This may be preferred over a constant low-level anxiety at baseline for those individuals.[11]

MICRODOSING EFFECTS ON COGNITION, CREATIVITY, AND PROBLEM SOLVING

In Silicon Valley there is always a desire to find the newest and best way of maximizing creativity. There was an era when most people in the land of high-stakes techno-creatives were focused on art, creativity, mindfulness, meditation, and open floor plans to maximize creative collaboration. Lately, psychedelics have entered the rarefied halls of the technorati. For instance, it's been reported that former Google president Sergey Brin occasionally takes psilocybin mushrooms. Product retreats encourage psychedelics to break through old ideas. Microdosing is used frequently to improve creativity, cognition, and overall performance.[12] Users who take psilocybin for these purposes often find that they have greater clarity and insight. They report that their use of psilocybin, and in some cases LSD, provides support for the demanding intellectual work of the technology world.

While Silicon Valley may be abuzz with psychedelics,[13] there are benefits for anyone who is looking to improve their day-to-day performance as it relates to cognitive tasks and self-awareness. Some researchers use the word *enhancement* to describe the effort of individuals who use psychedelics for performance. It is common to find opinions in the literature that individuals may be taking psychedelics to overcome a state of deficiency. If a person uses a substance to overcome some perceived or real psychological, cognitive, personality, or emotional deficiency, is the microdosing an enhancement or a *treatment*? We will need more research to definitively answer these questions. In our culture we are not in the habit of thinking of therapeutic treatments and psychedelics as existing in the same category, even if that is the direction that the use of these medicines is moving toward.

Another performance area that is sometimes discussed is in novel ways of thinking. Psychedelic experiences tend to connect areas of the brain that are not in regular communication. As a result, psychedelics are reported to help propel novel ideas and foster solutions in both convergent and divergent thinking. Convergent thinking is usually associated with logic. It presumes that there is a singular correct answer. Mathematics is one discipline where we often find convergent thinking. Science too, often will focus people's creative abilities into constrained boxes with convergent thinking as a model. By opening new connections that are outside of the well-worn brain circuitry, even someone who is engaged in a discipline that is very logical can have access to novel solutions.

Creative thinking happens in every discipline. But it is more difficult to address in more traditionally logic-based disciplines, as people have been trained in often rigid ideas and structures. Divergent thinking, on the other hand, is where there might be multiple answers to a problem, and there could be several that are "correct." Divergent thinking can best be summed up by things like brainstorming or abstract art. There isn't a singular "right" way of doing something. In creative disciplines this is often considered a benefit. As you might expect, psilocybin is sometimes used to help with creative problem solving across any of these disciplines. A high-level computational engineer faces certain constraints that could benefit from divergent thinking in the same way that a painter does, though they may not be used to engaging their brain in that way.

Research participants who were interviewed about microdosing for performance reasons reported results that included having greater focus, a calmer mind, and greater "fluidity" while navigating the day.[14] Respondents were generally effusive about the effects, indicating that their experience was overall beneficial. However, some respondents reported mistiming their doses, or sometimes overdoing a microdose, which took them more toward a low to moderate dose. These instances were seen as negative, and sometimes embarrassing or worrying. Researchers weren't able to discern the reasons for the miscalculations. It could have been outside of the control of the respondent, as individual mushrooms can have different concentrations of psilocybin. One of the downsides of these substances being verboten is that there is no standardization to help create predictable results. Despite the negative reports from some participants in these studies, most reported that the effects were worth the risk. They found themselves feeling calmer, more engaged, more energized about their tasks, and capable of coming up with solutions to difficult problems more easily.[15]

There is one caveat about performance as it relates to microdosing. While the reported benefits are consistent in areas of innovation, concentration, and divergent thinking, clinical studies frequently find that microdosing does not correlate with improvement in strictly cognitive tasks. In some studies researchers indicate that lack of success in cognitive tasks may be because of experimental conditions, or it could be that success during the cognitive task state is overestimated by the subject. In other words, microdosing may make someone feel like they're performing a cognitive task better than they actually are.[16] It's a good idea to consider the possibility that enhancing an experience doesn't always require or produce successful task-oriented outcomes. It could be that when there is active psilocin at work, there is too much activity or focused activity in a particular area of the brain to allow for coordination of cognitive efforts in the prefrontal cortex—the part of the brain that is most engaged when performing a cognitive task. It could also be that the default mode network (DMN) is rendered less effective because of what Robin Carhart-Harris calls cognitive entropy in his entropic brain hypothesis, which means that there is less organization and coordination of the different brain regions during a psychedelic state. Research is still new in this area, and we will no doubt learn more as the field continues to grow and expand.

MICRODOSING EFFECTS ON OCD

One of the most promising areas of research into psilocybin, especially as it pertains to microdosing, is in the treatment of obsessive-compulsive disorder (OCD). The default mode network or DMN is believed to be overactive in people who suffer from OCD. Currently the go-to pharmaceutical treatment for OCD is a daily selective serotonin reuptake inhibitor (SSRI) like fluvoxamine, also known as Prozac. Research into SSRIs and OCD has shown that after several weeks of treatment, SSRIs can help calm the intrusive thoughts that are characteristic of this disorder. Psilocybin and SSRIs work at the same 5-HT2A receptors, but psilocybin works much more quickly and without taking weeks of treatment. Because of their role as an agonist for 5-HT2A receptors in the brain, it is believed that psychedelics may influence the stream of intrusive thoughts associated with OCD. There haven't been any extensive trials as yet, but based on theoretical understanding of psilocybin's effects, a handful of clinical examples, and reports from those who are self-medicating with psilocybin, this appears to be a promising application. There is currently a trial underway at the Yale Program for Psychedelic Science investigating the efficacy of a combination of psychotherapy and psilocybin treatment in the treatment of OCD.[17]

HOW TO MICRODOSE

Based on the work of James Fadiman, most people create a dosing schedule that consists of a set of dosing days followed by one or more nondosing days.[18] There is no set schedule that is universally accepted, though two observations remain consistent. The first is that microdosing is generally undertaken for a discrete period of time, usually one to six months. Most people do not microdose in perpetuity, as with a statin or insulin. The second is that due to the brain becoming habituated to psilocybin and its effects, which happens with multiple psychedelics, it is best to give the brain a break so as to prevent habituation and thus a decrease in efficacy. You might remember that the brain has a set point for serotonin and other neurotransmitters, and it is recommended to work with the body's natural rhythms and patterns rather than against them.

Most people plan a course of microdosing for a set period, say two months, and then they stick to a schedule of something like three days on, and two days off. Others microdose on weekends only and have their weekdays without any psilocybin. Still others microdose Monday, Tuesday, and Wednesday, and then take the rest of the week off. If you choose to experiment, remember to start at the lowest possible dose on a day when you can observe the unique effects psilocybin has on you. Don't start a course of microdosing in parallel with your first day on a new job! Also, most people report that it is best to take a dose at a consistent time each day. You'll need to do a little experimentation to decide what works best for you. Some microdosers affirm that mornings are best because any possible effects are less noticeable when you're moving around through the course of your day. Still other folks swear by evenings or bedtime so as to not experience any possible side effects, however mild they may be at this dose. It depends wholly on your unique biochemistry. You may need to be quiet or occasionally lie down. Some people report experiencing headaches; others report feeling a bit antsy and cranky. The sensations differ for each person. Some people report sleeping well after microdosing, while others report that microdosing in the midafternoon is best for them because it acts as a pick-me-up. Experiment when you have some flexibility in your schedule and few demands on your attention.

Decide in advance whether you will be using fresh or dried mushrooms. You might consider pulverizing dried mushrooms and filling empty capsules (which can easily be found online or in most health food stores), with 0.1 mg each. This will give you a consistent dose. Even if you aren't sure about the concentration in the mushrooms that you pulverized, you'll at least be sure that each capsule has roughly the same weight. A small electronic kitchen scale is sufficient to help make this possible. Also, mushrooms tend to lose their efficacy over time. They should be stored at room temperature and in a dark place, even after they've been pulverized and placed in gel capsules. Once they are a few weeks old, they may start to lose their efficacy, depending on the species and strain, so store only a small amount at a time.

ADVERSE EFFECTS AND PHYSIOLOGICAL CONSIDERATIONS

Some adverse symptoms associated with microdosing psychedelics have been reported. These include anxiety on dosing days, headaches, and drowsiness. Some people find that depending on how they are storing and serving themselves their mushrooms, they may overdo it and give themselves more than a microdose.

There hasn't been enough research into the long-term effects of microdosing. However, given the research into the general lack of toxicity in most *Psilocybe* species, it is unlikely that there is a long-term health risk associated with microdosing. Still, there is concern in the scientific community that psilocybin has an affinity for the 5-HT2B receptor. This receptor is implicated in helping to build the tissues in the valves of the heart,[19] so one concern that is repeated in nearly every study on psychedelics is that there needs to be more research into long-term exposure to these compounds as it pertains to the possibility of bulking of the heart valves (cardiac valvulopathy) and resulting tissue fibrosis (hardening of the heart muscle).[20] These very specific forms of heart disease were found in the drug known as fen-phen. It helped people lose weight, but its affinity for the 5-HT2B receptors caused hardening of the heart and bulking of the heart

valves.[21] Build-up of the tissues in the valves of the heart can cause blood regurgitation inside the heart and surrounding vessels. This can be very dangerous, leading to cardiac problems that don't resolve, even after stopping the administration of the 5-HT2B agonist. No cases of psychedelic-related cardiac valvulopathy have been reported in the medical literature. However, the medical establishment has provided ample discussion of their concerns over long-term exposure to any substance that activates this particular neural pathway.[22] Exposure to psilocybin either in microdoses or therapeutic doses should be considered an occasional treatment and taken with an abundance of caution.

Journeying

Tripping, journeying—the way that we talk about the psychedelic experience is definitively grounded in the world (and language) of travel. Where are we going? If you have ever had a psychedelic experience, you probably already know the answer. You're headed to the depths. You are traveling through the terrain of the Land of You. Whether or not the mystery of life can be found in these hallowed caverns of self, I cannot say. I can only tell you that people from all walks of life and in every culture who have experienced psychedelics will offer similar descriptions: "I learned about myself. I saw myself, how ridiculous it was to worry about the things that I was so invested in." "I realized that I am everything and everything is me." "I learned that we are all connected. Every. Thing. Is. Connected. There is no separation."

People who use psychedelic mushrooms to see fractals and colors are often surprised when they come out of the experience having been moved by something profound. The more intention you go into a trip with, the more likely you are to come back with something meaningful. The most important message I have for anyone preparing for a psychedelic experience is to have a direction but not a destination. Those of us who work in the field of psychedelic therapy often use certain language that I personally find annoying, but I have yet to find better words. We use the term *inner healing intelligence* to describe allowing the psyche to lead. As someone who has a specifically psychodynamic orientation in my psychotherapy practice, I believe I am working at a deep and profound level with a patient's unconscious (psychodynamic therapy is focused on the relationship between the conscious and the unconscious). In my training, the unconscious is that part of the ground of being that we are not and cannot be in contact with because of the personal ego, which is necessary for emotional and psychological safety in our complex world. The ego protects us from all the unconscious content that bubbles up in our lives and our minds via symbols and strange associations. Without the ego to act as a filter, we would struggle to make sense of the material world around us.

But when you ignore the unconscious completely, or pretend it doesn't exist, then you really get in trouble. The ego can only work to protect us when it is allowed flexibility. When the ego becomes overidentified with the conscious mind or the material world and shuts off its connection to the unconscious, the unconscious starts to seep in through any available cracks in the psyche. Stay focused on the conscious mind alone, and pretty soon it's all conspiracy theories and satanic panic. It doesn't matter if any truth exists in those concerns. By denying the unconscious, anything that lives there has the possibility of being transformed into a monster. By denying any unconscious aspect, the mind risks turning even a positive trait or memory into a demonic force, simply by denying its existence.

Which brings us back to the psychedelic journey. While I do not claim to know the objective truth about what any of us encounter as a result of using a psychedelic substance, I can assert without hesitation that the remnants, roots, and connections will act on the individual unconscious of the person taking the trip. Healing typically takes place where there is a wound. Therefore, imagery and direction as a result of a psychedelic experience can feel like it's taking the form of a wound. In fact, the journey is simply revealing a wound that already exists, and directing your conscious attention toward it so that healing might be possible. Journeying asks us to consider healing as a natural and organic process. It can be facilitated physically, psychologically, emotionally, and, I dare say, spiritually. In our culture, we don't hesitate to consider that someone on a spiritual journey to Lourdes, Jerusalem, or the Kaaba is hoping for a spiritual awakening or healing. Sometimes the voyage to our deepest selves forces us to examine painful truths about our lives, histories, or traumas. Be respectful of your own history and experiences and go slowly.

If you were hiking the Pacific Crest Trail you wouldn't *plan* to get lost or hurt, but you would take precautions to reduce the risk. You'd have a map, wear hiking boots, and carry a basic first aid kit. Preparing for the psychedelic journey is the same. Inner healing intelligence is the same force in your body and central nervous system that knows how to activate your immune response when you get a cold. It is the same aspect that knows how to heal a cut if you accidentally slice your finger cutting vegetables. Just because we don't usually connect the dots between the physical injuries and the psychological ones doesn't mean that their healing isn't mitigated by the same internal function. In the West we've cut ourselves off from anything that isn't "materialistic," meaning that our culture has advocated for logic above reason, loyalty over love, and use over connection. We think about bringing value. We treat our bodies like machines. We treat nature like a toy box to plunder. But we are more than mechanical. The part of you that heals a physical wound is the same that can heal a psychospiritual one. If you're not a spiritual person, please don't dismiss the healing that is available to you. Your journey is the trip to yourself, the deepest part of you that knows the next steps you need in order to become the most complete version of *you*.

PREPARATION

To get ready for your journey, let's take an inventory of what you'll need. Act as though you're planning an actual voyage, headed for unknown territory, and hoping to have a meaningful experience along the way. You'll want to know where you're headed, or at least a general direction. You'll want a healthy body, the right companion(s), and as much safety as necessary while engaging in the goal of the trip, and you'll want to document your experience so you can reflect on it later.

SET AN INTENTION

It's always better to have a general idea of where you're going rather than having either a strict map to follow or a vague undeveloped idea that allows you to just float on the wind. No doubt you've heard the idea of having an intention before. It's a popular idea in some New Age circles—everything starts and ends with intention. But in this arena, I want to ask you to think about intention a bit differently. Allow yourself to develop an intention, not as a question seeking a discrete answer, but as a direction looking for context. Think of it like saying "Well, I want to go to New York." If you're headed to New York, you should point yourself in the physical or metaphorical direction that will get you there. If you're in California, point to the east and ask for guidance. If you're in Germany, point west and ask for guidance. Ask "What do I need to know to get me to New York?"

Not everyone has an intention as clear as "I want to go to New York." In fact, most of us don't have such clear intentions. If you aren't sure about a direction, then ask a question about how you got to where you are, how to decide what's next, or how to get unstuck. The question could look something like this: "How can I understand my stuck-ness better?" Or maybe you're struggling with a sadness or an emotional wounding that you can't figure out. "What is it that I need to do to acknowledge and move forward from this place?"

You'll notice that in none of these questions did I use the word *why*. There is a specific reason for this omission, and it has to do with our earliest anxieties. The first time the word *why* is directed toward human beings, we are about two years old. We've probably done something that annoyed or angered a parent or a caregiver: "Why did you color the white carpet with my red lipstick?" When *why* is hurled our way at this young age, we have the cognitive capacity to understand the question, but we lack the capacity to respond with words and explanation effectively. The ability to explain doesn't come until we're somewhere between four and five years old. In a two-year-old, this question creates anxiety, because they cannot perform a task and get their caregiver's support and affection. It initiates activation in the amygdala in the toddler, and we don't grow out of it. For most people, the word *why* initiates an anxiety response from the amygdala, and anxiety typically leads to defensiveness. So, in preparing for a psychedelic trip, I usually ask my clients to avoid using the word *why*. You can understand the reasons for something's origins without using the word itself. Here are some other options:

- What happened in my relationship with [important person] that I need to understand better?
- How can I use this experience to understand my history of [event, trauma, etc.] better?
- What do I need to know about the experience of [event, trauma, etc.] to help me move forward?
- What is blocking my path in [job/romance/career/creativity]?

You get the idea. Reframe your intention so that there are fewer defenses set up in advance of your arrival. Get a notebook and write your questions down, then forget about them. You'll be surprised how your psyche will bring you back to these questions as part of your journey.

PREPARING YOUR BODY

Most people preparing for a psychedelic experience will abstain from certain foods and substances before a journey. These are usually meat, cheese, alcohol, wheat products, and sugar—basically anything that might be heavy on the liver. You need to be well hydrated, so drink lots of water in the days leading up to your trip. I have found that most people will begin to reduce their grain, meat, cheese, sugar, and alcohol consumption a week before dosing, and eat only veggies, fruits, and maybe a tiny bit of cultured products like yogurt in the three days before and inclusive of the journey day itself. Going easy on the liver helps reduce the strain on the body and makes it easier for the liver to translate psilocybin into psilocin. In traditional journeys with Indigenous elders, some people are instructed to abstain from sex for several days before and after the journey as well. This is a good idea on multiple levels, including psychological, emotional, and neurological.

You should also do your best to be quiet and well rested before your journey. If you are focused on the to-do list at your stressful job, your psyche will have to do more work to clear out the job junk so that it can get to the real issues that keep you working so hard. Take a day off before and after journeying if possible. If your only option is a weekend, then go into preparation mode as soon as you get home that Friday, allowing yourself only light entertainment, staying as low stress and easy as possible before your journey on Saturday. After your journey on Saturday, spend Sunday in reflection and quiet with gentle music, wholesome food, art supplies, and a journal ready to receive any insights. Be prepared for the insights to flow for several days following your experience. From a neurological perspective, this is because of the serotonergic action occurring in your brain. As the neurotransmitter load comes back down to baseline, the active insights will start to diminish. The good news is that you'll remember them. And if you've kept a journal or other record, you'll be able to refer to the details, which you may find to be important as you engage in the integration process. Integration is a critical aspect of working with psychedelics. Don't treat the journey like an amusement park ride. If you don't work to make sense (integrate) any awareness, images, memories, or feelings from your experience, then your trip was about as useful as a ride on a roller coaster or merry-go-round.

Psychedelics should never be consumed with alcohol, cannabis in any form, or any other substance or drugs. The interactions are unpredictable. Mixing substances is a big *NO* in psychedelics. Alcohol is a disinhibitor, and psychedelics redefine the barriers of the psyche. The combination of alcohol or THC with psilocybin often causes panic because people don't feel safe on an existential level. Alcohol will cause some people to feel things that they usually have carefully ensconced behind psychological barriers. Adding a psychedelic is kind of like throwing a stick of dynamite at the barrier. Cannabis and its active ingredient, THC, will usually activate similar parts of the brain as psilocin—the amygdala, hippocampus, and prefrontal cortex. However, the cannabinoid system tends to work on dopamine receptors, while psilocybin works on serotonin receptors. This competition for neurological resources can make the person experiencing these effects feel disoriented, agitated, and fearful. Anyone is almost guaranteed to have

a "bad trip" when mixing cannabis or alcohol with psilocybin.

As it is, the psychedelic experience is likely going to challenge some of the ego structures that you consider normal aspects of your being. These may be protections, habits, or other aspects that have served you well throughout your life. Introducing other substances to the process only guarantees that you'll have a more challenging experience than necessary. Abstain from cannabis at least five days prior to your journey and alcohol at least three days prior. Maintaining a light diet and abstaining from alcohol and cannabis (or other substances) two days afterward will assist in helping you process and make the integration of your journey more meaningful. As you're making sense of the information, symbols, and feelings from your experience, it's best to have your senses and attention fully available and not dulled.

SET AND SETTING

If you've been around psychedelics at all or seen documentaries like *How to Change Your Mind* or read books like *Nine Perfect Strangers*, then you've certainly heard the phrase *set and setting* already. The idea behind set and setting is that you want to make sure to give yourself the best possible environment for your journey, both inside and out.

Set refers to your mindset—the way that you are approaching the journey itself. Having the right mindset looks different for each person, but there are some common threads, like knowing your intention, spending some time in reflection in advance so that you can approach your journey seriously but not dourly, and being in control of your mood, or at least not feeling erratic are important aspects of the proper set for the journey. Not feeling pressured or coerced is also critically important. If you feel pressured to do the journey, it is probably not the right time for you.

For most people, the journey with psilocybin lasts anywhere from three to six hours, and this makes the setting critically important. Because of the visual and auditory experiences that are common when using psilocybin, it is important to be somewhere you won't be disturbed, preferably in a calm and quiet environment with few intrusive sounds or visuals. Some people believe that a place needs to be comfortable and pleasing to look at, but I find that it is more important that your location isn't too busy or visually stimulating. Things like soft colors and rooms with limited art or symbolism are more important than being somewhere with an expensive couch and a Zen waterfall. Low external stimulation should be the goal. For some people it is important to change environments. If your home is charged with emotion or is generally or historically unsafe, it is not the best place for your journey. It would be better to be at a trusted friend's house where you feel safe and well cared for.

For almost everyone engaging in a psychedelic journey, blindfolds are recommended to reduce visual stimulation coupled with gentle but thoughtful music to accompany them on their journey. Part of set and setting that has come to be more discussed in recent years is the influence of music. I create playlists for my clients that are timed to the peaks and valleys expected on their journeys. There are hundreds of playlists on streaming services created by professional guides and therapists. Psychedelic music applications are even being developed by neuroscientists to help maximize

the experience for the voyager. Music should never include lyrics, and the pieces shouldn't switch mood or style too abruptly, but neither should they be boring and monotonous. Think about the music as though it is the soundtrack to an important voyage. If you are creating your own playlist, you're going to want to have peaks or changes in tempo and tone around 25 minutes into the session, and again at the 1-hour, 2-hour, 2.5-hour, 3-hour, and 4-hour marks. After the 4.5-hour mark, some people can begin to journal or converse about their experience, but this should be determined by the voyager. As much as possible, a person should be encouraged to sit with their experience and commit it to their journal or to another artistic outlet like a sketchpad.

COMPANIONS ON THE JOURNEY: THE SITTER

If you are not working with a professional psychedelic therapist or sitter, then it is critical, especially if you're a beginner, that you have someone who can sit with you during your journey. This should be someone you trust without hesitation, someone you know will respect your boundaries and who will have no interest in taking advantage of you while you're in a vulnerable state. In recent years there have been several scandals in the psychedelic community of people who were, at the very least, taken advantage of and, in many instances, sexually assaulted or raped while they were in the very vulnerable space of being "in the medicine."

Because of this vulnerability I highly recommend working with a professional therapist who is trained in psychedelics. That doesn't mean that there aren't unscrupulous therapists out there, but when there is a regulatory body that can take someone's license away or cause them to lose their livelihood, there is at least some pressure to maintain professional boundaries. If you have ever been taken advantage of while in a vulnerable state, it is always appropriate to report it to the proper authorities. Know that for psychotherapists and doctors, there are regulatory boards where you can report bad conduct. There are more options than just calling the police.

If you have a trusted sitter, that person should also understand things like preparation and set and setting. They should be prepared to sit and give you their attention while you're experiencing your voyage. They shouldn't need to distract themselves with the television or games while you're on your journey. The sitter should be prepared and well grounded to help you stay calm should you encounter something challenging during your journey. A traditional phrase of reassurance a sitter can say to the voyager is something like "You're okay. You took some mushrooms, and you're in the middle of your journey. I'm right here. You're completely safe." The sitter should be prepared to occasionally help you to the restroom, which may happen once or twice. You'll want to wear comfortable, uncomplicated clothes to make this easy. Your sitter should expect to help keep you steady and to hold you by the arms anytime you're moving as you will likely be unsteady on your feet. You shouldn't move too much during your journey, but if you need to, someone should be there for physical support.

The sitter shouldn't need to engage or direct you on your journey. If you're concerned that you'll find yourself feeling lost, you can work out some safety plans in advance. Return to your intention. Lightly hold the idea of your intention like a compass. Your sitter can remind you of that, saying something like "Remember you wanted to better understand [insert subject]? Hold that idea lightly; just follow the experience. You're safe. I'm right here with you." At the end of a journey, I find that sometimes it's helpful for the sitter—whether a friend or professional—to do something creative like drawing or writing in a journal while sitting next to the voyager.

One of the rules of working with psychedelics is to be very careful about touch. Some people will want to be touched, and others will not. It is up to the voyager to decide if they want to be touched, not the sitter to decide if the voyager needs it. Sometimes inexperienced sitters will reach out to touch their friend in a gesture of consolation and as a reminder that they are there for their friend. This is great so long as it has been worked out in advance. Be sure that you both discuss the possibility of touch in advance, as well as how to engage in it safely or disengage if desired. If the voyager is someone who generally likes the reassurance of touch, then it is safe to discuss what that might look like and how to withdraw touch if the voyager is uncomfortable. If the sitter is uncomfortable with the kind of touch that the voyager is engaging in, then the sitter needs to enforce gentle but clear boundaries. It is possible that the voyager will want to be held, or they may have sexual feelings while they are in their journey. The sitter should know this in advance, so they know to deter those feelings and emotions without causing shame or fear.

Hopefully, it's obvious that you shouldn't drive for several hours after your psilocybin journey. In addition, there should always be a back-up sitter in case of an emergency. Cell phones should be charged, and both you and the sitter should know your location's address in case of an emergency. You should know where the nearest hospital is, so that you can be transported there if necessary. While a trip to the hospital is unlikely, it is not impossible. Above all, the voyage should be safe, well controlled, and meaningful. It should be free from unnecessary stress, visual stimuli, intrusive sounds, and psychological pressure. Doing what you need to do ahead of time to have a productive journey may seem like a lot of work, but it will definitely be worth it on the other side. Anyone who has had a challenging experience at a rave or in any kind of unfamiliar environment can tell you firsthand how important it is to get the planning right before you embark on a psychedelic journey.

INTEGRATION

If I learn a new word and then add it to my day-to-day vocabulary, that is a form of integration. Psychedelic integration is similar. If you are taking a psychedelic journey looking for meaning, healing, or a better understanding of yourself, then integration should be considered the most important part of your experience. The goal of psychedelic integration is to examine the symbols, feelings, and memories that emerge in the psychedelic session (sometimes also referred to as the medicine session) and make sense of how the voyager sees their relevance and meaning. The time "in the medicine" refers to the four to six hours when you're actively under the influence of psilocybin, or "tripping."

I had a client who had an encounter with a whale during a psychedelic journey. I would normally consider this a positive experience, but the voyager felt that it was a symbol for her overbearing parent, who also happened to be a diver. In her journey she felt small and powerless in the presence of the whale. She feared being alone with it. The journey had her swimming and trying to find her own "ocean," and the whale kept silently showing up and suddenly taking up her "new" space. This opened a deeper level of discussion about her relationship with her family. My client reached a level of feeling that we had never touched before the psychedelic experience. The direction was determined by her medicine session, and her interpretation of her mother as a whale taking up all the space in her psyche was a critical part of integrating her journey.

By examining the symbolism that came up, we were able to more deeply understand her relationship with her mother and how my client could give herself permission to take up more space, own her decisions, and reconsider her relationship with her mother and sisters. This was especially relevant for how her mother's thought process had infiltrated her own. The whale showed her that even her internal thoughts were often based on her mother's opinions. After this experience, the client started to question if a feeling or thought originated with her mother or if she had come to a particular understanding on her own. Thus began a practice of my client examining her experiences, thoughts, and beliefs and questioning the lens through which she saw them. Within two months of her psychedelic session, this client had identified critical beliefs that she could attribute to her mother that had held her back for more than a decade. She couldn't see the pattern until she encountered the whale.

Even before the medicine session is complete, preparing for the integration of any material that comes up should be considered. It is much easier to integrate the contents of a session that has gone well (even if that content is challenging) if preparation, set, and setting have been considered. As the medicine session comes to a close, and the voyager is making their way back from an altered state of consciousness, they should be encouraged to document the experience. This doesn't require the voyager to be capable of complex thought or words; they can draw or scribble in a sketchbook. Another voyager might find themselves singing a song; if they cannot write it down, perhaps the sitter can help write down the name of the song or record it if it's something the voyager is creating on the spot.

The work that happens after the medicine session is centered on integration. What comes up in the medicine session and in the five or six days following it is extremely important content that can be used for understanding what the inner healing intelligence wants the voyager to understand. The medicine session itself is not where healing takes place; it is in the connections that are made after the session has ended. Indeed, research has repeatedly shown that the quality of postmedicine session integration is the greatest predictor of success with regard to psychedelic experiences.

Creating a symbolic dictionary that is unique to your experience is one way to help this process. This doesn't have to be a complex undertaking, but it should unfold organically as you engage with your psyche across multiple domains. Take note of the symbols and images that came up during your journey. Pay attention to animals, settings, and characters that appear in your dreams, and notice what songs, art, and media you feel drawn to both before and after your journey. Jot down

important memories or relationships that might be floating around in the back of your mind while you're driving or taking a shower. Take brief notes. Doodle in a journal. Make bulleted lists with dates. Your journal entries don't have to be long or perfectly constructed narratives of the "dear diary" variety. Simply a date, what you're experiencing, a few bullet points, a single descriptive sentence, a feeling—these are enough.

You can have a breakthrough in a single psychedelic session. You might experience the eureka moment that you long for, and the meaning and interpretation of this experience might connect to other deep experiences over multiple months or years. I have a client who has been adding to—and finding deeper meaning from—a psychedelic session they had more than five years ago. From a psychodynamic therapy perspective, this makes perfect sense. Each time the symbolism from the original psychedelic journey surfaces, my client reflects on how the old meanings of those symbols make sense in his current state. He is in relationship with the old meaning and with the new awareness. Together, they form a continuity across a challenging period in his life, and he frequently engages with the symbolism that came forward in that particular psychedelic session to make sense of his present moment.

Allow the integration process to unfold over time, and you will find that your journey has layers of meaning that are additive rather than reductionist. A journey doesn't "mean" just one thing in one moment. Its meaning is there as a guide to the sojourner, to help make sense of what has been as well as what can be in the present and in the future. If you had an experience that you can't explain straightaway, that's okay. There's no prescription or one-size-fits-all method to interpretation and integration. Your journey is meant for the exploration of the terrain of your deepest self. If there are still mysteries in the landscape, that just means that there is complexity there. Your journey may be asking for you to return and explore some more. Whether you engage in that exploration through another psychedelic journey, through psychotherapy, or through artistic endeavors doesn't necessarily matter. The journey is there to serve as a metaphorical postcard between the person who works, goes to school, walks the dog, reads books, and dreams, and the deepest self who is at the center of your existence, the you that was you before you knew who you were. That self wants to be in dialogue with the one who takes the subway home late or cries when they watch commercials with dogs in them. That is the gift of the journey: it's a message (or a postcard) from the outside you to the inside you, and it is meant to bring both sides of your self closer. You get to know one another on a deeper level, and from that depth you get to direct your life with more authenticity and authority.

PSYCHEDELIC-ASSISTED PSYCHOTHERAPY

There is a boom in psychedelics going on around the country, indeed around the world. Soccer moms are going off to the jungle to do ayahuasca. People are learning how to be shamans so that they can sit with others in the sacred space of possibility. There are also predators taking people's money and promising them psychedelic experiences and then giving them illicit drugs rather than sacred medicines. This happened to a client of mine, and it was one of the reasons I got trained to

become a certified psychedelic therapist. My client was a seasoned journeyer. She had done mushrooms, MDMA, ayahuasca, and DMT more than once. She was a spiritual person who regularly did yoga and meditated every day. She was an educated person who had a PhD in a challenging discipline. And one weekend she spent several hundred dollars to participate in a ceremony with people she had met in the psychedelic scene. She had been in ceremony with almost all these people before and felt safe. But on this occasion, she got very ill from whatever medicine she'd been given. It was supposed to be ayahuasca, but when the group took her and another woman to the emergency room, a drug test revealed that what she and the rest of the group had taken was actually methamphetamine. My client was furious. She felt betrayed, and she had every right to feel that way.

There are currently far more people who are curious about psychedelics than there are trained providers. Further, some companies are looking to make a quick buck and sending people ketamine or other substances by mail. This is done with little support or education on how to stay safe, and with very little guidance on how to maximize the potential of the medicines in order to have a safe and meaningful journey. You don't have to work with a person who is certified in psychedelic-assisted psychotherapy to get meaning from your experience, but please be sure to work with someone who has your best interest at heart and who isn't looking to take advantage of you on a physical, financial, or sexual level. Working with a licensed person gives you the benefit of knowing they have some training and standing in the discipline of psychotherapy. If you have trustworthy, emotionally stable friends with whom you can plan in advance, then you are just as likely to have a good experience. Don't go on a journey if you don't feel safe. You are the expert in *you*; trust your inner healing intelligence about what you need.

Psychedelic psychotherapy will be similar to the journey described in previous sections, but it will be structured differently in order to make it easy for the therapist to help the client make sense of their journey. Typically, this will include an interview where the client and therapist meet to see if they are a good fit. The therapist will be curious about your experience with psychedelics. They will also want to know about significant trauma in your life and any psychiatric diagnoses you may have received. A psychedelic therapist will want to discuss your preferences for touch, and they should ask about your reasons for seeking psychedelic therapy. Depending on the type of medicine being used—if you're in a place where the medicine can be prescribed—the therapist will ask for a medical clearance to make sure that you don't have any contraindications, like severe cardiac issues. If you're working with an underground therapist (someone who is engaging in psychedelic therapy outside of the rules and regulations of the state or country where you live), they should still ask you about your health in order to rule out any serious concerns.

There will usually be at least two preparatory sessions before the medicine session takes place. These preparation sessions are meant to help bring forward any therapeutic issues and to see how you have dealt with trauma in the past. A responsible therapist will not just drop you into a psychedelic session and hope for the best. The therapist will want to make sure that they are acting as a guide on a healing journey

and not injuring you further in the process. After the preparation sessions have been completed, your therapist will schedule your medicine session. They will come to you for the session, or perhaps it might take place in an office or space that is designed specifically for psychedelic sessions.

It is typical for the medicine session to feel like it has a sacred or religious tone. The ritual nature of a medicine session is there for the psychological safety of the client. Ritual has a way of helping the psyche make sense of the kinds of encounters that one experiences while under the influence of these medicines. For most people, ritual is calming and reassuring. It communicates to the psyche that there is a person anchoring the experience for everyone else and supports the sense that you're in a unique situation, not just taking a pill or getting on a merry-go-round. Don't be alarmed if the therapist or trained guide adopts a ritualistic tenor as part of your session.

A trained psychedelic therapist or guide will be with you the whole time. They may bring another person to the session to ensure that you are never alone, so that the sitter or therapist can have a break from time to time. This is normal. During and after your session, it is typical for your therapist or guide to take notes. Importantly, a therapist may receive impressions or ideas while you are having your experience. Sometimes these are very meaningful and insightful. We don't have a good explanation for why this is, but some of us believe that there is something in the interaction that takes place between a therapist and a journeyer during a session that communicates symbolically from psyche to psyche. I don't know if this is objectively true, but I've experienced it enough to know that it is real. Don't be freaked out by it; it's a form of communication that happens all the time, and we just aren't used to indulging it. When the session is over, you'll be driven home by someone you trust (no rideshares or taxis), and you should make every effort to be quiet and thoughtful. You may continue to have deep emotions or feelings for the next 24 hours. That's okay and normal, too. Let yourself laugh or cry as necessary. Draw, play music, write, do anything creative that you can in the 24 hours after your medicine session. The images and insights that crop up during this time are an important part of the experience. They aren't residual aftereffects—they are the point!

Within 24 hours of your journey, your therapist should check on you. Within 48 hours you should meet again for your first official integration session. In this session you'll discuss what came up during the experience and highlight important images, symbols, and themes. Your therapist will likely ask you to continue to explore and engage in your creative practice. You'll schedule a follow-up integration to continue discussing the themes and insights that occurred during and after your medicine session. It is normal for there to be at least two integration sessions. I have clients with whom I have had years of therapy and integration to work through material that first appeared in just two or three medicine sessions.

If you have a regular therapist and would prefer to bring your integration work to them, ask the psychedelic therapist for a brief report (they may charge you for this extra step). You should prepare to bring your intention and integration materials or content to your regular therapist. A word of warning though: therapists who haven't been trained in psychodynamic techniques or who focus solely on cognitive behavioral therapy may struggle with the contents of psychedelic sessions. Don't be afraid to talk to your regular therapist in advance about their point of view with regard to dreams, psychedelic experiences, or other alternative forms of consciousness. If they respond warmly and have some expertise, they'll be delighted to work with you on your psychedelic content. If they're skeptical or dismissive of the unconscious or the value in working with images, then perhaps your integration would be best kept with the psychedelic therapist.

FINAL THOUGHTS ON JOURNEYING

Now that you are planning or have taken a journey, you've earned the title of psychonaut, a person who explores the depths of the psyche. To be a psychonaut is to be unafraid to face the deepest fathoms of the self. Don't be afraid of the depths. Almost everything down there is meant to help or protect you. Even the scary bits are usually protective forces that we've exiled because they're powerful. A wise clinical professor of mine once told me that all therapy was about helping people learn to be comfortable with being uncomfortable. I think that working with psychedelics is the bravest form of this effort. In psychedelics we dive into the unknown to bring treasures up from the depths. Sometimes we don't know what the treasure is worth. We have to polish it and clean it up a bit before we can see how beautiful and valuable it is. Treasure your journey. Be unafraid of your fears. Your deepest self is longing to guide you toward the life you desire and deserve. Welcome that relationship with open arms, and you will live a life filled with awe and understanding beyond what you ever thought possible.

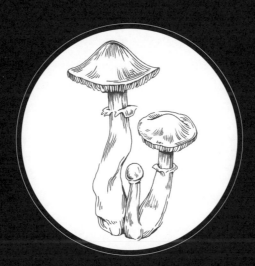

ORISSA INDIAN

Nature is not our enemy, to be raped and conquered. Nature is ourselves, to be cherished and explored.

—TERENCE MCKENNA

CHAPTER 6

Varieties of Mushrooms

The World of Psychoactive Fungi

There are more than 180 different species of mushrooms that cause psychoactive or psychedelic effects in human beings. Other fungi that aren't mushrooms, like the parasitic ergot, can cause psychedelic effects, too. Ethnomycologists—people who study mushrooms and fungi in the context of culture—believe that mushrooms spread across the world by traveling via human and animal caravans. Mushrooms often grow in decomposing substrates or layers of earth, like animal dung and rotting wood. If a horse or a yak eats mushroom spores in Siberia and migrates over into what is now Alaska, pooping out spores along the way, those spores will land in the soil, the mycelium of those spores will create networks underground, and eventually fruiting bodies or mushrooms will grow from those networks of mycelia. People and animals have brought mushrooms along various travel routes for millennia. Mushrooms have been our companions in the development of humanity just as much as domesticated animals.

Psychoactive Mushrooms and Their Relationship to Neurotransmitters

The psychedelic renaissance has been made possible by advances in neuroscience and our understanding of how neurotransmitters work within the structure of a neuron. Neuroscientists have also discovered in the last 10 years that the receptors for different neurotransmitters have very different affinities based on what the neuron's job is and where it is found in the brain and other places in the body, like the heart.[1] These advances in neuroscience have dovetailed with recent research into psychoactive substances like psilocybin and LSD. In addition, there is increasing interest in psychoactive fungi and their potential to provide healing compounds that can aid in the development of new drugs to treat everything from depression to Alzheimer's disease.

The new research into different mushroom species has generated scientific and commercial interest because of the various psychoactive substances found in psychedelic mushrooms. Together, these compounds are referred to as amyloid tryptamines, and they can function in vivo (in living cells) as either neurotransmitters or neuromodulating compounds. The best understood of these in vivo relationships is the relationship between serotonin and psilocybin. When psilocybin is ingested, it acts as a prodrug, a biologically inactive compound that can be metabolized inside the body to produce a drug. The body transforms psilocybin into a more usable form called psilocin, and it does this by removing one of the psilocybin molecule's phosphate groups. The resulting psilocin derives its psychoactive power from its structural similarity to the neurotransmitter serotonin. Their similar structures mean that the receptors in the brain where serotonin is processed (in biological parlance these are called "agonists") are filled very easily with psilocin molecules.

Serotonin is one of the most important neurotransmitters in the brain. It is responsible for regulating multiple functions in your body. Serotonin is necessary for regulating mood and many other physiological functions. Despite the body's ubiquitous need for serotonin, it is not the most prolifically produced neurotransmitter. It is manufactured in a part of the brain called the raphe nuclei and stored in different vesicles until it is needed. An important note: serotonin is critical for functioning in other parts of the body, including the liver, and it plays a vital role in the functioning of the nervous system, digestive system, reproductive system, and other areas of the body. This may explain why some serotonergic substances from medications to mushrooms can sometimes have unexpected effects on the body.

In some conditions, the serotonergic systems don't work as robustly as they should. The mechanisms inside the brain are fairly complex, and the brain's functions depend on the presence of special receptors that can take in different types of neurotransmitters. These neurotransmitters are like keys that unlock different neuron behaviors. When there aren't enough neurotransmitters or specialized receptors for them to bind to, or if for some reason they don't work very well, then the associated brain structures do not function as well as they should. The most well-known example of this phenomenon surrounds the mechanisms involved with depression. We know that when someone experiences depression, sometimes they lose synapses or have damage to the area of the brain that produces serotonin.[2]

The flow of neurotransmitters is complex. It is far too simple to say that psilocybin is translated into psilocin and that this then affects a person's mood. Psilocybin introduced into the body also initiates the release of other neurotransmitters and proteins and resets the DMN, as we discussed earlier. Many other mechanisms are affected by a cascade of neurotransmitters traveling through the brain and body because of the introduction of psilocin. The visual cortex—the area of the brain that processes visual information—has some of the most robust development of serotonin receptors, and the introduction of psilocin activates these receptors, which is why visual phenomena and hallucinations are often reported by those taking psilocybin. In addition, there are effects on the system that regulates glutamate, which is the most prolific of the neurotransmitters in the brain. In the presence of psilocin and serotonin, glutamate also cascades through the central nervous system.[3] As the primary excitatory neurotransmitter in the brain, glutamate is active in learning, memory, and synaptic health. Additionally, glutamate and its antagonist, GABA, are critically important in the development of an individual brain's neuroplasticity, the crown jewel of healthy brain function.[4]

In addition, other proteins and neurotransmitters, like brain-derived neurotropic factor (BDNF) and dopamine, are released and mediated in the cascade of neurotransmitters that results from taking psilocybin. The protein BDNF has been studied frequently in the last decade, and it has been shown to play an important role in mood, as well as in the health of neurons.[5] It helps ensure the proper distribution and use of neurotransmitters like glutamate and serotonin. Increases in BDNF have been correlated with a higher subjective sense of well-being. Low concentrations of BDNF are associated with increases in depression and poor cognitive function and higher instances of challenging mental health problems like psychosis.[6]

Depending on their species and strain, different psychoactive mushrooms have shown varying ratios of chemicals that affect brain function. Some psychoactive species have higher concentrations of psilocybin; some have additional, but often smaller, concentrations of direct psilocin; yet others have even more compounds that appear to impact the activation of other brain chemicals like BDNF or dopamine. Of these species, the most important combination to search for will be that of psilocybin and psilocin. If a mushroom species produces psilocin as well as psilocybin, that mushroom will be faster acting than one that doesn't have psilocin. This is because psilocin will act directly on the brain, while psilocybin must be digested so that the liver can translate the psilocybin into psilocin. Then,

the psilocin will make its way to the brain. This is why, for most people, the strongest effects of taking mushrooms don't occur until a half hour or more after the mushroom has been ingested.

The concentration of the psychoactive compounds in psychedelic mushrooms has been studied using multiple methods over several decades. The most reliable method for examining the relevant compounds is liquid chromatography–mass spectrometry. In this method, samples are crushed, and the relevant parts, like psilocybin, psilocin, and baeocystin, are separated from the other fungal compounds.[7] The extracted parts are submitted to a process that allows a mass spectrometer to measure ionized compounds that have been isolated. This measure then allows a researcher to compare the extracted compounds to the weight of the mushroom used in the sample. The sample's concentration is then compared as a percentage. Most psilocybin mushrooms contain less than 1% psilocybin. The most potent psilocybin mushrooms, *Panaeolus azurescens*, can contain almost double the amount of psychoactive compounds, typically around just under 2% psilocybin.[8] These mushrooms were discovered just a few decades ago, and they are not very easy to find. They can also contain other substances that can cause the dangerous muscle spasms and rigidity known as wood lover's paralysis.[9]

As we explore the varieties of psilocybin mushrooms in the rest of this chapter, please note that the science on these species is still emerging. The last time that there was this much interest in the science of psilocybin was in the 1950s and '60s. We have learned a great deal in the last 20 years thanks to the pioneering research of scientists like

Robin Carhart-Harris, Roland Griffiths, Paul Stamets, and Franz Vollenweider, but there is still much to discover. Psychedelic research is advancing quickly, and many more details may be uncovered as you develop your own research and practice. Staying up to date on all the latest research is a critical part of maintaining a responsible psychedelic practice.

Taxonomy: How We Describe the Living World, and How We Identify Mushrooms in the Wild

Mushrooms, like other living organisms, are described according to scientific language called taxonomy. The goal of scientific taxonomy is to help people understand different species of flora, fauna, and fungi by aligning them according to their form, function, and behavior. By organizing the other inhabitants of our world this way, researchers can better understand the natural world and its various families, groups, and subgroups. This can be important when coming across something new. For example, you have likely seen many dogs in your life, but it's possible that you have never seen a wolf in person. So, if one day you're hiking with your family and see a wolf, your brain would make certain assumptions automatically. You'd likely notice that the wolf is bigger than a dog, and then you would understand how powerful it is in comparison. You'd know to expect that the wolf has big canine teeth, and that, like dogs, it can probably be very dangerous if provoked. Marking the similarities between a wolf and a dog will help keep you safe.

Similarly, using a classification system for understanding fungi, plants, and animals

helps us to understand which members of these groups might be beneficial to humans and which ones might cause damage. This is especially important in understanding the taxonomy of mushrooms and other fungi. Several species of mushroom are deadly. One serving of these species is all it would take for the body's protein synthesis process to be interrupted, thereby causing fatal liver, kidney, and digestive damage.

What's more, several mushroom species look remarkably alike. This makes it imperative that you know your shrooms! If you are a beginner, it's of paramount importance that you learn from others who are knowledgeable in the world of mushrooms before you begin your journey. Reading books and looking at photographs are both great steps, but you will be much better served by joining a local group and going on forays into the landscape with experienced mushroom foragers. They will help show you the small—sometimes minuscule—differences that will tell you whether a mushroom is safe to ingest or not. The most important thing to remember when searching for mushrooms in the wild is that while the vast majority of psilocybin-producing mushrooms have very low toxicity, there are several poisonous and even deadly mushrooms that are almost indistinguishable from the ones you want.

Finally, sourcing mushrooms from a controlled environment is preferred for psychedelic purposes. One of the most amazing gifts of mycelia and mushrooms generally is their ability to create networks that help clean up toxins and metals from the soil. Mycelia are remarkably skilled at filtering and concentrating substances that are dangerous to living things. While we don't know why this happens—perhaps it is some kind of protective measure for the health of an ecosystem—we do know that mycelia are very effective at it. Thus, mushrooms that are foraged in the wild may contain toxins that you wouldn't want to take a risk with. If you want to have a positive experience with psychedelic mushrooms, it is best to grow them yourself or acquire them from a person who is skilled at growing them in a controlled and sterile environment.

Species versus Strain

Taxonomies organize different living things into scientific groups that help us to understand them better. When reading the scientific names of organisms, you're reading the names of specific species based on a longer list of organizing principles. In modern taxonomy the organizing principle flows from the top of the hierarchy—moving from the largest group down to the specific level of a type of individual, in the sequence of kingdom, phylum, class, order, family, genus, species. Humans belong to the kingdom Animalia, meaning animals, and the phylum Chordata, meaning all the animals that share the feature of a spinal cord. We belong to the class Mammalia, meaning mammal, and this is where things start to get a little more complex. Mammals give birth to their offspring, rather than laying eggs. Mammals also have endothermic, or self-regulating, systems for managing body temperature (rather than lying on a rock to warm up). Skipping down to the species level, modern human beings also have our own species name: *Homo sapiens sapiens.* The word *Homo* means "man" in Latin. Our genes are compatible with other members of our species.

The word *sapiens* means "intelligent," and describes us as beings with particularly large brains. This is especially noticeable in the area of the frontal cortex, compared to historical examples of other extinct members of our species who did not have large brains. The second *sapiens* is there to further denote the "modern" part. We have discovered in recent decades that our nearest extinct relative, Neanderthals, were not a separate species. We know this because we have found Neanderthal DNA in modern human populations, which means that tens of thousands of years ago, there were children born from groups of Neanderthals who mated with groups of anatomically modern humans. I could go on and on, but you see how this works.

Fungi belong to their own separate kingdom. They are neither plants nor animals. They are a unique type of organism and organize differently from plants or animals. Interestingly, some are dependent on plants, and some fungi help to break proteins down so that they can be recycled and used again. New research shows that mushrooms communicate along networks of mycelia—the threadlike structures that connect beneath the root systems of plants. These perform a critical function that supports the health of both other kingdoms: animal and plant. Research into mycelial networks in old-growth forests has shown that trees and fungi use mycelial networks the way humans use phone lines. Trees send signals along the networks to let other individual trees know about, and send nutrients to, young or sick trees. They use the mycelial network to warn of toxicity in the soil. Fungi break down the once living tissue of plants and trees and return it to basic molecules like nitrogen that can be recycled in the ecosystem. Mycelia process and store heavy metals and toxins, breaking them down and concentrating them away from where they can do harm to other living things.

To tell the difference between mushroom species, we must make sense of each fungus and its form and function, and then we organize them according to characteristics like whether or not they have gills, or the ways in which their fruiting bodies (the literal mushroom itself) develop. The naming of different mushrooms includes the genus name, and sometimes the species name reflects the place where it was found, the characteristics that make it different, or the person who discovered it. Sometimes scientists just want to introduce a little fun into their work, as reflected in names like *Spongiforma squarepantsii*, which was recently named after the popular cartoon character SpongeBob SquarePants. This name was chosen because the fungus's fruiting body looked similar to a sea sponge.

While species names denote the members of the group that can breed within that species, strains are a different type of taxonomic description. They reflect different lines of breed types, kind of like a family name. Strains aren't used in every scientific discipline. You find them in mycology, microbiology, agriculture, and virology, especially in the realm of public health. Strains are particularly well known in the cannabis industry, and they are very popular in the world of psychedelic mushrooms as well. A strain typically refers to a unique line of a particular species that has been developed and reproduced to highlight certain features of that species. If we were talking about dogs, French bulldogs would be their own strain that has been bred for their smushed faces. In the case of psychedelic

mushrooms, strains are typically developed for concentrations of psilocin, psilocybin, or co-occurring molecular components like aeruginascin, which is believed to aid in the sense of well-being that can be felt during the psychedelic experience.

There are three primary genera of psychedelic mushrooms: *Panaeolus*, *Psilocybe*, and *Copelandia*. There have been some taxonomic changes with regard to the genera *Panaeolus* and *Copelandia*. In some instances, these genus names are conflated; in others, they are being reviewed in the taxonomic literature. Another well-known genus is *Amanita*, and while some of the mushrooms in this group do have psychedelic properties, most of the mushrooms in the *Copelandia* and *Amanita* genera are toxic and should be avoided. The most prolific of the psychedelic-producing mushrooms are members of the genus *Panaeolus*. However, the most cultivated of the psychedelic-producing mushrooms come from the genus *Psilocybe*. Of these, the most frequently cultivated species is the first one in our list, *Psilocybe cubensis*. This species is easy to grow and generates generous flushes (crops) of mushrooms. Because of its robust, reliable growth, *P. cubensis* is one of the most frequently used mushrooms for creativity and experimentation for developing new strains.

PSILOCYBE CUBENSIS

This species is the most cultivated among the known psilocybin mushrooms. It has been widely shared and creatively developed over the last 50 years. There are multiple strains, some of which you will find in the coming pages. The hallmark of this mushroom is its golden color that sometimes can lean toward deep orange. Like all mushrooms containing psilocybin, *P. cubensis* will bruise blue if it is blemished or pressed. Variants of *P. cubensis* can be found all over the world, from the southeastern United States to Mexico, Cuba, Central and South America, Asia, and even in parts of Australia. This mushroom does well in hot, moist climates, but it can grow almost anywhere. It is particularly fond of dung substrates, so in natural habitats you'll likely find it in horse, cow, and other large animal droppings. The fruiting bodies can become quite large, making them easy to spot.

In comparing the potency of psilocybin-producing mushrooms, researchers have reported variations from as low as 0.15% psilocybin up to 1.8%, and from 0.11% to 0.60% psilocin. Cultivated mushrooms—those grown intentionally in controlled environments—tend to have higher concentrations of psychoactive ingredients. The *P. cubensis* mushroom typically contains both psilocybin and psilocin, which may help to explain why it is particularly well tolerated. The direct psilocin content helps to transition the voyager into the deeper phases of the psychedelic experience without the acute nausea that is often reported with other species. Theoretically, the body has access to the active psilocin already present in the mushroom and uses it first after the mushroom has been ingested. Meanwhile, the body is simultaneously working to translate the psilocybin found in the mushroom into a second round of usable psilocin via metabolization in the liver, where it removes a phosphate group on the psilocybin molecule. Because of this translation from psilocybin to psilocin, psilocybin is often referred to as a prodrug. Psilocybin is the initial substance that must be metabolized in order to be of use to the body in the form of psilocin.

There are many strains of *P. cubensis*. Some have been around for decades, and others are relatively new. As mentioned at the beginning of this chapter, cultivated mushrooms tend to produce greater and more reliably consistent concentrations of psilocybin and psilocin. The other strains of *P. cubensis* in this list have been developed by cultivators—ranging from scientists to amateurs—for their tolerability, reliability, and high concentrations of psychoactive compounds.

GOLDEN TEACHER

This strain of *P. cubensis* is the most prolifically grown and distributed. It is one of the best known and most widely used strains of psychedelic mushrooms. This is due to Golden Teacher's ease of cultivation and its ability to reliably produce a positive psychedelic experience. Golden Teacher mushrooms are distinguished by their golden to orange cap, which retains its color even when the mushroom is dried. They have relatively thin stems that grow to about 3 to 4 inches in length. This strain has a moderate measured comparative potency of both psilocybin (0.5–0.6%) and psilocin (0.35–0.6%).[10] The effects of this strain come on relatively quickly, after about 30 minutes, due to its high psilocin content. The subsequent journey can last between two and four hours, which is shorter than most strains. The more manageable duration is likely due to the ratio of psilocybin to psilocin that exists within this strain. The Golden Teacher strain is considered to be gentle on the psyche,[11] offering users intuition and insight with less jarring images and/or anxiety that can sometimes occur with other strains.[12] The mushroom experience with Golden Teacher is said to unfold in a meaningful rather than a haphazard way, which explains the name's origin. This experience may be related to the fact that Golden Teachers are most typically used by psychonauts who are intentionally seeking insight, thus priming the psyche for an educational or spiritual experience.[13]

B+

The B+ strain was reportedly discovered in Florida, which distinguishes it from many of the other strains of *P. cubensis*, whose origins are typically in Mexico and Central America. This strain is considered hardy and easy to cultivate, and it tends to grow larger than other strains.[14] The stipes of the B+ strain are thick and long, and their caps typically turn a caramel color as they mature. Their caps also often have a distinct umbo, or bump, at the center. They favor the warm and humid climates connected with their natural habitat. They often appear rapidly after a sharp increase in warmth and humidity. Anyone who

has ever lived near the natural habitat of the B+ strain may wake up one morning to see mushrooms appearing as if by magic across cow or horse pastures. This strain has moderate potency of psilocybin (0.59–1.0%) and psilocin (0.11%).[15] Self-reported experiences from users suggest that these mushrooms tend toward a relatively mild psychedelic journey, similar to the Golden Teacher strain. Anecdotal evidence has found that some users who already tend toward anxiety or persistent negative cognition might experience similar overthinking when using this strain.[16]

ALACABENZI

Anecdotal reports about the Alacabenzi strain assert that it is a hybrid of other strains, specifically the Golden Teacher and Mexicana strains. Other reports suggest that the Alacabenzi is a hybrid of the Alabama and Mexicana strains.[17] However, there is no published research to support these claims. Genetic testing would be the most accurate way of determining the truth, but no such testing was found at the time of this book's writing. The Alacabenzi strain is reported to have effects similar to some cannabis strains, featuring physical sensations often called a body high. Self-reports include numerous experiences of relaxation and feelings of being soothed, consistent with experiences

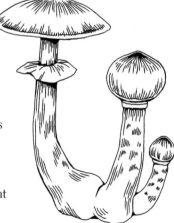

of the *P. mexicana* species.[18] When taken at moderate doses, fewer visual experiences and a higher frequency of well-being and euphoria are reported. At higher doses, some psychonauts report visual experiences and synesthesia (like hearing colors and tasting music) with this strain. Like most *P. cubensis* strains, Alacabenzi has a moderate level of tryptamines, with moderate psilocybin (0.67%) and lower levels of psilocin (0.02%).[19]

PF CLASSIC

This strain was developed by the famous Robert McPherson, who created the PF Tek method for growing mushrooms.[20] This relatively simple procedure revolutionized amateur cultivation of psychedelic mushrooms. The "PF" in PF Classic and PF Tek stands for Psilocybe Fanaticus and was his protective pseudonym. This strain, like others of *P. cubensis*, has a moderate amount of psilocybin (0.62%) and psilocin (0.05%).[21] However, despite the similar percentage of psilocybin to other mushrooms in this species, aficionados often refer to the PF Classic as an "advanced" mushroom.[22]

It is well known for providing an intense psychedelic experience. Experienced sojourners report that there is a profound difference between a Golden Teacher and a PF Classic journey.[23] Where the Golden Teacher journey is gentle and methodical, the PF Classic journey may be disjointed and demanding. The psyche may respond to the presence of the PF Classic by serving challenging imagery and memories. If a psychonaut is resistant to facing their issues and does not respond to gentle therapeutic techniques, this strain may be the best choice. It will push them deeper but will likely do so with images and symbols that might be frightening and dramatic. Experienced sojourners praise it, but all caution that PF Classic is not for beginners.[24] Sojourners report that the consumption of this mushroom often ends with nausea.

ORISSA INDIAN

As you might guess by the name, this strain is native to India. It was discovered in Odisha, which is India's eighth-largest state. The region was formerly known as Orissa, but is now known as Odisha; however, the mushroom kept the English transliteration as its name. The region's namesake mushroom was discovered growing in elephant dung, and like its preferred substrate, it grows very large. It is one of the largest of all the *P. cubensis* strains.[25] Unlike other strains in this species, this mushroom is very potent. The reported tryptamine content is extremely high, with the combined content of both psilocybin and psilocin typically measuring greater

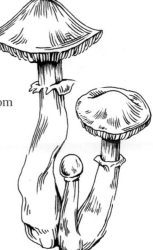

than 1.5% and sometimes measured as high as 3.0%.[26] Self-reports of those who have journeyed with these mushrooms include a deeply introspective journey with significant insights, visual phenomena, and profound emotional experiences.[27] It is not a surprise that this strain also can induce a feeling of ego dissolution or universal oneness, feelings that are often reported at high doses of psilocybin and psilocin. Voyagers say that the experience of taking Orissa Indian is similar to those had with strains like B+ and Penis Envy, but more intense.

PENIS ENVY (VARIOUS)

Ever since the introduction of the Penis Envy strain, substrains have been developed and given similar provocative names. As its title suggests, this strain is known for its unique morphology resembling, yes, a penis. It boasts a thick stem and a smaller compact cap. Its substrains have followed the model with names like Penis Envy Uncut, which boasts a very potent level of psilocybin (1.36%) and psilocin (0.62%).[28] Albino Penis Envy is a little milder with lower levels of psilocybin (0.97%) and psilocin (0.15%).[29] With multiple different substrains, it is best to understand whether you are working with classic

Penis Envy or one of its newer descendants. Most Penis Envy mushrooms are considered to be very potent.[30] They require more intense efforts to grow, and they take longer to cultivate. They aren't very prolific at dropping their spores because of the closed cap typical to this strain. As a result, Penis Envy may be more difficult to find. Sojourners report that the experience of these mushrooms is notably different, especially with regard to the visual effects experienced while under its influence.[31] Penis Envy's visuals tend more toward waves in comparison to the more typical geometric visuals that are usually reported by people taking other strains. Effects of Penis Envy include synesthesia (hearing colors, tasting sounds), intense feelings of joy or euphoria, and auditory distortions or intensity. Some voyagers also report ego dissolution and deep mystical awareness.[32] Reports on this strain also seem to focus the experience on the psyche, affecting insights and emotions as opposed to the physical experience sometimes aligned with a body high. Psychonauts report that this strain is better for more experienced sojourners. It can set voyagers on an intense wave of emotions that can be both positive and challenging.[33]

Z STRAIN

This is a cultivated strain that was developed to be larger and more potent, and it is described as a powerful colonizer. The mycelia grow robustly, and the fruiting stage comes quickly, with multiple flushes or crops.[34] This strain is also reported to drop lots of spores, which makes it popular with cultivators. The experience of this strain tends toward intense visual phenomena, somatic involvement like body sensations, and, at higher doses, feelings of euphoria and mystical experiences.[35] This strain is believed to have been isolated and developed from the Golden Teacher strain, and so it may offer a similar effect. It has been cultivated for at least the last 20 years. Because it is easy to grow, it is a common strain to find among professional and amateur cultivators. The Z Strain has a moderate amount of tryptamines. It has a moderate amount of psilocybin (0.67%) and a higher amount of psilocin (0.17%) than most.[36] This higher-than-average psilocin content means that the psychedelic experience will likely begin within 30 minutes of consumption.[37]

TIDAL WAVE/ENIGMA

Amateur and professional mycologists often experiment with crossing strains in an effort to unite and elevate the best qualities of particular mushrooms. This variety—which was developed from the B+ and Penis Envy strains—is one of the best examples of engineering for increased potency and effect. The Tidal Wave strain won the 2021 Psilocybin Cup with more than 3% total tryptamines. However, on average, samples haven't tested that high consistently. Typical Tidal Wave measures from moderate to high amounts of psilocybin (0.68–1.3%) and psilocin (0.30–0.60%).[38]

When developing Tidal Wave mushrooms, sometimes a mutation called Enigma is produced. Enigma mushrooms are strange, alien-looking blobs.[39] They can look like cauliflower or like truffles. Because this mutant version doesn't drop spores, they are created only by experienced growers. They must be developed with hand-gathered spores and then injected with a needle into a cultivator's substrate like the one used in the PF Tek method. They are extremely potent, sometimes testing at more than 3% overall tryptamines (combined psilocybin and psilocin), but they grow slowly. They must be monitored to protect them against contamination. Experienced voyagers report that the journey on Tidal Wave/Enigma is very intense and reminiscent of MDMA, with waves of feeling, an increased sense of openness, euphoria, synesthesia, profound emotional experiences, and deep insights. Because of their potency, you should consume much less of these mushrooms when preparing for a journey.[40]

FUZZY BALLS

This privately developed strain was entered into a contest for mushroom growers called the Psilocybin Cup in 2021. This strain tested at a very high potency, about 3% tryptamines, with approximately equal parts psilocybin (1.67%) and psilocin (1.32%).[41] Because it is a relatively new strain, information on it is extremely limited. It is in high demand because of its potency. The high ratio of psilocin to psilocybin implies that the psychedelic experience would start within 30 minutes of ingesting, and it would likely last for several hours.

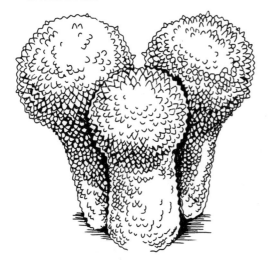

SUMMING UP *P. CUBENSIS*

This is a very limited list of *P. cubensis* strains, which are the most prolific of all the psychedelic mushrooms. *P. cubensis* are found in nature in multiple parts of the world. Because this species is easy to cultivate, it is also experimented with by growers in almost every climate and environment. Because of its flexibility, potency, and reliability, this species is one of many that is being used to advance research in the development of medications that can be made from psilocybin and psilocin. There are easily another 30 or so varieties of *P. cubensis* that have been developed by cultivators over the years but are not listed here. Some are easier to find than others. This list includes descriptions of both the most well known and the most interesting strains that have been developed in the last 20 to 30 years. If you want to experiment with magic mushrooms, you should give yourself the benefit of learning about the different strains and species that you are likely to encounter. For anyone wanting to experiment with psychedelic experiences or therapy, understanding the types of experiences that can result from different strains is a helpful way of preparing for your journey. Not all strains are equal.

Next, we'll look at different species of magic mushrooms. While the mushrooms most frequently used for psychedelic experiences come from the *P. cubensis* species, they are by no means the only (or the most powerful) naturally occurring psilocybin producers. Different species have evolved all over the world. These mushrooms have very different appearances and may include other psychoactive substances that can contribute to or mediate their effects.

A World of Psychedelic Species

It is well known in psychedelic circles that the first modern shaman to reintroduce *Psilocybe* mushrooms to the world was a Mazatec woman named Maria Sabina. Without her, and her collaboration with R. Gordon Wasson, we might never have rediscovered the power of psychedelic mushrooms. The most important person in the world of mushrooms today is mycologist Paul Stamets. There have been many other important researchers, writers, mycologists, and voyagers, but Stamets is a living legend. If you have watched a

Table 1. *Psilocybe cubensis* comparison

P. CUBENSIS STRAIN	% PSILOCYBIN	% PSILOCIN	EXPERIENCE LEVEL 1–5*	NOTES
Golden Teacher	0.5–0.6	0.35–0.6	1–2	Tends to be gentle, intuition and insight are hallmarks
B+	0.59–1.0	0.11	2–3	Mild journey, similar to Golden Teacher
Alacabenzi	0.67	0.02	3	Moderate journey
PF Classic	0.62	0.05	5	Intense, sometimes unpleasant/challenging
Orissa Indian	1.2–2.5	0.08–0.95	4	Deeply introspective journey
Penis Envy	0.97–1.36	0.15–0.62	5+	Very potent, lots of visuals, synesthesia, joy euphoria, auditory hallucinations
Enigma	0.76–2.5	0.07–0.5	5	Confronting, deep, often very clear
Z Strain	0.67	0.17	3	Intense visuals, euphoria, mystical experiences
Tidal Wave	0.68–1.3	0.3–0.6	4	Openness, euphoria, deep insights, synesthesia
Fuzzy Balls	1.67	1.32	?	Unknown

* lower experience level is better for beginners

documentary, seen a TED Talk, or heard a podcast about mushrooms, you surely have heard his voice or, at the very least, his name.

Stamets has discovered and named several species of *Psilocybe* mushrooms. He is also a consummate scientist, learning and sharing all the ways that various fungi engage with their environment. He has discovered fungi that can clean up oil spills, reduce heavy metals in soil, act as natural pesticides, and improve how we build homes.[42] There is no one living person who more eloquently and lovingly talks about mushrooms and how they connect the different biological kingdoms we inhabit. He writes eloquently about his relationship with the living earth, and about our interconnectedness as part of a great network of creation, insights he received through his relationship with mushrooms. Stamets's work continues to inspire me as I engage in my own research in neuroscience, consciousness, and the gifts that the earth shares with us to bring us closer to her and each other. Many of the following references come from Stamets's work. In the next few pages, you will read about mushrooms that contain psilocybin, psilocin, baeocystin, and aeruginascin. These mushrooms have been spread across the world, their spores riding on the legs of domesticated animals, lumberjacks, and college students.

In his book *Psilocybin Mushrooms of the World*, Stamets tells the story of one of his first experiences with *Psilocybe* mushrooms. In it he recounts how in the 1960s and '70s *Psilocybe* mushrooms weren't very easy to find in the woods of the Pacific Northwest.[43] But as more people started to look for them, they would appear in the places people populated, mostly in the suburbs. The spores traveled into the suburbs with the wood chips that entered the landscaping of suburban terrain. They colonized parks, college campuses, roadsides, police stations—anywhere that enjoyed fresh landscaping. The mycelia and spores had stayed with their host substrates, even after these had been turned into mulch or landscaping timbers and transplanted into tony suburbs.[44]

As you look through these pages, consider that these species of mushrooms have been around for thousands or even tens of thousands of years. People all over the earth, during every human time period, have ingested these mushrooms to come closer to understanding the mystery of being. Why are we here? What is it all for? How do we meet our fellow humans along the path? What's it all about, anyway? The unique mystery of working with these fungi is that the answers aren't in the mushrooms; they are in us. The mushrooms unlock doors deep within ourselves.

The Genus *Panaeolus*

There are several psychedelic mushrooms in the genus *Panaeolus*. Many in this group do not have psychedelic properties. One of the most important features of this genus, however, is how closely it resembles other genera of mushrooms. Just because you see small brown mushrooms doesn't mean you've found psilocybin-containing mushrooms. Mushrooms in this genus look very much like *Psilocybe* mushrooms and like highly poisonous *Galerina* mushrooms. They have black gills, a concave cap that will open and flatten a little bit as they mature, and a long, thin stipe. The way to tell the difference upon visual inspection is by the color of the spores. The mushrooms in the *Panaeolus* genus have black spores, while *Psilocybe* have purplish-brown spores, and *Galerina* have brown spores.[45] There are at least three poisonous varieties of *Panaeolus*, and there are many more poisonous varieties of the similar-looking *Galerina*. If you find little brown mushrooms and can't tell the difference between them, err on the side of caution, and leave them alone!

Another confusing feature of working with mushrooms in the *Panaeolus* genus is that some taxonomic issues in the mycological sciences have introduced confusing nomenclature to the scientific descriptions. This genus, *Panaeolus*, is sometimes referred to as *Copelandia*. This nomenclature was created to honor naturalist Edward Bingham Copeland, who sent samples of these to his friend Abbé Giacomo Bresadola. The nomenclature distinguishes the tropical psychedelic mushrooms in this genus from other *Panaeolus* mushrooms. The *Copelandia* nomenclature distinguishes psychedelic from nonpsychedelic species. This distinction is not considered scientifically relevant in some mycological circles, and there are mycologists who simply reject or ignore it.[46] This introduces confusion into the naming of this genus, but these terms can simply be treated as synonyms. If you should happen upon any mushrooms referred to as *Copelandia cyanescens*, for example, know that they are the same as *Panaeolus cyanescens*.

CAMBODIAN: *PANAEOLUS CAMBODGINIENSIS*

As the name suggests, this species was first discovered in Cambodia but has also been found naturally occurring in other parts of Asia and as far from its home turf as Hawaii.[47] Like many of its psilocybin-containing relatives, its preferred substrate is animal dung. The mushroom bruises blue when handled, an indicator of the psilocybin and psilocin present. This strain is relatively easy to cultivate and produces rich flushes with multiple specimens. Voyagers report that the psychedelic experience with this species is introspective, without the visual phenomena often attributed to mushroom journeying. Be mindful that this species is not terribly potent. It has lower psilocybin (0.45–0.57%) and psilocin (0.06%)[48] content in comparison to the popular *P. cubensis* strains.[49]

BLUE MEANIES: *PANAEOLUS CYANESCENS*

This species is highly sought after because of its reputation as a highly potent psychedelic.[50] In most measurements, these mushrooms tend to have a moderate to high amount of psilocybin (0.71–1.3%), low psilocin (0.05–0.16%), and some baeocystin (0.01%).[51] The familiar name Blue Meanies comes from their tendency to bruise blue on handling, even turning gray as the fruiting body (the mushroom itself) matures. The "Meanies" part of the name is a reference to the intensity of the experience for most voyagers. The ratio of psilocybin to psilocin is likely the culprit here, with the psychedelic effects showing up intensely after ingestion.[52] The measurable presence of baeocystin may not be relevant, though new research has demonstrated that baeocystin may be a prodrug (precursor) to another tryptamine called norpsilocin, which in recent experiments has been reported to have varying effects.[53] Some tests show that it may act as a mild psychedelic, and other tests report that it may act as a serotonergic antagonist that enables greater uptake of translated psilocin.[54] Blue Meanies are also well known because of their confusing name. Their bluish-gray color, easy blue bruising, and psychedelic effects have meant that they have been conflated with other psilocybin-producing, easily bluing psychedelic mushrooms, such as *Psilocybe cyanescens* (*cyanescens* means "bluing"). The Blue Meanies of the *Paneolous* genus are much stronger than other strains that are sometimes mistakenly referred to as blue meanies, but which are typically either a version of *Psilocybe cubensis*, or *Psilocybe cyanescens*, which are also called Wavy Caps.[55] If you find yourself with Blue Meanies, it would be useful to know what the actual genus and species of your strain is to know what kind of journey to expect. If you are working with *Panaeolus cyanescens*, you can expect a strong trip with deep insights, rich imagery, sometimes

challenging images, and lots of introspection.[56] If your Blue Meanies are *Psilocybe cyanescens*, you can expect a moderate trip with introspection, visual phenomena, and euphoria. If you are working with *Psilocybe cubensis* Blue Meanies, the experience will be similar to that of *Psilocybe cyanescens*.[57]

TROPICAL: *PANAEOLUS TROPICALIS*

This species, like other psychedelic mushrooms, is often found in animal dung of both domesticated animals and wild animals living in more tropical environments. This mushroom has been found in environments as disparate as Hawaii, Africa, and Asia. Paul Stamets notes in his book *Psilocybin Mushrooms of the World* that the differences between the *Panaeolus tropicalis* and *Panaeolus cyanescens* are so minute that they may not warrant *P. tropicalis* being categorized as a separate species.[58] The only distinctions found between the two species are microscopic differences that Stamets argues may be environmental rather than genetic. Like most psilocybin-producing mushrooms, this one bruises blue when handled.

The Genus *Psilocybe*

About half of the species in the *Psilocybe* genus (as of this writing, approximately 117 of the roughly 200 known species) contain sufficient tryptamines to be considered psychedelic mushrooms. Compared to other genera and species, the *Psilocybe* genus is a smorgasbord of psychedelia (for example, there are 19 known members of the *Panaeolus* genus that are known to have psychedelic properties out of approximately 100 different members, about 19%). The *Psilocybe* genus has relatives all over the world, with representation on almost every continent.

The genus *Psilocybe* consists of many species known for their psilocybin and psilocin content. Of these two tryptamines, psilocybin is the most stable. The presence of psilocybin and psilocin account for the bluing reaction of most species in the *Psilocybe* genus when they are handled. There are other mushrooms in this genus, though not all are psychoactive.

In the next several pages you will read about many different *Psilocybe* mushrooms from different parts of the world. What all of them have in common is the ability to connect us to something greater than ourselves. Mushrooms will not do the work for us. The sacred act that they enlist us in is the act of becoming aware. By facilitating our growth, awareness, consciousness, and connection, *Psilocybe* mushrooms give us an incredible gift. On a more mundane level, these mushrooms create substances that may help people heal debilitating mental health conditions, almost all of which can be characterized by disconnection. The research in this area stretches back more than 60 years, and in almost every report we see the efficacy of using these psychoactive substances to help people heal their traumas and thereby reconnect to their lives. As a therapist, I know that the biggest impediment to connection is trauma. When people have a psychological or physical trauma, the central nervous system responds by taking protective measures. These almost always take on a defensive appearance, breaking the psyche into smaller, compartmentalized pieces that can be managed for survival.

Mushrooms from genus *Psilocybe* first reintroduced those of us in the West to the healing possibilities that come along with working with these particular fungi. Every single one of these mushrooms has a story to tell you about yourself. Every species could also tell you a story about the people who discovered it, revered it, and used it to connect to a deeper existence. If you are hoping to investigate the depths of human experience, working with *Psilocybe* mushrooms will not disappoint.

BOTTLE CAPS/KNOBBY TOPS: *PSILOCYBE BAEOCYSTIS*

This species was first discovered in the Pacific Northwest of the United States, and as you might expect from a species native to this environment, it is very fond of fir trees, wood chips, and wood substrates.[59] This mushroom is one of the most popular strains because it is a very potent *Psilocybe*. It boasts a mixture of psilocybin (0.85%), psilocin (0.59%), and baeocystin (0.10%).[60] Sojourners report that this particular species is known for

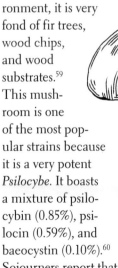

intense visions and experiences of color during the journey. *P. baeocystis* mushrooms have a white stem that can blue when bruised or handled, and sometimes the stem also has blue mottling or veining. The cap looks gelatinous and unappealing. These mushrooms don't preserve well, and they tend to lose their potency within a few days, even if dried.[61] These mushrooms were once considered rare, but they have thrived in the Pacific Northwest in mulch, turf, and wood cut from the forests. They will sometimes appear with other mushrooms. If you are working with a therapist or guide who has collected or cultivated these mushrooms, know that if they are dried, they won't be very potent. If they are fresh, you will want to make sure that they have been properly cleaned and sterilized. If fresh, they will be very powerful.[62]

WAVY CAPS: *PSILOCYBE CYANESCENS*

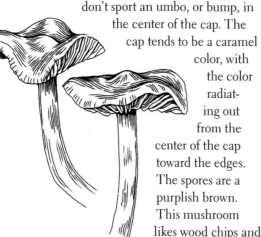

These are one of the most potent *Psilocybe* species measured. These mushrooms fall into the "little brown mushroom" category. They have a distinctive cap that is, yes, wavy. They don't sport an umbo, or bump, in the center of the cap. The cap tends to be a caramel color, with the color radiating out from the center of the cap toward the edges. The spores are a purplish brown. This mushroom likes wood chips and other mulch-type substrates. It often grows with other mushrooms, including the deadly *Galerina* species, so please be very careful if you come upon these in nature. Don't assume a patch of mushrooms is made up of individuals of the same species just because they are found growing next to each other. Wavy Caps tend to have a very powerful effect on voyagers. They typically have a high tryptamine content with psilocybin (0.3–1.68%) and psilocin (0.28–0.51%) ranges making for intense journeys.[63] This mushroom will bruise blue when handled. When they appear in nature, Wavy Caps usually occur in wildly rich flushes, with hundreds of individuals showing up in a flush at once. It is unlikely to find one or two of these mushrooms on their own, so be advised that if you see a single individual, you probably don't have a wavy cap specimen but something a bit more dangerous. These mushrooms can be found in the United States and in Europe.

LIBERTY CAPS: *PSILOCYBE SEMILANCEATA*

Considered to be the common type of the species, the *Psilocybe semilanceata* is the typical example of the *Psilocybe* species. It is one of the most prolifically distributed psychedelic mushrooms in the world, and you can find it in grassy areas. It is a small, warm reddish- to caramel-brown mushroom. The edges of the cap tend to be lighter than the center.[64] This species is one of the best for drying and storing. This *Psilocybe* mushroom has a high psilocybin count (1.0–2.38%), little to no psilocin, and a relatively high measure of baeocystin (0.21%).[65] Unlike most *Psilocybe* mushrooms, the Liberty Cap is less likely to bruise bluish when it's handled. This is probably due to its low to no psilocin content. If it does bruise blue, it will likely be at the base of the stem only. Liberty Caps like pastures and grass, especially rich grass associated with grazing animals.[66] This mushroom is also one of the first whose effects were described scientifically, in 1799. The name Liberty Cap is often associated with the freedom of mind that comes from ingesting this mushroom, but the name is actually related to the Phrygian cap, a hat that symbolized someone as a free person during the age of antiquity. During the French Revolution, descriptions of this mushroom likened it to seeing the Phrygian cap on a pole, which was a common sight at the time.[67] These mushrooms aren't easily cultivated, because they are delicate and a bit challenging to maintain, and finding them in the wild is often perilous, as they look very similar to poisonous *Galerina* mushrooms, especially *Galerina marginata*. Be cautious if you find these while you're foraging. The Liberty Cap experience is also "typical." Voyagers describe audio and visual phenomena, euphoria, and deep insights. The experience with these mushrooms will begin within 40 minutes of ingestion and can last up to six hours.

FLYING SAUCERS: *PSILOCYBE AZURESCENS*

This mushroom was named and described by Paul Stamets and his colleague Jochen Gartz.[68] It was discovered in the Pacific Northwest and grows in timber detritus and sandy soil. These mushrooms are small and brown in appearance, and like most psilocybin mushrooms, they bruise blue when handled. The name *azurescens* means bluing. This species will blue into deeper colors from a light blue to almost black when handled or bruised. Its spore print looks purple to black. This mushroom does well in flower beds, especially those of woody flowers like roses. It is easier to cultivate these mushrooms indoors with a wood substrate rather than other substrates. There are some reports of voyagers using Flying Saucers experiencing a frightening problem called wood lover's paralysis, which is associated with mushrooms grown on a wood substrate. The experience produces temporary paralysis, with loss of muscle tone, muscle control, and general incapacitation that can last approximately 24 hours. This can be very challenging for anyone, but it is especially alarming for anyone unfamiliar with psychedelic experiences. This mushroom is one of the most potent ever measured, containing high levels of psilocybin (1.78%), psilocin (0.38%), and baeocystin (0.35%).[69] As such they are not recommended for those who are new to psychedelic experiences. Voyagers describe intense visual experiences, deep insights, vivid imagery, and in higher doses increased anxiety.[70] This mushroom stores fairly well once dried because of its high psilocybin content.

BLUE LEGS: *PSILOCYBE STUNTZII*

This mushroom is named after mycologist Daniel Stuntz, who was a professor at the University of Washington, on whose campus the mushroom was first discovered.[71] It gets its popular name Blue Legs from the presence of a blue ring around its stipe. As a mushroom matures, the area around the gills separates as the cap opens to spread its spores. This is called a veil, and it is common for many species to have a residual ring around the stem that once protected the gills. In this species, the veil itself becomes a ring and turns blue. This mushroom is not very potent, with about three times more psilocybin (0.36%) than psilocin (0.12%).[72] Because of its low psilocybin content, this mushroom is not cultivated very often. A person would require a very large serving of these mushrooms in order to generate a strong psychedelic experience. Blue Legs, more than any other *Psilocybe*,

is often mistaken for the highly poisonous *Galerina marginata*.[73]

BOHEMIAN: *PSILOCYBE SERBICA*, SOMETIMES CALLED *PSILOCYBE BOHEMICA*

Found in deciduous forests, this *Psilocybe* mushroom likes rotting wood substrates. When genetic testing became more widely available, it revealed that this specimen is likely the same as *Psilocybe serbica*.[74] The Bohemian mushroom has reportedly high concentrations of psilocybin (1.38%), and relatively lower concentrations of psilocin (0.11%) and baeocystin (0.02%).[75] This mushroom has a white stipe, and a lightly colored cap. When dried, this mushroom gets lighter in color, and it has a specifically high concentration of psilocybin that makes it good for drying and storage. Like most *Psilocybe* mushrooms, this species produces purple spore prints.[76] This mushroom is found more frequently in Europe, and it is not commonly found in North America, though many mycologists suspect that it might be more widely distributed than currently reported.

LANDSLIDE: *PSILOCYBE CAERULESCENS*

This mushroom is found in Mexico and Central America. It is also found sporadically in the Southeastern United States. This *Psilocybe* mushroom often appears after landslides or other devastating changes to the landscape. This mushroom seems to fruit when exposed to air after these major events, taking advantage of the newly exposed terrain to expand and colonize.[77] This is believed to be one of the mushrooms introduced to R. Gordon Wasson in a ceremonial valada,[78] though the next entry is a more likely candidate. Wasson introduced *Psilocybe* mushrooms to the West thanks to his work with Maria Sabina in the 1950s. He wrote about his work in a now infamous article titled "Seeking the Magic Mushroom," which appeared in *Life* magazine in 1957. *P. caerulescens* mushrooms are likely moderately to highly potent. Desiccated samples have been measured at low psilocybin (0.20%) and little to no psilocin.[79] As of this writing, I could not find an updated study of their tryptamine concentrations. All the research available suggests that these mushrooms are likely more potent than reported based on the desiccated samples. Some voyagers report that this strain tastes like a cucumber. If we rely on the reports of Wasson and others, this mushroom produces rich visual experiences, deep insights, and feelings of euphoria.

PAJARITOS: *PSILOCYBE MEXICANA*

One of the species used in traditional Mazatec ceremonies, Pajaritos is one of the most well-known mushroom varieties. The name means "little birds." This species is famous for inspiring Terence McKenna's book *Food of the Gods*.[80] This mushroom is one of the possible candidates for carrying the mantle of the Aztec mushroom called teonanacatl, sometimes translated as "flesh of the gods," or just "sacred mushroom." Anthropologists believe that this is one of the species used by the Aztecs for thousands of years before the arrival of the colonizing forces of the Spanish Crown.[81] During the period of the Spanish colonization, with the influence of Catholicism and the subjugation of native religion and culture, mushrooms and their ceremonies were driven underground.

These mushrooms contain low to moderate concentrations of psilocybin (0.25%) and psilocin (0.15–0.25%).[82] They are best consumed while still fresh. Though these levels are considered relatively low, there may be variability in native populations that are dependent on the richness of the substrate. They tend to develop in humid, grassy areas along the edges of the woods. They also have an unusual capability to develop a sclerotia, a hard, seedlike body. The mushroom desiccates and dries out on its own to protect itself from intense heat.[83]

When the environment is more favorable, it will rehydrate into a hard, seedlike body that dries until it is time to rehydrate and start colonizing the mycelia. In a journey, these mushrooms are reported to bring insights and are accompanied by visual phenomena. It is from the *Psilocybe mexicana* mushroom that Albert Hofmann first isolated psilocybin and psilocin.

PHILOSOPHER'S STONES: *PSILOCYBE TAMPANENSIS*

These rare *Psilocybe* mushrooms are called Philosopher's Stones thanks to their fascinating origin story. During a mycology conference that had become painfully boring, mycologists Steven Pollock and Gary Lincoff left the conference for an impromptu foray.[84] They found a lone specimen in a Florida sand dune. When they cultivated new specimens from the original, they saw the development of sclerotia. They tried several names, and the one that stuck was Philosopher's Stones.[85] Since its discovery it has not been found again in Florida, and rarely anywhere else in natural surroundings. One other specimen was found in Alabama in a similar sandy substrate. This mushroom is considered low

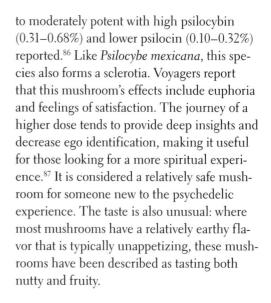

to moderately potent with high psilocybin (0.31–0.68%) and lower psilocin (0.10–0.32%) reported.[86] Like *Psilocybe mexicana*, this species also forms a sclerotia. Voyagers report that this mushroom's effects include euphoria and feelings of satisfaction. The journey of a higher dose tends to provide deep insights and decrease ego identification, making it useful for those looking for a more spiritual experience.[87] It is considered a relatively safe mushroom for someone new to the psychedelic experience. The taste is also unusual: where most mushrooms have a relatively earthy flavor that is typically unappetizing, these mushrooms have been described as tasting both nutty and fruity.

BADO: *PSILOCYBE ZAPOTECORUM*

This species of *Psilocybe* mushroom is believed to have been an important mushroom to the Indigenous people of the Oaxaca region of Mexico.[88] It is found in central Mexico and in South America, especially in subtropical environs. Anthropologists believe that some of the mushroom statues typically found in Oaxaca and in some areas of Guatemala may represent these mushrooms.[89] This species is considered very potent, and it blues easily when handled. Like most *Psilocybe* mushrooms, *P. zapotecorum* produces purple-black spores. This strain

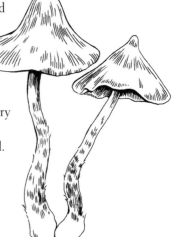

is often found in muddy and swampy environments, especially where there are rich substrates filled with leaves and wood debris. The psilocin (1.0%) content is greater than the psilocybin (0.30%) content.[90] This implies that the Bado mushroom would be most effective if consumed as a fresh specimen rather than a dried one. The caps are asymmetrical. These mushrooms are similar in appearance to Liberty Caps but with a more subdued yellowish-ochre color. They will darken and blacken as they age and bruise bluish green when handled.[91]

DR. WEIL'S: *PSILOCYBE WEILII*

This mushroom was discovered in the US state of Georgia and is named for Andrew Weil to honor his contributions to promoting mushrooms for health.[92] It is rare to find this mushroom in the wild, but it has been successfully cultivated. This mushroom is considered moderately potent with a strong presence of multiple alkaloid tryptamines: psilocybin (0.61%), psilocin (0.27%), and baeocystin (0.05%).[93] It was originally found in an area with pine forests in red-clay soils. If found, it will frequently be located in a robust flush with clusters of many individual specimens. *Psilocybe weilii* also have a strong bluing reaction to handling or bruising. These are

easy to cultivate for psychedelic purposes. Voyagers report that they have a pleasant taste. They typically don't grow in soil but beneath mulched leaves.[94]

More Psilocybin Mushrooms to Know About

More psilocybin-producing mushrooms are discovered every year. In addition, cultivators are constantly developing new strains to concentrate and amplify the best aspects of other strains and species. The lists provided so far are meant to offer descriptions of some of the most popular and historically important strains. As psilocybin therapy is more widely accepted and legalized, new strains will be developed, and new uses and practices will emerge from new settings, new compounds, and discoveries in the fields of anthropology, psychotherapy, neuroscience, and pharmacology.

The rest of the psilocybin-producing mushrooms in this list are species you may encounter in your psychedelic journey, but they likely won't be as widely available. Perhaps a new variant of the species will be discovered, and this book will be the place you saw it first. Regardless, the previous list of mushrooms was organized by common name, but this list is organized by the scientific names of different species. Most of the mushrooms that you will encounter through cultivators or by growing them from your own spore prints will be found in the previous list. However, it is still good practice to be well versed in other varieties, especially if you are interested in the science and research going on in the field.

Table 2. Selected species comparison

SPECIES	% PSILOCYBIN	% PSILOCIN	% BAEOCYSTIN	EXPERIENCE LEVEL 1–5 *	NOTES
Panaeolus cambodginiensis (Cambodian)	0.45–0.57	0.06	~	3	Introspective, unlikely to include visual phenomena
Panaeolus cyanescens (Blue Meanies)	0.71–1.3	0.05–0.16	0.01	5	Intense experience, deep insights, challenging images, introspection
Psilocybe baeocystis (Bottle Caps or Knobby Tops)	0.85	0.59	0.10	4	Best fresh, lose intensity even when immediately dried; intense visions, experience of colors, synesthesia
Psilocybe cyanescens (Wavy Caps)	0.3–1.68	0.28–0.51	~	3	Best fresh; intense euphoria, introspection, hallucinations, synesthesia, visually intense
Psilocybe semilanceata (Liberty Caps)	1.0–2.38	0.0–0.1	0.21	3	Audio and visual phenomena, euphoria, deep insights
Psilocybe azurescens (Flying Saucers)	1.78	0.38	0.35	5	Risk of wood lover's paralysis if foraged wild; intense visuals, increased anxiety at high doses

* lower experience level is better for beginners
~ = either no reported data, or zero %

Table 2, continued

SPECIES	% PSILOCYBIN	% PSILOCIN	% BAEOCYSTIN	EXPERIENCE LEVEL 1-5*	NOTES
Psilocybe stuntzii (Blue Legs)	0.36	0.12	~	1	Beware the little brown mushroom—easily confused with poisonous *Galerina marginata*; not very potent
Psilocybe bohemica (Bohemian)	1.38	0.11	0.02	2	Found mostly in Europe; insights, mild visuals, euphoria
Psilocybe caerulescens (Landslide)	0.20	~	~	3	Rich visuals, deep insights, euphoria
Psilocybe mexicana (Pajaritos)	0.25	0.15–0.25	~	3	Best consumed fresh; visuals, insights
Psilocybe tampanensis (Philosopher's Stone)	0.31–0.68	0.10–0.32	~	2	Euphoria, feelings of satisfaction, at higher doses reduced ego identification and mystical experiences
Psilocybe zapotecorum (Bado)	0.3	1.0	~	unknown	Unknown
Psilocybe weilii (Dr. Weil's)	0.61	0.27	0.05	2	A pleasant taste, relatively easy journey, mild visuals and insights

PSILOCYBE ARGENTIPES

This is one of the most widely available psilocybin-producing mushrooms that is native to Japan. It is not found growing indigenously outside of Japan. It has been called the "laughing" mushroom and the "dancing" mushroom. While it is considered related to *Psilocybe zapotecorum* genetically, its effects appear to be markedly different in some respects, though the mechanisms of action are not well understood. The word *argenti* refers to the silver color, and *pes* is Latin for feet, referring to the silvery-colored threads that extend from the middle to the bottom of the mushroom's stipe.[95] There have been reports of this mushroom causing food poisoning in some cases.[96] This species was identified with novel research into the use of psilocybin-producing mushrooms in the treatment of obsessive-compulsive disorder.[97] Researchers compared the effects of *P. argentipes* and pure psilocybin in mice that engage in OCD behaviors and found that *P. argentipes* produced a significant positive result, while pure psilocybin did not. This implies that there is some biochemical difference in the *P. argentipes* species versus the pure psilocybin molecule. The *P. argentipes* specimens positively engaged the central nervous system to calm OCD behaviors in animal experiments.[98]

PSILOCYBE AUCKLANDII

This *Psilocybe* mushroom is native to New Zealand. In recent decades wood and forest products have been exported from New Zealand, making it more likely that this species will find its way into other environments. This mushroom is considered moderately potent, though there were no available results of testing as of this writing. This mushroom,

like *Psilocybe argentipes*, also appears to be a relative of *Psilocybe zapotecorum*.[99] It will blue when bruised or handled, and it has a punctuated umbo, or bump at the top of the cap.[100]

PSILOCYBE AUSTRALIANA

This species is native to Australia and Tasmania. It thrives in lands with pine debris. It can also be found near eucalyptus groves. The distribution of timber from regions of Australia near Sydney that are rich in pine and eucalyptus has helped this species to colonize and flourish in other areas in Australia.[101] This mushroom is described as mild to moderately potent, though I could not find any published reports on its tryptamine content. It will blue when handled or bruised.[102]

PSILOCYBE AZTECORUM

Ethnomycologists believe that this species is one of the likely candidates (along with *Psilocybe mexicana*) for the Aztec teonanacatl, sometimes translated as "flesh of the gods" or "sacred mushroom." This species prefers higher altitudes, and it is often found in pine forests that are part of the trans Mexico volcanic belt. This *Psilocybe* species is native to the tallest mountains of central Mexico. It has been added to the Global Fungal Red List,[103] a list compiled by conservation scientists in response to the lack of inclusion of fungi in the study of endangered or compromised species on Earth. The conservationists report that while it is possible to find this species in other habitats (like Colorado, for example) the original native species is at risk due to climate change, wildfires, and illegal cultivation and trade. There are no official reports on its potency, but based on *Psilocybe aztecorum*'s use as a cultural entheogen by the Indigenous peoples of the region, it is presumed to be moderately potent.[104]

PSILOCYBE BRASILIENSIS

As the name implies, this *Psilocybe* is native to Brazil. Though it was first documented in the late 1970s, this mushroom has not been the subject of significant scientific research. Because it has not been deeply or widely studied, it may have multiple habitats, local strains, or subspecies that have yet to be documented.[105] This speculation is based on the distribution of samples of these fungi that have been found and the dense, unexamined world of flora, fauna, and fungi that exist in many areas of Brazil.[106] Tryptamine testing results for this mushroom were not available as of this writing, but the mushroom produces very strong bluing when handled or bruised, indicating high psilocybin or psilocin content. It has a similar appearance to other little brown mushrooms from Mexico. It is important to note that there is a strain of *Psilocybe cubensis* that is named Brazilian; these are not the same mushrooms. The Brazilian mushroom that is sometimes consumed in North America is a strain of *P. cubensis*. It is not clear if that strain was developed from *P. cubensis* in Brazil, or if a professional cultivator or mycologist was able to develop a hybrid with *P. brasiliensis*. This mushroom should be relatively easy to cultivate from spores outside of its natural habitat if it is given the tropical conditions that help promote its growth in the wild. It is very hardy and colonizes easily.

PSILOCYBE CYANOFIBRILLOSA

This mushroom is found natively in the Pacific Coast region of the northwestern United States. It is distributed from Northern California into Washington State and parts of Western Canada. It favors estuaries and other areas that experience patterns of waters meeting waters, like streams of rivers flowing into each other, or rivers flowing into lakes or the ocean.[107] This mushroom hasn't been found to maintain its active tryptamine content when dried. When fresh, it is considered mild to moderately potent, with samples testing under 1% of total tryptamines, typically psilocybin (0.21%) and psilocin (0.06%).[108] Stamets reports that this mushroom has a tendency toward a strong bluing reaction, and while this is usually a sign of a moderately or highly potent psilocybin-producing mushroom, this species is the exception, not the rule.[109]

PSILOCYBE FIMETARIA

One of the original "fairy ring" mushrooms. This species has a wide distribution; it can be found in Great Britain, Scandinavia, Eastern Europe, the Pacific Northwest region of the United States, parts of Canada, and sometimes in South America. It tends to grow well in dung or areas where animals have recently left droppings. It is believed to be moderately potent, though I could not find any tests reporting the tryptamine content. Most psychedelic mushrooms of the little brown mushroom presentation are associated with Mexico or Central America. This one is primarily associated with Europe.[110] As always, little brown mushrooms deserve a word of caution. In the wild, it is easy to confuse the presentation of dangerous toxic mushrooms with psychedelic mushrooms. Mushrooms in the genus *Galerina* tend to closely resemble psychedelic mushrooms.[111] Be VERY careful. *Psilocybe fimetaria* has a reddish-brown cap and bluish-green tones in the stem. The spores of this mushroom resemble the spores of poisonous mushrooms. This has purple-brown spores, whereas the toxic imposters will be brown only. Use caution when foraging. Should you happen upon mushrooms in the wild, it is best to examine them with someone experienced, and always examine every individual specimen in your find, as different species will often fruit together.

PSILOCYBE HERRERAE

This rare fungus is another one of the little brown mushroom types found in Mexico. It is related to a small subspecies called *Psilocybe fagicola*.[112] These mushrooms are very delicate and have long, elegant stems. There are eight known mushroom species in this family. Most of these subtypes have what is called a pseudorhiza, a root-looking structure that distinguishes these mushrooms from other fungi in that the pseudorhiza pushes the immature mushroom up from beneath the ground to the soil surface. Upon examination, the pseudorhiza may look like roots from a plant rather than a mycelial structure. These structures allow the mushroom to participate more directly in the nutrient network of the trees associated with the substrate in which they grow. This structure has evolved independently several times.[113] This species is found only in two places in Mexico: Veracruz, and Chiapas. It will blue when handled, which may indicate psychedelic potency, but as this species has not been deeply examined, its actual strength as a psychedelic is unknown.

PSILOCYBE HOOGSHAGENII

This little brown mushroom was named after American anthropologist Searle Hoogshagen, who was instrumental in helping R. Gordon Wasson in his quest to find the mushrooms featured in the 1957 *Life* magazine article "Seeking the Magic Mushroom." This mushroom is moderately potent, containing both psilocybin (0.30–0.60%) and psilocin (0.10–0.30%). The cap is conical and looks like a fairy cap. The mushroom is a light brown color, and it is found only in Mexico. *P. hoogshagenii* will blue when handled or bruised. It is one of the most potent of the native fungi, though less intense than many of the cultivated strains. The Mixtec people indigenous to the region where it is found used several species of mushrooms in their ceremonies and rituals. There is some history of this mushroom having likely been misidentified as *P. zapotecorum* in the 1950s when Wasson and Roger Heim were cataloging the different psychedelic mushroom species in the region. It is not easily cultivated. Like most little brown mushrooms, it is easily confused with toxic species, so use caution.[114]

PSILOCYBE LINIFORMANS

This mushroom is found in different habitats around the world. There is a form that grows in the United States, and one that is found more frequently in Scandinavia and Eastern Europe. Specimens have also been reported in England and the Netherlands.[115] There have been some reports of this species found in South America as well. This *Psilocybe* is not frequently used as a psychedelic mushroom because of its low and/or inconsistent levels of tryptamines. When studied, the rates of various strains were different depending on whether the researchers tested European or American samples. In the European varieties, the rates of psilocybin were very low (0.16%). The psilocybin levels were a little higher in the American varieties (0.59–0.89%). Neither showed any psilocin. The stipe will sometimes bruise blue when handled.[116]

PSILOCYBE MAIREI

Almost all of Africa's countries are considered mycophobic, which means their population avoids mushrooms except under certain conditions (familiar species growing in familiar surroundings at specific times of year). This mushroom, *Psilocybe mairei*, is one of only a handful of species of mushroom that is well documented in North Africa.[117] There is now renewed interest in African mycology for multiple purposes, including the fact that edible mushrooms might offer people low-cost sources of protein that are available year-round. Medicinal mushrooms could also be cultivated to assist with health issues in remote areas. Ethnomycologists and food scientists point to a lack of folk knowledge regarding mushrooms as an ongoing problem, and there is an effort underway to promote better knowledge in both remote settlements and scientific communities in different African areas. The lack of knowledge may be due to changes in ecology, rapid culture change over the last 200 years, or other co-occurring factors. As such, there is not a robust understanding of mushrooms generally or psychedelic mushrooms in Africa specifically.[118]

There is some anthropological evidence that in earlier times, when the sands of the Sahara were verdant grasslands, there may have been some cultural practices around psychedelic mushrooms. Cave art in Algeria includes mushroom-shaped images protruding from the hands and body of a masked character, possibly a shaman. The cave art appears in Tassili n'Ajjer, a national park in the southeast region of Algeria, and researchers like the late Terence McKenna have proposed that the image depicts a practitioner of a mystical tradition that used psychedelic mushrooms in their practice.[119] Paul Stamets reported in his book *Psilocybin Mushrooms of the World* that the cave where the Tassili n'Ajjer "bee" man was depicted would have been an area rich with alluvial soil during the Neolithic period, which would make it ideal for the growth of psychedelic fungi.[120]

This mushroom blues when handled, especially the cap, and it tends to be found in soil that has significant mulch or woody debris. It is often conflated or confused with *Psilocybe serbica*. Indeed, there are some intense discussions online arguing that *P. mairei* is the same species. Mycologists appear to have settled that it is a separate species as of this writing.[121] There are no available reports on its tryptamine content. It can be found in Algeria and Morocco, and it is the only known bluing wild mushroom native to North Africa. An important caveat: there has not been enough scientific research into the different species of fungi native to Africa. Thus, the emphasis on "lack of known" species should focus on the "known" part.

PSILOCYBE OVOIDEOCYSTIDIATA

This mushroom is distributed along the East Coast of the United States, but it is particularly plentiful in the Ohio River Valley. It is typically found in woody substrates and wood chips. It is especially fond of areas where water ebbs and recedes. This mushroom is sun averse, preferring shady areas. There have been some descriptions of this mushroom appearing in the western United States, from California up to Washington. It is believed that mycologist Richard Gaines introduced the mushroom to the West Coast (Mandrake 2022). It has proliferated without much assistance. It has also recently been found in Europe. This mushroom will blue when handled or injured, implying psilocybin content, and it will turn bluish green as it ages. The caps have a distinctive ovoid shape, reflected in the name. It is very prolific and will fruit in abundant flushes. There are no testing results as of this writing, but the tendency to blue and the substrates it prefers implicates moderate potency.

PSILOCYBE PELLICULOSA

This mushroom's species name *pelliculosa* means "filmy" in Latin. These mushrooms grow in woody debris substrates, and they are one of the types of mushrooms that have been associated with wood lover's paralysis. The symptoms of wood lover's paralysis are well known and frightening, including full motor paralysis in some cases or partial paralysis in others. The symptoms typically pass within 24 hours. This mushroom is mildly potent, with samples testing positive for psilocybin (0.41%), and very low baeocystin (0.04%), but no psilocin (Stamets, 1996). This species is a very close relative to *Psilocybe silvatica*, with the only notable difference being the measured length of their spores. This species is found in the Pacific Northwest, ranging from Northern California to Western Canada. It blues at the base of the stem rather than the cap. This little brown mushroom tends to fruit in clustered flushes, and it is particularly easy to find in forest areas where there is new expansion due to felled trees or abandoned human development, like old homesteads or newly developed trails or roads.

PSILOCYBE QUEBECENSIS

This species is native to Eastern Canada and most notably found in Quebec. It has also been reported in Michigan and Cape Breton. This mushroom is tiny, and it grows in small flushes of one or two individuals, in woody debris or desiccated wood. It blues when bruised. It prefers sandy substrates and was first discovered in the Jacques Cartier River Valley in Quebec, a forested area where there is ample flowing water. A singular specimen was reported from Nova Scotia, though there is only one report. This *Psilocybe* is described as having been discovered at the highest latitude in North America (Stamets, 1996). This mushroom is considered mildly to moderately potent, though there are no clear testing results as of this writing due to its low distribution. It has not been the subject of much scientific or clinical inquiry. It is very tiny, and it may be more widely distributed than is currently known or observed. The small size of the fruiting bodies may make this variety difficult to spot, and it is not considered easy to cultivate.

PSILOCYBE SERBICA

This mushroom is a small, wood-loving mushroom with purplish-brown spores. Its cap tends toward a yellowish-red hue, and it will become darker in color as it ages. Its stipe is white with mottled bluish-green coloring. This mushroom is believed to be the same species as *Psilocybe bohemica*. Some samples of *Psilocybe serbica* contain high levels of psilocybin (as high as 1.3%), which makes it one of the most potent *Psilocybe* species in the world. Despite this finding, testing has also yielded disappointingly low levels (0.11%).[122] Samples gathered from the wild test at very different levels, indicating that tryptamine concentration is very likely dependent on the health of the substrate. The taxonomy of *P. serbica* and other apparently related species has been a topic of scholarly debate. As such, its taxonomy may eventually go through a reclassification process. Historically it has been included in the *P. cyanescens* family, but recent studies describe *P. serbica* as its own separate species.[123]

PSILOCYBE SILVATICA

A close relative of *Psilocybe pelliculosa*, with similar shape and coloring, *Psilocybe silvatica* tends to be more of an ochre color than its cousin, the dark mustard–colored *Psilocybe pelliculosa*.[124] The name *Psilocybe* comes from Latin and roughly translates as "bald." This refers to the fact that most *Psilocybe* mushrooms have a thin layer on their caps called a pellicle. In almost all of the *Psilocybe* genus, this pellicle is easy to peel off of the cap, leaving the head of the mushroom "bald." One of the features of this species is that the pellicle is not easily peeled off. This *Psilocybe* mushroom is most frequently found in the Pacific Northwest of the United States, though it has been sparsely reported in other forested areas like Michigan and New York,[125] hence the name *silvatica*, which means "of the forest" in Latin. It has little to no bluing on handling or bruising, though mild bluing is sometimes observed upon separating the stipe when the mushroom is collected.[126] This mushroom has been kept in the *Psilocybe* genus despite its apparently low production of psilocybin and psilocin content. A recent paper that examined several species of *Psilocybe* resulted in reordering the taxonomy slightly.[127] This subspecies was grouped with another low-psychoactive version called *Psilocybe medullosa*.

In the taxonomy study, *P. medullosa* and *P. silvatica* were kept in the *Psilocybe* genus but reorganized into a separate clade (a branch sharing a common ancestor) from the *Psilocybe* species that produces tryptamines easily. The researchers examined the genetic sequences and performed gas chromatography–mass spectrometry on these and three other species. Using these techniques, the researchers hypothesized that this clade may have an epigenetic reason for lowering or ceasing tryptamine production. (More research is required.) As might be expected from its low psilocybin and psilocin content, it is not very potent as a psychedelic.[128]

PSILOCYBE STRICTIPES

This mushroom grows wild in parts of the Pacific Northwest of the United States, and it is widely found across much of Europe, including France, Holland, Slovakia, Czechia, Sweden, and Germany. This species is usually found in rich, grassy landscapes. It is not coprophilic, so you won't find it on animal dung, though the presence of dung in grass will not impede the fruiting of this species. It doesn't blue when handled or bruised, implying low psilocin content. *Psilocybe strictipes* gets its name from the Latin words *stricti* (narrow) and *pes* (foot). It is easily mistaken for another little brown mushroom, the potent *Psilocybe semilanceata*. The best way to tell the two apart is that the *P. strictipes* lacks a papilla or umbo, whereas *P. semilanceata*, or Liberty Cap, has a clear circular demarcation at the top of its cap. Testing results were not available at the time of this writing, though Stamets believes this to be a potent mushroom due to its apparent relation to other *Psilocybe* mushrooms.[129]

PSILOCYBE SUBAERUGINOSA

Though this mushroom and *Psilocybe subaer-uginascens* have similar appearing names, they are not the same mushroom. This species is widely distributed in many parts of Australia, and it has another close relative, *Psilocybe cyanescens*.[130] Like its relative, *P. subaeruginosa* is a potent psilocybin producer. It is found only in the areas of Australia and Tasmania, and usually in forest areas, especially eucalyptus groves. Some mycologists believe that this species is actually a new introduction to the region, while others identify it as closely related to other mushrooms indigenous to the region like *Psilocybe australiana*, *Psilocybe eucalypta*, and *Psilocybe tasmaniana*.[131] The species name comes from the feminine Latin *aeruginosa*, and it is used to describe the green oxidation of copper that is similar in color to the bluing of these mushrooms when handled or injured. This mushroom has been described as moderate to strongly potent. The measured psilocybin (0.45–1.93%) content ranges from moderate to very high.[132]

PSILOCYBE SUBAERUGINASCENS

This species is found in parts of Japan and in Java in Indonesia; it has also been reported in South Africa.[133] It can vary in color from white to orange to gray green. This mushroom can be found in soil rich in rotting wood.[134] Sometimes fertilized wood chips act as a substrate. Like other *Psilocybe* mushrooms, this species can fruit in places where woods have been cleared, and it is common to find it on footpaths and roadsides. Considered moderately potent, this mushroom will blue when handled or injured. It generates purplish-brown spores. There were no reports on its potency as of this writing.

PSILOCYBE WASSONIORUM

This tiny mushroom blues easily when handled. Its cap can often take on a dark rusty-colored hue. It is distinguished by a long pseudorhiza. It was discovered near Veracruz, Mexico, and has not been found outside of that area. This mushroom prefers high elevations, and the fruiting bodies are likely to grow in small numbers. It is believed to be similar to related species native to the area. This mushroom is named after R. Gordon Wasson and his wife, Valentina Pavlovna Wasson, in honor of their work, which brought the potent "magic mushroom" to Western ethnomycological studies. As of this writing there are no published reports on its potency or the characteristics associated with ingesting it.[135]

PSILOCYBE YUNGENSIS

The *Psilocybe yungensis* mushroom's cap is conical or bell shaped and quite appealing to the eye. Like *P. silvatica*, this mushroom has a pellicle that doesn't peel from the mushroom's cap. *P. yungensis* grows in wood substrates, sometimes at the base of tree trunks.[136] It is a dark orange-ochre color, and it will age into a dark brown, with splits and frays in the cap. One of its distinguishing characteristics is that it tends to fruit in abundant flushes. It can be found in Mexico, Colombia, Ecuador, and Bolivia. It is believed to be moderately active, due to its tendency to bruise blue, and its proximity to related species in the area.[137]

Other Genera That Matter

CONOCYBE/PHOLIOTINA

This genus is in the midst of taxonomic changes. In some articles and texts, it is listed as *Conocybe*, and in others it is listed as *Pholiotina*. In this text, we will use the older description of *Conocybe* so that enthusiasts and researchers can easily find references. Though the newer *Pholiotina* designation is likely to persist, genetic tests and the resulting taxonomic and phylogenetic discussions will continue.[138] The genus *Conocybe* includes a mixture of psychedelic, inert, and poisonous mushrooms. The individual species in this genus share a long thin stipe and a conical cap. They grow in a variety of substrates from dung to rich soil filled with decayed wood. They look very similar to mushrooms in the *Galerina* genus. The psychedelic species in this genus will blue when handled, but only after a little time has passed. There are more than 240 species of *Conocybe* mushrooms; of these, only four have psychedelic properties: *C. kuehneriana*, *C. siligineoides*, *C. cyanopus*, and *C. smithii*. Some of these look identical to deadly *Galerina* mushrooms, so caution is advised.

CONOCYBE CYANOPUS

This delicate, caramel-colored mushroom is tiny but has a heavy concentration of tryptamines. Testing reveals a very strong presence of psilocybin (0.90%), lower percentages of other psychoactive substances like psilocin (0.17%) and baeocystin (0.16%), and small amounts of norbaeocystin (0.053%) and aeruginascin (0.011%).[139] This mushroom likes grassy substrates. It is found in many parts of the world, including North America and Northern and Central Europe. It will blue on the base of the stem when bruised, and it produces rusty-brown spores.[140]

CONOCYBE SMITHII

This mushroom is small and easily overlooked like its cousin, *Conocybe cyanopus*. This mushroom has an ochre cap that often becomes cinnamon colored as it ages, and it favors mossy and humid substrates. It will bruise blue when handled. It is almost identical in macroscopic appearance to *Conocybe cyanopus* and can only be differentiated microscopically. Like all little brown mushrooms, there are far too many toxic lookalikes, and thus caution is always advised where this mushroom is concerned. Eating wild mushrooms, especially small brown ones, is not advised.[141]

Poisonous Genera

There are more species of mushrooms that produce psychoactive compounds than just *Psilocybe*. Because so many of the other psychedelic mushrooms have more individual species that are dangerous, it is imperative to be able to distinguish the other mushrooms from the ones that are known for their psychedelic properties. Mushroom poisoning can be very dangerous, to the point that some species can be deadly after only one bite. Knowing a bit about the other genera of mushrooms can help you develop a healthy understanding of what to look for if and when you encounter mushrooms in the wild or mushrooms provided by someone you don't know. For example, there was a recent incident of mushroom foragers in France selling toxic mushrooms at the farmers market! Luckily, French food authorities check the local markets regularly and often test wild-collected mushrooms. In another case a woman served deadly mushrooms to several lunch guests in 2023 in rural Australia. Three people died from being served the Death Cap mushroom, *Amanita phalloides*.[142] If you want to really know mushrooms, you are best served by knowing more than just one type or species.

AMANITA

This genus of mushrooms has one of the most recognizable members in all of the mushroom species. The Fly Agaric, or *Amanita muscaria*, is one of the most iconic images of mushrooms. When concerts want to portray their sounds as "psychedelic" or when an artist wants to represent the fairy rings of Ireland or Great Britain, this mushroom—with its easily recognized white spots on a fleshy red cap—is *the* image of choice. It is quite striking to see these mushrooms in the wild. Their color bursts from the brown and green of the forest—the red and white color palette strikes the hiker or traveler. They are quite beautiful to look at, and they are hard to miss. If you see this mushroom in the forest or emblazoned on a T-shirt, you know immediately that it is a magic mushroom.

The iconic Fly Agaric is only one of many members of the genus *Amanita*. And while this species is not typically poisonous, there are many members of this genus that are highly toxic, and some are even deadly. You're far more likely to get a severe case of gastroenteritis or kidney problems from ingesting most *Amanita* mushrooms, however. While uncomfortable, the active compound that causes these symptoms (allenic norleucine) rarely causes fatal poisoning. Many *Amanita* genus mushrooms produce toxins called amatoxins and phallotoxins. These toxic substances are incredibly dangerous. They can interrupt RNA replication or destroy the lining of the intestinal tract. Some of these toxins attack the liver, which can lead to death. One of the most challenging aspects of mushroom poisoning is that it can sometimes take up to 24 hours before the person who ate them becomes symptomatic. By this time, most people don't realize that the mushrooms are the culprit in their illness.[143]

The dangerous *Amanita* species include the Death Cap mushroom (*Amanita phalloides*). This mushroom looks innocuous enough; indeed, it can appear downright appetizing.[144] There are many harmless lookalikes that fool even the most experienced foragers. But the Death Cap is one of the most lethal of all mushrooms. At first, the typical Death Cap poisoning looks like a case of food poisoning. The patient will find themself with cold sweats and nausea that leads to vomiting and diarrhea. The heart is sometimes weakened, especially in patients who already have heart problems. As the poison continues to affect the body, the liver and kidneys begin to shut down. In recent years there have been fewer deaths, but the risk is very real. Lives have been saved through liver transplants, demonstrating the seriousness of the poisoning. Another deadly *Amanita* mushroom is called the Destroying Angel (*Amanita virosa*), with similar symptomatology after ingestion. Both of these *Amanita* species have an ovoid whitish-yellow cap and white gills. They grow in wooded areas. The Destroying Angel smells rather unpleasant, while the Death Cap smells slightly of roses.[145]

FLY AGARIC: *AMANITA MUSCARIA*

Despite its role as the iconic psychedelic mushroom, this species doesn't contain the same profile of tryptamines—psilocybin, psilocin, and baeocystin—found in the other psychedelic species highlighted here. Amyloid tryptamines have similar structures to the neurotransmitter serotonin, and thus have the potential to interact directly with the body's central nervous system. The psychoactive compounds in the Fly Agaric mushroom are completely different. The active components in this mushroom are ibotenic acid and muscimol.[146] These compounds tend to cause central nervous system depressive or excitatory effects, dependent on the individual's brain chemistry. They can include delirium, agitation, hallucinations, and occasionally seizures.[147]

This mushroom derives its name from the fact that historically it was used as an insect repellent. The Latin species name, *muscaria*, means "fly." In the common name, Fly Agaric, it's obvious. Ibotenic acid in particular is both attractive and a dangerous poison to insects, so it makes an ideal insecticide. People used to cut this mushroom into small pieces and soak them in a small pan of water or milk.[148] The active compounds dissolve into the water or milk; when insects ingest the toxins, they get confused and drown, or they die. There are also stories of reindeer eating these mushrooms and looking drunk; maybe that is the source of the stories of Santa Claus's flying reindeer![149]

A. muscaria is not considered a "true" psychedelic mushroom; however, the ibotenic acid and muscimol found in this species do act in ways that are similar to traditional tryptamines. Ibotenic acid is an NMDA receptor agonist, which means that it will encourage the uptake of glutamate in the central nervous system. Meanwhile, muscimol is structurally similar to the neurotransmitter GABA, which is the antagonist of glutamate in the central nervous system. Muscimol acts as a GABA inhibitor in the central nervous system. Agonists will encourage neurotransmitters to engage receptors, while antagonists will inhibit receptors, allowing more of the internally produced neurotransmitters to be paired up with the receptors.[150]

GALERINA

An important directive in this book is "Beware the little brown mushroom!" That is because while a great many of the *Psilocybe* species are tiny or small brown mushrooms, there is an entire genus of little brown mushrooms of which many are toxic: *Galerina*.[151] The most conclusive way of distinguishing between *Psilocybe* and *Galerina* mushrooms is the color of the spores. *Psilocybe* spore prints will be some hue of purple. They may have a purple-black hue, a purplish-brown hue, or even a light purple or lavender tone. But *Galerina* mushrooms will almost always have a rust or brown spore print.[152] There is one rare and novel member of the species that bruises blue and does produce psilocybin: *Galerina steglichii*. But this species is exceedingly rare and unlikely to be encountered outside of the place where it was discovered in Germany.[153] The majority of *Psilocybe* mushrooms will bruise blue when handled or injured, while all but one *Galerina* will not. Don't touch little brown mushrooms with your bare hands to test for bluing reactions. Wear gloves to protect yourself from toxins and to protect specimens from contaminants.

Galerina and Psilocybe often grow together. As a result, if you are gathering wild mushrooms, it is critical that you examine each specimen individually, examining spores and overall morphology. Just because the mushrooms look like they are all from the same flush doesn't mean that they are the same species. Galerina marginata is frequently mistaken for Psilocybe cyanescens by mushroom foragers. This Galerina species, which is also known as Autumn Skullcap, or Deadly Galerina, is a poisonous mushroom found in temperate regions around the world, including Europe and parts of the United States. It is fond of rotting wood and can be found in multiple types of habitats, from forests and woodlands to suburban parks or urban trails.[154]

But don't limit yourself to the Galerina covered in this book. Wherever you find rotting wood you can encounter Galerina.[155] Always beware the little brown mushroom! It cannot be overstated how critical it is to be careful of these little brown mushrooms. A Galerina sulcipes found in Indonesia was recently reported to be responsible for several deaths. It has been reported to be more toxic than Amanita phalloides, the infamous Death Cap mushroom.[156] Many Galerina mushrooms contain amatoxins, which can cause dangerous symptoms that include kidney and liver failure after an unpleasant bout of gastroenteritis.

GYMNOPILUS

A yellow stem or stipe is one of the common characteristics of the genus Gymnopilus, which has more than 200 colorful species. A handful of species in this genus produce psilocybin, baeocystin, or other tryptamines, including G. aeruginosis, G. braendlei, G. junonius, G. liquiritiae, G. luteofolius, G. luteoviridis, G. luteus, G. purpuratus, G. validipes, and G. viridans. This genus is distinguished by its red-orange color and its orangey-rust-colored spores.[157] Because of the presence of psilocybin, many of these mushrooms will develop a dark blue to green hue when injured or handled. Though these mushrooms may contain amyloid tryptamines, several also contain other toxins that render them poisonous. These include G. junonius and G. spectabilis. The poisonous G. spectabilis is distinguished by its larger size and its tendency to be found on conifer trees. It has a cap that is striking, ranging in color from yellow to yellow-orange to a deep orange. It has yellow gills with orange spores (Strauss et al., 2022). If you come across an orange mushroom or one with orange or rust-colored spores, it is best to leave it alone.

INOCYBE

There are a handful of psilocybin-producing Inocybe mushrooms, but there are also several poisonous species in the genus. The genus is characterized by mycorrhiza that interact in a symbiotic relationship with local plant life. There are more than 1,000 species of Inocybe mushrooms. The Inocybe that contain psychedelic tryptamines include I. aeruginascens, I. coelestium, I. corydalina, and I. tricolor.[158] Notably, however, these mushrooms don't contain a great deal of active psychedelic tryptamines. Most are found in Europe, and some are also found in the northern United States. Their mycorrhizal morphology lends itself to aggregation in wooded areas like forests.

The poisonous members of this genus (*I. fastigiata, I. geophyllia, I. lacera, I. pudica, I. decipiens, I. napipes*) act primarily by muscarine poisoning. The concentration of muscarine in these mushrooms can be as high as 1.0% in some cases. This toxic alkaloid interrupts the processing of the excitatory neurotransmitter acetylcholine. Historically, muscarine poisoning could lead to death, but with contemporary medicine it is often treated successfully with atropine. One of the reasons that treatment is often successful is that the symptoms tend to come on quickly, within two hours of ingestion, giving people time to get to the hospital.[159]

Symptoms of muscarine poisoning include vomiting, gastroenteritis, sweating, crying, and bradycardia (slowing of the heartbeat). Patients may also experience coldness in the extremities and a tendency toward fainting or loss of consciousness (syncope). Muscarine ingestion is very serious and must be treated medically.[160] It will not resolve on its own without medical intervention. It can cause hallucinations through its action on the central and peripheral nervous systems. Though these may appear to be similar to the hallucinations experienced with other psilocybin mushrooms, these should not be mistaken for a typical psychedelic experience. If accompanied by these other symptoms, immediate hospitalization is required. Muscarine compounds are very powerful. Recent research indicates that muscarine may promote the expansion of cancer cells in colon and bile duct cancers.[161] Because the *Inocybe* genus mushrooms create so many negative outcomes by working on the acetylcholine channels in the central and peripheral nervous systems, they should be considered very dangerous.

PHOLIOTINA

The capacity to study DNA of different families of fungi is changing taxonomic classifications. New techniques enable species to be reclassified based on their DNA results and their relationship to other species, based on the sequences and placement of DNA sequences. This genus is branched off of the genus *Pholiota*.[162] Because of the dynamic nature of reclassifying the members of fungi species, several members of this species were previously classified in the genus *Conocybe*.

There is a critically notable member of this species called *Pholiotina filaris*. In some guides it will appear as *Conocybe filaris*. These are the same mushroom, and this individual species is highly toxic.[163] It is critical that anyone who wishes to learn how to identify wild *Psilocybe* mushrooms learn to distinguish this individual species. This mushroom sports a yellow to brown cap and rusty-brown spores. It contains phallotoxins and amatoxins on par with the Death Cap, *Amanita phalloides*, and *Galerina autumnalis* mentioned previously. Stamets found this species growing near psychedelic mushrooms like *Psilocybe baeocystis*, *Psilocybe cyanescens*, *Psilocybe pelliculosa*, and *Psilocybe stuntzii*.[164] Knowing that this dangerous species favors similar environments to *Psilocybe* species means that developing skills of observation and discernment are paramount.

�֍

As you no doubt have noticed by examining many of the varieties of mushrooms that contain psilocybin and related psychedelic tryptamines like baeocystin and psilocin (and maybe some that haven't been isolated as yet), there is a diverse array of fungi that can be used for medicinal and psychedelic purposes. These species vary in their properties and often in their appearance. However, mushrooms that exhibit toxic possibilities can be very similar visually to those that provide psychedelic experiences. The benefits of psychedelic mushrooms are many, from the deep psychospiritual experiences we have examined to cutting-edge medical treatments. The next chapter goes into detail about the latest developments in research. The world of psychedelics is changing. With research into treatments that expand from addressing depression to relief for chronic pain, psychedelics are opening a new frontier in medicine, health, and wellness.

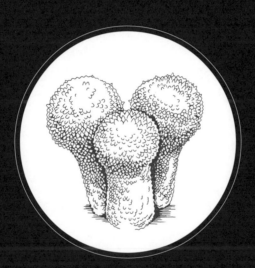

FUZZY BALLS

Look deep into nature and you will understand everything better.

—ALBERT EINSTEIN

CHAPTER 7

Medicinal Uses for Mushrooms

﹏﹏﹏﹏﹏﹏﹏﹏﹏﹏﹏﹏﹏﹏﹏﹏﹏﹏﹏

The nervous system is made up of neurons. Depending on where in the body these neurons are organized, they are considered part of different systems and subsystems. The central nervous system includes the neurons that make up the brain and spinal cord. The peripheral nervous system is composed of the neurons that extend from the central nervous system to the extensive innervated areas of the body. On a smaller scale, neurons are organized in the central nervous system and brain into important structures, and these structures are often organized into network systems.

Neurons aren't generic. Though they are flexible, they produce different neurochemicals, and individual neurons act in unique ways. In combination they may also act in different ways. It is kind of like when you get one sound from one musical instrument, but when you add a second and third instrument, the sound changes entirely. Neurons working in concert with one another are similar. Neurotransmitters are chemical compounds produced in the neuron and active in the neuron's synapses. The type of neurotransmitter tells the neuron what to do. But not all neurons produce equal amounts or types of a given neurotransmitter, and not every synapse can process every neurotransmitter. All neurons have receptors for specific neurotransmitters like serotonin, acetylcholine, and dopamine, to name just a few. Generally speaking, a neuron can produce only one type of neurotransmitter, but it can receive and use more than one.

We have already discussed the mechanisms of action for psilocybin. The way psilocybin works in the body is based on its likeness to serotonin. There are many variations of receptors for the serotonin molecule in the nervous system. Serotonin's chemical name is 5-hydroxytryptamine, abbreviated to 5-HTA. The receptors for this molecule are often referred to as 5-HTA receptors. They have different subgroups like 5-HT1A or 5-HT2A receptors. Sometimes an R is put on the end of the abbreviation to denote that the scientist is discussing the receptor.

The relationship between neurons and the neurotransmitters is critical for the body to function properly. When the body lacks sufficient types of a particular neurotransmitter, or if areas of the brain or body are damaged or struggling to process them, different disease processes can result. Whether there is too much of a particular neurotransmitter or a deficit, the nervous system will respond. Sometimes these experiences are overwhelming, and in other cases they are relatively minor. For example, we know that in some disorders like schizophrenia there is too much dopamine in the nervous system. The body cannot process the dopamine properly, and this overabundance is partially responsible for the symptoms we see in people who suffer from this debilitating disease.

Serotonin is implicated in many different mental health diagnoses, but more important, it is necessary for everyday functioning of the nervous system and gastrointestinal system. As a result, your brain and body have an abundance of neurons that have receptors for serotonin. Your brain, your gut, and your heart are the most common areas that use serotonin. Psilocybin and other related tryptamines are molecularly similar to serotonin, and therefore the body can process psilocybin and make it available in the nervous system almost immediately.

Mechanisms of Depression

There are several theories about how depression happens in the brain and body. In the last decade new theories about depression have been discussed at academic conferences and published in prestigious medical journals.

From discussions of the gut-brain axis[1] to the Research Domain Criteria framework,[2] which suggests that we rethink diagnoses altogether, the most common finding of psychiatrists, neuroscientists, and psychologists is that depression is an outcome, not a cause in and of itself. The experience of depression is often oversimplified. Those who have never suffered from a depressive episode think that depression is the same as being "sad" or "down." But depression begins with a cascade of possible causes and neurological feedback system activities, and it usually ends with easily recognizable symptoms like memory loss and the tendency to isolate from others, which is sometimes called social withdrawal. The symptoms of depression can also be more sophisticated, like anhedonia, the inability to feel pleasure, and can include problems of appetite and satiety that cause weight loss or gain.

We have discussed how the similarity of psilocybin and serotonin affects some brain structures, but in order to have a fuller understanding of the ways that psilocybin works on the brain, it is helpful to have a slightly more robust understanding of the current research into the neuroscience of depression, anxiety, and other disorders. This will help us understand why there is so much excitement in the addition of psilocybin to the pharmacological toolbox.

DEPRESSION AND ANXIETY

Chapter 2 includes a section on recent research into ways that psilocybin is being investigated to help treat various forms of depression. This section won't recap on that, but instead add to an understanding of how psilocybin is being investigated to treat depression, anxiety, and related disorders like postpartum depression. Before we continue, however, it should be noted that today many mental health practitioners categorize depression and anxiety similarly. Though the experiences of each feel different, medications to treat depression sometimes help alleviate anxiety, and vice versa. As such, there is a widespread opinion that there is a similar or related mechanism in the brain that causes different responses to the same brain activity or neural stimuli. What might initiate a depressive episode for me might create an anxious response in someone else, based on each individual's unique neural chemistry.

NEUROTRANSMITTER THEORY

This leads to one of the oldest and most common theories of depression and anxiety found in psychological and psychiatric research. It is also one of the most relevant for our discussion of how psilocybin can have an impact on treatment. For our purposes, we will call this the neurotransmitter theory.[3] In the last two decades, doctors have noticed that selective serotonin reuptake inhibitors (SSRIs) like Paxil and Lexapro help people who are suffering from both anxiety and depression. The implication of serotonin in both disorders is helping scientists to make sense of how psilocybin and other serotonergic substances might help develop new treatments for people suffering from anxiety and depression.[4] There are multiple serotonin-receptor-rich areas of the brain. Problems with regulating serotonin are connected to several disorders, including everything from anxiety and depression to Alzheimer's disease, sudden infant death syndrome, and restless leg syndrome.

Even before picking up this book, you may have heard of some of the brain structures that use serotonin, like the amygdala, hippocampus, and hypothalamus. Others may be less well known to you, like the raphe nuclei (where the majority of brain-produced serotonin is made), the nucleus accumbens, the ventral tegmental area, and the corpus callosum. In the neurotransmitter theory of depression, all of these (plus a few other areas) are affected by either not having enough serotonin or having too much.

An important caveat is that the neurotransmitter balance in the brain is not *only* serotonergic. That is, serotonin is not the only important neurotransmitter. In fact, one of the key things to remember when reading this section is that neurotransmitters and neural proteins like brain-derived neurotrophic factor (BDNF) will often stimulate the production and release of other neurotransmitters.[5] So, when there is a rise in serotonin there may also be an increase (or decrease) in BDNF or dopamine, depending on what part of the brain is being stimulated and by which neurotransmitter. I often talk about this kind of downstream action with my clients in terms of a shopping list. If you primarily eat cereal for breakfast, then your consumption and restocking habits are not linked to just the cereal. Few adults eat their Cheerios without milk. Some of us like to add strawberries and bananas as well. So, when you're restocking your cereal, you're probably also checking and possibly adding the downstream elements of milk, strawberries, and bananas to round out your shopping list. Your brain produces serotonin separately, but when it's being used it may cascade with or initiate other neurotransmitters, proteins, and hormones as a result.

Researchers studying the effects of psilocybin and other tryptamines have described impacts on the neurotransmitter system beyond serotonin, with glutamate, BDNF, and dopamine often entering the discussions of psilocybin's activity in the brain. What is critically important to take away from this discussion is the knowledge that all these different neurotransmitters will have an effect on mood, and they may even help to reset certain network systems in the brain.[6]

There are seven primary network systems in the brain: the sensorimotor system, the visual system, the limbic system, the central executive network (CEN), the default mode network (DMN), the salience network, and the dorsal attention network (DAN). While these networks are responsible for some functions independently of one another, the vast majority of brain activity is composed of inter-network connections and communications.[7]

The sensory motor system is responsible for processing and making sense of internal and external stimuli, and then responding to it. The visual system is self-explanatory: it takes in visual stimuli and then makes sense of and contextualizes what we see. The limbic system is responsible for multiple diverse activities in the brain, including emotion, memory, sex drive, hunger, and social behavior. The CEN is responsible for complex problem solving, logic, attentional control, cognition, inhibition, and goal-directed behaviors. We have spent a lot of time discussing the DMN, but to briefly summarize here, the DMN is responsible for self-referential thoughts and behavior. The salience network helps separate threats from friendly behavior. It attenuates, processes, and contextualizes information and helps prioritize responses. The DAN can be thought of as an extension of some or all of these systems. It helps maintain focus on important stimuli, and it assists in goal orientation and cognitive control. All of these networks work in concert with one another to help individuals make sense of and operate in the world.[8]

By now I'm sure you're starting to see why this area of research is so complex! Psychedelics have the potential to impact multiple networks as well as the integration and cooperation of those networks with one another. One of the most important findings of the last 20 years has been the discovery of the DMN, as was discussed in chapter 2. Research into the effects of psilocybin in this critical network area by Robin Carhart-Harris and his research teams at UCSF and Imperial College London have demonstrated that psilocybin reduces the activity of the DMN and may actually reset it.[9] All of the brain's networks are affected when someone is working with psilocybin. How they're impacted depends on context and on each individual's unique neurobiology.

CHRONIC STRESS THEORY

One of the ways that depression may occur is as a consequence of prolonged or chronic stress. Scientists have examined the brains and bodies of people who have been exposed to prolonged periods of stress via early childhood trauma, combat, or chronic health problems, and they have found that these folks often share a common set of biomarkers: increased inflammation, hypersecretion of cortisol, and often enlarged adrenal glands. These biological indicators are often described as complex problems of the hypothalamic-pituitary-adrenal (HPA) axis.[10] The HPA axis is responsible for helping to mediate activities of several related systems in the body; this includes everything from metabolism to immune response and heart rate.

Constant exposure to stress and dysregulation of the HPA axis often results in both neurochemical and structural complications. When the HPA axis is overstimulated, a person may have substantial difficulty regulating their emotions. This can be caused by the brain and central nervous system being flooded with cortisol. Researchers have also found that people who suffer chronic stress have reductions in volume of critical brain areas or network connections.[11] Sometimes prolonged stress can lead to neurodegeneration, meaning that neurons lose their capabilities. One neuron losing some function isn't that serious; the brain is by and large a redundant organ, meaning that some functions in the brain can move into new areas in case of injury or illness. But systemic interruption or depletion of synaptic activity, axonic growth, or neuronal activation will quickly show up as impaired brain function.[12]

Chronic stress has been shown to reduce the brain volume in areas of the brain critical to executive and emotional functions. The medial prefrontal cortex (mPFC) is necessary for proper executive functioning and the ability to regulate emotion. The seahorse-shaped hippocampus is necessary for learning and memory. Finally, the amygdala is implicated in emotional regulation, rumination, and threat detection. If neurogenesis is slowed down under constant stress, that means that the person suffering from stress has a more difficult time making sense of their experience and regulating their emotions around it. They genuinely lack the brain capacity.

When a person endures chronic stress, these areas of the brain sometimes atrophy or lose cortical volume. This is an evolutionary advantage. An organism that is constantly living under threat doesn't have the resources to dedicate to anything other than survival. As a result, resources are used to shore up defenses and ensure that a person's threat-detection system is the primary one getting the internal investments. Specifically, the complexity and density of neurons in these areas will sometimes reorganize their functions to remain in a state of vigilance. The neurons that help regulate emotions may be sacrificed in order for the neurons responsible for being attentive to threats to remain active. As a result, the brain's ability to process negative emotions or putative threats is elevated, as we see in people with post-traumatic stress disorder (PTSD). Soon, everything is a threat, because the neural systems that might have helped discern between threat and nonthreat are no longer operating properly.[13]

Psilocybin and other psychedelics have been shown in laboratory experiments to stimulate neurogenesis.[14] These substances assist the brain's own natural functions for developing new neurons, as well as neural structures like axons and synapses, in existing neurons. By initiating neurogenesis, psilocybin and other substances like DMT may be the key to healing complex disorders like treatment-resistant depression and PTSD, where brain volume has been diminished.

The activation of neurogenesis has multiple possible benefits. First, it communicates across the systems and subsystems of the central nervous system to make it clear that there is a window of nonthreat. This opportunity to relax, reflect, and take stock allows the brain to reduce its hypervigilance. In addition, and more important, neurogenesis literally gives the person new neurons to help rebuild the structures that can affect their psychological healing.

THE GUT-BRAIN AXIS

There has been a great deal of public interest in the relationship between the biology of the helpful bacteria in the gut—also known as the microbiome—and psychological well-being. Our understanding of the importance of the gut microbiome deepened profoundly in the last decade, as scientists studied the relationship between these bacteria and the human host's dependence on them for digestion, immunity, and mood. Meanwhile, we've recognized only in the last 20 years that the majority (95%) of the serotonin produced in the body is created not in the brain, but in the intestines. Besides being a critical molecule for brain health, serotonin is also necessary for the proper functioning of the intestinal tract, and there is ongoing research into the role of serotonin in satiety and hunger in both the gut and the brain.[15]

The connection between the microbiome and the brain is sometimes referred to as the gut-brain axis. Researchers into the relationship between the brain and the gut-brain axis have learned that bacteria in the gut promote the biosynthesis of serotonin. Serotonin impacts multiple physiological processes outside of the brain. In the gut, serotonin helps to manage the motility of the gastrointestinal tract. In blood serum, serotonin helps modulate immune response and platelet function, and it helps repair valves in the heart. In laboratory experiments, researchers have observed that gut bacteria produce enzymes that increase or decrease the serotonin levels in the gut biome. While there has been no research

into the impact of psilocybin on the gut-brain axis, there is a distinct possibility that psilocybin may have a similar effect there as it has in other serotonergic systems.[16]

One of the biggest concerns for patients taking antipsychotic medications is weight gain. It is not at all uncommon for people to gain a significant amount of weight within the first six weeks of taking medicines like olanzapine, clozapine, and risperidone. The weight gain is associated with the medications' actions at the 5-HT2A and 5-HT2CA receptors. In addition, these drugs have an impact on dopamine receptors. Depending on the patient's personal neurochemistry, the person prescribed these medications may always feel hungry, or their body may process sugars more efficiently, storing more of the sugars they take in as fat. There hasn't yet been enough research to understand the mechanisms at work. But we know that there is a clear correlation between serotonergic antipsychotic medications and the patients who take them experiencing significant weight gain.[17]

Regardless of whether the increase in serotonin results in more hunger or in a change in physiological process, patients who are prescribed these medications often stop taking them. In clinical jargon, this is called being medically noncompliant. Weight gain is one of the biggest reasons clients become medically noncompliant. Research into the ways that psilocybin affects these systems without causing weight gain would be a welcome transformation in the use of antipsychotic medications.

NETWORK DYSFUNCTION AND PSYCHOSTRUCTURAL CHANGES

Researchers who investigate ways that psilocybin can make positive impacts on depression are careful to make sure that we don't focus solely on biology and ignore psychology. If you have heard about the positive impacts of psilocybin on people struggling with PTSD or other chronic psychological problems, it is important to understand that the psychology and neurobiology at play are complex and deeply intertwined.

Psychology is often misrepresented as a soft science. This conceptualization is based on the fact that the brain and how it responds to stimuli is profoundly heterogeneous. No two brains operate in precisely the same way. The organ is too complex, and its structure too flexible, for there to be a 1:1 correlation between form and function. Despite this distinction, psychology has successfully identified ways that this complex organ sometimes exhibits symptoms or disease. It is best to think of neuroscience and psychology as two sciences that interact with one another to best describe the form, function, and mystery of the psyche.

Psychiatry and psychology began about 200 years ago as the study of the intersection of physiology and consciousness. At the time, science was in an early and decisively materialist stage. Mendelian inheritance, the precursor to modern genetics, was discovered in the 1820s, at the same time that psychology was first given a name. The structure of the double helix of DNA wouldn't be discovered until more than 100 years later, in 1953. The brain was considered a dense bundle of neurons, and though there was some basic understanding of the brain's function, its form and structures were not understood at all. The development of psychology as a discipline, by Wilhelm Wundt and William James, included the examination of everything from brain morphology to psychic powers. Because it had

become a catch-all for what was not understood in the human condition, many people treated psychology like a pseudoscience (and some still do).[18]

Psychological processes change more than *what* we think and feel. Trauma (and treatment) changes *how* the brain functions because it impacts the actual structure of the brain itself. When a traumatic event happens, the brain marshals the necessary resources for the defense of the organism. The frontal lobes, which are the parts of the brain needed for rational thought, are not important during defense-of-life actions, and so the connection to them is temporarily and significantly reduced. Instead, resources are sent to the parts of the body and brain necessary to save the life of the organism: the amygdala, the heart, the gut, the limbic system, and, to a lesser degree, the hippocampus.[19]

Constant trauma, or never processing trauma (and thus making it feel constant), keeps the brain in the mode of vigilant response. As noted earlier in the section on the HPA axis, this means that the parts of the brain necessary for more advanced or nuanced thought and action don't get resources. Any structure that doesn't get resources to keep it strong and whole will either atrophy or eventually die. That means that both the structures and connections may become compromised over time with exposure to traumatic or stressful stimuli.

So why do we care about psilocybin's role in all of this? If psilocybin can help regulate, promote, and facilitate the development of new neurons and the release of neurochemicals and neurotransmitters, and generally provide a bridge between the content of psychological processing and the structures that process the content, then it is a potential miracle substance. Thanks to ongoing neuroscience research we know that the structures of the brain are discrete and networked *and* that they can create redundancies when they have the capacity and time to do so. We also know that psychological and emotional trauma (and treatments) affect both the structure and function of the brain.[20]

As discussed in a previous chapter on psilocybin research and depression, it appears that psilocybin activates the brain and its pathways by helping people have a greater capacity for feeling. The standard treatment for depression and anxiety for the last 30 years has been SSRIs. In comparing the effects of SSRIs with those of psilocybin, the two seem to work in opposite ways. The SSRI acts to decrease the capacity for feeling, blunting both sadness and joy. This means that there is less of either type of emotion. By contrast, psilocybin appears to act to expand the range of capacity for feeling. Therapy assists in this process by expanding the capacity to allow and make sense of more extreme feeling, rather than blunting it entirely.[21]

It is important to note that this and other theories are not necessarily in competition with one another. Scientists don't know whether the mechanisms that produce depression are based on an integrated system that ultimately comes apart if you start having too many deficits, or if genetic or structural deficits in the system create the symptoms. The likely answer is that depression, as an outcome, has a multifactorial etiology. I would liken it to how systems in your car are interconnected. You wouldn't think that the alternator that keeps your car's battery charged would affect your air-conditioner, but if the alternator is

going out, you might first discover it by finding yourself getting uncomfortable in your car. In many cars there is a shaft in the alternator that powers the AC. When this mechanism stops working, multiple systems are affected, not only those that are the most obvious.

One final important note about the brain: there is a connection between autoimmunity and trauma. Poor communication between the brain and the thymus, which regulates immune response, will impact the body's ability to fight off disease.[22] This means that people who suffer from trauma or chronic stress are more likely to struggle with immune system disorders. It is a sad but predictable observation that people who have been exposed to prolonged trauma or stress are the most likely to develop disorders like fibromyalgia, rheumatoid arthritis, and other autoimmune diseases. There also appears to be a connection to diseases like cancer that flourish when the immune system is compromised. Restoring balance in the brain may help more than just your thought processes. Restoring balance to the brain can bring equilibrium to several other systems that are critical to life itself.[23]

Postpartum Depression

The experience of postpartum depression (PPD) is more common than it is discussed. For most women, the shift in hormones after birth facilitates a profound shift in mood. Sometimes this is pleasant, with mother and child bonding thanks to the assistance of big releases of a neurohormone called oxytocin. In other circumstances, this period is punctuated by mild depressive symptoms sometimes referred to as the "baby blues," which are caused by an imbalance in neural chemistry after exhausting the physical resources necessary for a successful birth. But PPD is more than a mild downward shift for many of the women who experience it. Postpartum depression can easily transition to psychotic depression and/or treatment-resistant depression (TRD).

The research into PPD is significantly lacking, especially when compared to other forms of depression and mental health conditions. The presentation of PPD may look similar to TRD or unipolar depression (once called major depressive disorder), but it has both a unique potential etiology (or etiologies) and unique dependencies and downstream psychosocial complications. The well-being of a newborn and older children and other dependents may be at risk when the primary caregiver cannot function. When I began the research for this book, I found three studies that proposed using psilocybin for PPD. As of this writing, those three proposed studies have not published any findings. Indeed, they may not be moving forward at all, as there are no updates on ClinicalTrials.gov.

I felt, though, that ignoring this unique area of psychological care was not in the best interest of my research. I have treated several women with PPD, including one whose postpartum depressive episode led to a particularly challenging case of TRD. One of the most frustrating aspects of providing psychological care to people who suffer from PPD is that obstetricians don't have adequate training in treating this frequent consequence of pregnancy. Obstetricians rely on psychiatrists, and psychiatrists either refer clients back to their OB/GYN or they treat PPD like a standard case of depression or TRD. There is desperate need for us all to do better. The long-term consequences and complications for both the women who suffer and their families are not insignificant. Women who suffer from PPD often report that they have little to no interest in caring for their children, or worse, they feel resentful toward their children. As a result, the children of a parent with PPD can suffer with their own negative consequences that may be life-long.

Epidemiologists estimate that 10–20% of pregnant people experience perinatal depression (depression around the time of birth, encompassing the weeks both right before and immediately after).[24] What's more, other risk factors for depression including but not limited to low income, previous mental health diagnoses, and intimate partner violence predispose women to experiencing PPD. The scant research that separates PPD from TRD shows some significant differences. In TRD the amygdala is activated, while in PPD it is blunted.[25]

Researcher Bochao Cheng led a study across multiple institutions that examined a large sample of women and compared brain images of postpartum women who had been diagnosed with either postpartum depression or postpartum anxiety against women who had no postpartum complications.[26] They found that the women who suffered from postpartum depression or anxiety had functional differences in the ways their brains worked. Specifically, the women who struggled with postpartum depression or postpartum anxiety had connectivity problems. Cheng and his colleagues found that these women had deficits in the areas of their brains that are necessary for the network connections between the hippocampus and the prefrontal cortex to work properly.

In their article in the *Journal of Psychopharmacology*, "Postpartum Depression: A Role for Psychedelics?" researchers Chaitra Jairaj and James Rucker wrote that there is likely a significant role for the administration of psychedelics for PPD.[27] They point to the possibility of resetting the default mode network (DMN) and changes in the amygdala as having the potential to make state changes in people suffering from PPD. They cite the low dependence risk and the low likelihood of transmission of psilocybin in breast milk as possible encouraging factors, and they cautiously offer that we need more research into these areas to determine if psilocybin is safe for women who have just given birth or may be breastfeeding.

One of my patients has been on a psychedelic regimen for several years, and it has been one of the few things that has helped her recover any function. Prior to the introduction of psychedelics—in her case, ketamine—she struggled with what most of us would consider the minimum requirements of life: getting out of bed, eating, spending time with her children. Since the introduction of psychedelics, she still suffers from TRD, but we have new tools in the toolbox. Some days she can get out of bed, make breakfast, and get the kids to school. Other days she can do that and do highly demanding financial work. And still there are days where she can do none of those things, but she can regulate her emotions enough to know that she needs to rest. Before psychedelics it wasn't possible for her to get dressed in the morning. She couldn't tolerate any negative emotion, and she would have days filled with hours of tearful episodes or

dissociation. I truly believe that ketamine saved her life and thus saved her children and family from a devastating loss that would have marked the rest of their lives. As hopeful as the research into psychedelics is, we need more tools to help this specific population. Perhaps this book will help inspire a neuroscientist, obstetrician, gynecologist, psychiatrist, or psychopharmacologist (or a combination!) to consider new research for treating PPD patients.

Post-Traumatic Stress Disorder

It wasn't until the 1980s that the medical profession named the concurrence of symptoms we now call post-traumatic stress disorder or PTSD. Before this the disorder was sometimes called "shell shock" based on the experience of soldiers in World War I. The soldiers who returned home from that conflict had seen and experienced traumas that they were unprepared for. Some of this was due to the sheer scale of the destruction they witnessed, but the introduction of deadly and efficient weapons of war created profound psychological problems for many soldiers. During and after World War II the term was refreshed. Soldiers were reported to suffer from "combat fatigue." After the Vietnam War it was given yet another name, post-Vietnam syndrome. After each conflict, there seemed to be a deeper and more profound set of symptoms and the experience was renamed. To complicate matters, these effects were considered the domain of soldiers alone. Sexual trauma survivors, those who had grown up dealing with systematic abuse, refugees, and others were not included in this group because the original term dealt only with those who had served in combat. We now know that the symptoms that define PTSD aren't limited to soldiers. Anyone who has suffered a trauma and who has lasting, disruptive effects can be given this diagnosis.[28]

If you've read an article or watched a film on psychedelics, it probably included the pioneering work of psychiatrists and psychologists treating people suffering with PTSD. In the last several years many articles have been written about the work of the Multidisciplinary Association for Psychedelic Studies (MAPS) and its efforts to change the perception of psychedelics by engaging in pioneering research to help people with PTSD and TRD. But before the work of Rick Doblin and his team at MAPS, research was done in the United States and Britain in the 1950s and '60s using psilocybin. Doctors like Humphry Osmond in the UK and Walter Pahnke and Stanislav Grof in the US were some of the first physicians to engage in research into LSD and psilocybin.

Beginning with the end of World War II and lasting into the 1980s, a pioneering Dutch psychiatrist, Jan Bastiaans, used psilocybin and LSD to treat people who suffered with what we would today call PTSD. The term *PTSD* hadn't been codified yet, but Bastiaans treated hundreds of people successfully for what he called KZ syndrome (KZ was an abbreviation of Konzentrationslager, the German word for concentration camp) with techniques he developed.[29]

Psychological terms and diagnoses are very popular in common parlance these days. It is not uncommon for me to hear a patient report that they have PTSD from a brief encounter with a negative colleague or rude waiter. It is not in their best interest for me to correct them. For our purposes, though, it is important to understand that while PTSD has some correlation with other mental health diagnoses, it is a unique condition that is complex in both its etiology and severity. Though we will discuss the official diagnosis, the key to understanding PTSD is through fear and fear extinction. Fear is easy to understand; we all know what fear feels like. Fear extinction is the ability to address fear rationally at first and ultimately change the pattern in the brain. Fear extinction happens when the person suffering from fear is able to train their brain, specifically the medial prefrontal cortex (mPFC), to understand that a perceived threat is not the kind of risk that involves life-and-death actions.[30] A healthy brain can easily distinguish between a threat condition and a safe condition. The brain's inability to experience fear extinction, and thus to discern between a threat and a nonthreat, is the hallmark of PTSD. Fear extinction is mediated by the mPFC sending a signal to calm the amygdala.[31] If the amygdala never stops firing, it means something in the system is not working. If the signal isn't working, it could be the connection itself, the amygdala, or the cortical structure of the mPFC.[32]

The *Diagnostic and Statistical Manual of Mental Disorders* defines PTSD as a specific disorder. To fit the definition, the person being diagnosed has to have been exposed to or witnessed torture, serious injury, a death, or actual or threatened sexual violence. This can be either their own direct experience or vicarious trauma through a threat to a loved one or someone in close physical proximity. As a result, the person struggles with one or more forms of intrusive thoughts or memories. These can come in the form of nightmares, flashbacks, and physical reactivity to related or similar stimuli. This disorder is categorized by the person engaging in some sort of avoidance behavior and having at least two alterations in cognition or mood. These alterations are wide ranging but may include everything from the simple "negative affect" to full or partial amnesia about the traumatic events. Finally, for a diagnosis of PTSD, a person's symptoms can't be due to a substance, a drug, or any other organic mental illness, and the person suffering has to have endured the symptoms for at least one month and have experienced significant distress or inability to function in daily life.[33]

As you can probably assess based on just the criteria for a diagnosis, PTSD is a serious illness that has a profound effect on the person struggling with it and on all of their loved ones. We often focus on the stress of soldiers and survivors of war-related trauma. It's only in the last 15 years or so that we have understood that PTSD also affects people who have experienced car or work accidents, terrorist attacks, sexual trauma, and physical abuse, to name just a few. Sadly, there are new criteria for diagnosing childhood PTSD specifically related to the experiences of children in abusive situations, trafficking, and gun violence.

Few pharmacological treatments have been helpful in the treatment of PTSD. Sometimes patients are given sedatives or SSRIs for anxiety and depression, but studies performed since the 1980s have shown that these medications often prove to be ineffective, with less than 50% efficacy for most patients. Sedatives tend to be abused, and SSRIs sometimes have as low as a 30% response rate in treating PTSD. As a result, patients who are diagnosed with PTSD often struggle to remain in treatment because medications don't provide much relief. They lose hope and find themselves engaging primarily in coping behaviors, usually self-medicating with alcohol, cannabis, or opioids.[34]

Some treatments like exposure therapy or eye movement desensitization and reprocessing therapy (EMDR) have proven more helpful than medications for PTSD, but they require specialized training for psychotherapists and psychiatrists. Further, these treatments are not without risks. Exposure therapy in particular can retraumatize patients if done by someone who is not trained or who may be inexperienced in the techniques, with even some professionals thinking that exposure therapy is as simple as forcing a person to relive or confront traumatic events head-on. True exposure therapy helps a person struggling with PTSD to create alternative pathways of understanding their trauma, with a therapist then slowly and gently exposing them to memories or related stimuli over time. An untrained professional or caregiver reexposing a traumatized person to the traumatic stimulus while adding encouragement is cruelty, not therapy.

Throughout this book I have reflected on neuroscience research specific to different mental health conditions. I hope you notice that as the mental health conditions get more complex, the neuroscience gets more complicated. This is one of the primary reasons that research into psychedelics is so exciting. Conditions like PTSD involve multiple areas of the brain that are activated in different configurations or sequences. Science, medicine, and imaging are catching up, but we currently have an insufficient understanding of the mechanisms of PTSD. This makes developing new medicines a challenge.

The pathophysiology of PTSD is more complex than that of treatment-resistant depression, and consequently even more challenging to treat. Imaging studies have improved our understanding somewhat. As mentioned in other sections of this book, one of the brain-level hallmarks of depression, PTSD, and other similar disorders is that the brain's structure changes as a result of these conditions. We don't completely understand the mechanism behind why this happens, but we have already discussed some of the prevailing observations, like the HPA axis impacting the flow of certain neurochemicals like glucocorticoids (cortisol).[35] These keep the brain focused on its duties as a threat detector, and as a result, they prevent the brain from investing its precious resources into neurogenesis and neuroplasticity. Imaging studies such as functional magnetic resonance imaging have shown that patients suffering from PTSD have reduced brain volume in critical areas like the hippocampus and amygdala compared to healthy people. Researchers also report that PTSD patients who tend toward hyperarousal/hypervigilance have less density in the connections *between* neural structures in the brain. This implies that the impacts of PTSD on the brain affect multiple functions simultaneously or in a downstream fashion the longer the brain is exposed to either trauma or the expectation of trauma.[36]

One recent development in our understanding of PTSD is that one of the first areas of the brain impacted by trauma is the capacity for social cognition and empathy. Social cognition's neural correlates have been the subject of many studies in the last two decades. As you might discern from the name itself, social cognition refers to the ability to discern the feelings of others, predict behavior, and act on social cues. It requires that an individual be capable of considering someone else's motivations, thought processes, and experiences, and that they subsequently make decisions based on these perceptions. Basically, social cognition refers to the ability to put ourselves in someone else's shoes.[37]

Some of the relevant areas of the brain (the neural correlates) that have been identified in studies of social cognition include the posterior cingulate gyrus, the left temporal gyrus, and the amygdala. Patients who suffer from PTSD often demonstrate impaired activation of these areas of the brain. They struggle to make sense of social cues, and their threat detection and hyperarousal may add to the agitation experienced in not understanding what is happening in the social milieu. For many of these patients, their frustration grows because there was a time in the past when the person didn't struggle with this skill set. They often are very much aware that their brain functioned differently prior to being exposed to the trauma that initiated their PTSD.[38]

In previous chapters we've discussed ego dissolution—the experience of oneness, oceanic consciousness, or realizing we are all connected is a common feature of psilocybin journeys. It is often reported by sojourners that the experience of ego dissolution leads to feeling more connected to other people (and life itself), even weeks after a single psilocybin journey. Indeed, research into these states has demonstrated that ego dissolution plays an outsize role in healing. The presence or absence of this feature in someone's journey is predictive of their outcome.

One of the key mechanisms lies in the reduction of the self-referential thought processes associated with the default mode network (DMN). When someone takes psilocybin, the research indicates that the DMN goes offline in favor of less-hierarchical cognitive processes. Researchers like Robin Carhart-Harris and his team have published findings that show that not only does the DMN go into a greater state of disorganization or entropy, but it also likely resets after taking or being administered psilocybin.[39] This offlining of the DMN means that there is at least a momentary break in the cacophony of negative affect associated with PTSD and similar disorders. The addition of ego dissolution and its resulting sense of connectedness engages the parts of the brain necessary for the experience of social cognition and empathy, the medial prefrontal cortex (mPFC) and the temporal-parietal junction. The mPFC has turned up quite a bit in this chapter. It is necessary for mediating a number of processes required for turning down threats and turning up connection. It also has a profuse area of 5-HT2A receptors, as does the temporal-parietal junction. You're hopefully seeing the connectedness yourself! The brain has structures, networks, connections, growth, and pruning happening all the time. But the constant is the ubiquity of neurotransmitters; for our purposes we are most interested in the 5-HTA receptors and serotonergic processes, because psilocybin maps so easily to these networks.

Anxiety Disorders

Anxiety can be diagnosed in many forms. From generalized anxiety to social phobias and panic disorder, we recognize anxiety in our culture, but often we don't treat it as seriously as we should. Anxiety disorders are serious and can be debilitating. They cause very real social, economic, and family consequences, like lost wages and difficulties in relationships.[40] The mechanisms of anxiety look very similar to those associated with depression. While the experience may feel different, the neural mechanisms are affected by the same medications, implying a shared origin and/or mechanisms of action.

When someone struggles with anxiety, it's not the same as having a little worry here or there, which is normal. Most people have experienced anxiety about something simple, such as an upcoming event like a job interview or a wedding. But to be diagnosed as suffering from an anxiety disorder means that the same kinds of feelings and racing thoughts that might turn up around an upcoming first date or medical diagnosis are happening to a person all the time, without an obvious thing to worry about.

People who suffer from generalized anxiety often complain that they can't stop their minds from constantly giving them problems that beget more problems. In recent years research has found that worry and problem solving activate dopamine release in the brain as a means of trying to calm the amygdala.[41] However, dopamine is a neurotransmitter whose effects are strong, positive, and short lived. So, if your brain realizes it can get dopamine by worrying, then having more worries gives you more dopamine. It becomes a vicious cycle. Your brain gets addicted to the dopamine, which for someone with anxiety looks and feels like being accosted by uncontrollable worries and negative thoughts constantly racing through the brain.

Clinically, to be diagnosed with an anxiety disorder, the worry a person is dealing with must be consistent, it has to cause disruption in their daily life, and it cannot be associated with another disorder where anxiety is a feature, like anorexia. Nor is something considered an anxiety disorder if it's the result of taking a specific medication or an adverse drug interaction. There are other types of anxiety disorders, too, where anxious feelings are connected to a context, like social anxiety, when the anxiety appears only when in a social situation or thinking about a social situation.[42] We will discuss some of these, but they all have a number of things in common: mainly, the amygdala and threat circuit activation.

Many of the studies on depression covered in chapter 2 also included data on anxiety, as these two disorders often overlap. Recent research into the efficacy of psychedelics by Robin Carhart-Harris's team at Imperial College and the University of California, San Francisco, and the late Roland Griffiths's team at the Johns Hopkins University Center for Psychedelic and Consciousness Research has had compelling results. The Johns Hopkins team in particular has researched the effects of psilocybin for people who have a diagnosis of a serious life-threatening illness and found that a deep journey with a relatively high dose of psilocybin (as opposed to microdosing) provides patients with a significant reduction in anxiety.[43] In the next few paragraphs, we'll examine some of the more common anxiety-related diagnoses and the research into how psilocybin may be of use in treating them.

When discussing anxiety, it is useful to discuss how psychology measures different aspects of personality. Psychologists, doctors, and therapists conducting research to examine diagnoses like anxiety and other psychological and psychiatric concerns regularly study five personality traits: openness, conscientiousness, extroversion, agreeableness, and neuroticism.[44] These are often called the Big Five. Of these, neuroticism is usually associated with anxiety. Neuroticism refers to traits that are negative in psychological testing. People who score high in neuroticism tend to be those folks who are expecting disaster or bad luck. They are the worriers, the ones who always answer "Yeah, but . . ." Neuroticism is a key trait in personality tests and psychological experiments because it is associated with conditions like anxiety and depression. When researchers want to test whether or not a particular treatment had an effect on someone's thought process, they will include tests to measure neuroticism as either a state or trait attribute of personality.[45]

A trait attribute reflects a feature of the personality, like narcissism or openness, that exists regardless of circumstances. Trait attributes are considered permanent or semipermanent parts of someone's inborn personality. State attributes are ones that are dependent on circumstances like health, relationship status, employment, or other external indicators. When we are conducting research into whether or not a treatment is effective, we often want to understand whether it is affecting the state or trait attribute being measured. With diagnoses like generalized anxiety disorder, neuroticism is generally considered a trait attribute. A medication or intervention that can help alleviate trait symptoms is more valuable than one that can address only state conditions. This is because the trait attributes generally don't change very much over the course of someone's life.

When someone scores high in trait neuroticism, they may show a tendency toward negative feelings and behaviors like anger, self-consciousness, irritability, anxiety, emotional dysregulation, discomfort with change, and depression. Typically, people who score high in openness tend toward being more interested in novelty, feel ease in adapting to new situations, have an easier time with change, and frequently don't feel an overwhelming need for control. In a study by Katherine MacLean et al., researchers found that some individuals who scored high in neuroticism before psilocybin treatment experienced increases in openness and decreases in neuroticism after treatment.[46] The researchers also discovered that the predictor of these outcomes was whether or not the participant had a mystical experience on their psychedelic journey. The quality and depth of this experience also predicted the importance of the reduction in neuroticism and the increase in openness for the participants.

Similarly, in a study by Maggie Kiraga et al., researchers worked with a group of self-selected participants who were participating in a psychedelic retreat.[47] Participants were given personality tests before the retreat, one day after psilocybin was ingested, and again one week after the retreat's conclusion. The researchers worked with a group who were attending a legal psilocybin retreat in the Netherlands. In this retreat, participants were encouraged to work with the material that came up in their journeys as part of the retreat experience, but no therapeutic interventions were conducted by the organizers.

Researchers found that there was a distinct decrease in neuroticism both one day and one week following the retreat. Participants reported that they had fewer negative thoughts after administration of psilocybin. Personality tests captured scores confirming lower neuroticism scores after receiving psilocybin. Researchers believed that they would see an increase in openness, as had been reported in other studies. But instead, researchers reported no change in openness scores, though they did see a small increase in scores of agreeableness after the retreat as compared to scores prior to the psilocybin experience. Researchers also asked participants to complete questionnaires that measured their capacity for mindfulness as part of the study. They found that after psilocybin treatment, participants had a greater capacity for mindfulness, indicating an ability to separate their experience of negative affect from their decisions and judgments about whatever was causing their negative feelings.

SOCIAL ANXIETY DISORDER

Social anxiety disorder (SAD) is one of the more challenging forms of anxiety to treat. It doesn't respond well to SSRIs or short-term treatments like benzodiazepines (e.g., Valium), which are prone to abuse. Social anxiety affects people in situations when they have to be around others or when they have to perform tasks or skills in the presence of others. The impact of this disorder on work, relationships, school achievement, sports, and overall quality of life is real and challenging. This disorder is one that often first shows up in childhood. Because of its early onset, people who had SAD as children may find themselves prone to other mental and overall health problems in adulthood.

Most people who struggle with SAD have an overactive DMN and are constantly reflecting, revising, and reconsidering how other people are evaluating their behavior or performance. As a result, these patients often exhibit a high degree of apprehension about social situations, especially those where there will be a greater number of people by whom they might be judged.

Potential psilocybin treatments for SAD were considered by researchers Kim Felsch and Corinna Kuypers in an article in *Neuroscience & Biobehavioral Reviews*.[48] They note that in one study, psilocybin and meditation, when paired together, produced an acutely positive experience of ego dissolution that interrupted the constant self-referential thought process associated with SAD. The authors linked this to a decoupling of two key brain structures, the medial prefrontal cortex and the posterior cingulate cortex. Researchers used functional MRIs to measure the activities of these structures one day after psilocybin administration and found that their connectivity was far lower than the baseline measures prior to psilocybin. The potential to combine a meditative practice with psilocybin treatment might make both more effective.

EXISTENTIAL DISTRESS

There has been a great deal of research in the last several years on the impact that psilocybin can have for those who are suffering with a serious illness or who are facing death as a possible near-term outcome. Palliative care medicine developed out of hospice care, and it can be provided from the moment of diagnosis; it also often accompanies treatments that are intended to be lifesaving or prolonging. The World Health Organization defines palliative care as "an approach that improves the quality of life of patients and their families facing the problems associated with life-threatening illness, through the prevention and relief of suffering by means of early identification and impeccable assessment and treatment of pain and other problems, physical, psychosocial, and spiritual."[49] It is noteworthy that the spiritual element is highlighted in the definition. In the domain of palliative care, spirituality is a core component.

People who receive a diagnosis of a debilitating condition or disease describe anxiety and demoralization as some of the most frequent psychological experiences. Anxiety often appears as questioning whether one's life has had meaning and whether they have taken care of the people they love, and worrying about not being in the world to participate in important events involving those they cherish. Demoralization can show up as anger, nihilism, hopelessness, or a feeling of powerlessness. Often people in this state describe wanting to hasten an ending rather than prolong their suffering. These complex feelings are often too much for the person with the diagnosis to deal with, and they may withdraw from their loved ones or otherwise become emotionally distant as a defensive mechanism. Other people may completely deny their own mortality, reaching for a miracle cure or thinking they can outrun their diagnosis. If they have not confronted their fears, the end of life can feel like a betrayal of the patient and their loved ones by God, life, karma, or whatever the patient considers greater than themself.

In the last decade there has been an interest in better treatment options for people who face a life-threatening illness. Traditional psychotropic medications like SSRIs haven't proven to be very effective for patients with existential distress. In a study by Gabrielle Agin-Liebes at Palo Alto University and the NYU Langone Center for Psychedelic Medicine, researchers found that psilocybin-assisted psychotherapy provided profound positive changes for cancer patients.[50]

The study reported that after the first follow-up, which took place around six months after the psilocybin treatment, between 60% and 80% of patients continued to feel positive effects. More shocking still was that more than four years after a single administration and psychotherapy, patients described sustained reduction in anxiety, depression, hopelessness, demoralization, and death anxiety. The study's researchers reported that the patients in the study all survived the multiyear duration of the study, and that 15 of the 16 patients agreed to continue being part of the study over time. Researchers reported that the participants were overwhelmingly positive in their feedback, stating that psilocybin-assisted psychotherapy had been beneficial and that they found profound personal and spiritual meaning in the experience.

Roland Griffiths at the Johns Hopkins University School of Medicine was one of the founders of the current movement to reengage science in the application of psychedelics for medical research. He was the founding director of the Johns Hopkins University Center for Psychedelic and Consciousness Research. His research spanned applications of psychiatric care with psilocybin, including research into addiction and end-of-life care. His group was one of the first to study the effects of psilocybin on patients facing life-threatening cancer. The group conducted a double-blind study in more than 50 patients who had a life-threatening

illness and were struggling with symptoms of depression and/or anxiety. In their study, patients weren't the only ones asked to assess their mood and well-being. Their caregivers and attending medical staff also provided assessments of any changes in the patients' demeanor, attitude, and outlook pertaining to all of the possibilities before them, even death. The results were very encouraging.[51]

This study profoundly affected how the medical community considered psilocybin's effects on mood and well-being, and it has been cited in more than 1,600 other scientific papers. The study included two possible types of administration: a low and a high dose. The high dose produced the best results. Depression and anxiety decreased for most participants in the large dose group. The same group saw increases in positive attributes like quality of life and optimism. Most important, anxiety about death decreased significantly. The effects were durable after six months, with more than 80% of the study participants reporting they felt that the quality of their life increased and that their death anxiety had decreased significantly. The patients who reported the greatest improvement were those who had experienced a typical "psychedelic trip" after receiving a high dose of psilocybin.

Roland Griffiths passed away in October 2023, following a diagnosis of stage IV metastatic colon cancer. In a *New York Times Magazine* article published before his death, the researcher and the journalist discussed his scientific legacy. Griffiths was reflective about his own prognosis, but not dour. He reported that, at first, he avoided having his own psychedelic experience after receiving the diagnosis. He was feeling grateful for the life he had lived, and he felt joy at examining his life and the meaning he had created. As a scientist, he was curious that there might be something unconscious he was avoiding, so he went ahead with a psychedelic (LSD) experience, holding the specific intention of asking if he was avoiding something. In his psychedelic experience he came back with a clear sense that his joy was appropriate. His love of life and his desire to be grateful rather than depressed was a great gift, one that he should continue to explore.[52]

Griffiths was one of the first scientists in the 21st century to petition the scientific community and its regulatory bodies to study psilocybin for its potential as a medicine, not just as a recreational drug. His love for life and the experiences he has had are palpable while reading the article. He did not appear to be depressed or rueful about any aspect of his life. He appeared appreciative and expressed his gratitude with the creation of an endowment at Johns Hopkins to continue research into psychedelic medicine. His experience as someone who has both studied the effects of psilocybin and other psychedelics from a scientific perspective *and* had his own experience in comparison is remarkable. To me, this reflects a turning point in the 19th-century materialistic model of medicine and science. The experience is no longer forbidden to those who study the effects or power of medicines. Knowledge is not only gathered from the outside, but from our own individual experiences as well. We need both. I am deeply grateful for Griffiths's work and contribution.

Eating Disorders

Disordered eating is a pernicious problem in Western culture. For many years disordered eating was found mostly in adolescent girls. Today disordered eating can be found in all genders across all age groups and social classes. Anorexia in particular is very dangerous, with one of the highest mortality rates in psychiatric care.[53] Despite what most of us think about when we hear the word *anorexia*, the motivation behind this disorder is not specifically "thinness." Anxiety about weight and appearance are the main focus, but the real culprit beneath that anxiety is a desire for control. People who suffer from anorexia often are demonstrating a deep need for control over the most basic and fundamental aspect of life: eating. Sometimes anorexia isn't obvious because a patient looks like they have a normal body weight, or they might even appear to be overweight.

Bulimia nervosa and compulsive eating organize around different fears and concerns, though the obsessional focus on body weight and appearance is shared. These are subtle differences that may never become clear to those who don't treat people with these disorders. People presume that anorexia is just about being skinny, and bulimia is just about eating and then throwing up. But the neural correlates of these disorders show profound changes in the brain, especially with reference to the DMN.[54]

Some therapists consider eating disorders to either be a type of obsessive-compulsive disorder or adjacent to it. Anorexia nervosa and OCD share some genetic markers; this may point to an epigenetic component, so that when the conditions are ripe for stressors or anxiety, a pattern of rigid, self-referential thought is engaged.[55] The connection of both disorders to the gene has been established, but its expression in this way is purely speculative.

As of this writing several studies are underway to investigate how psilocybin affects patients with eating disorders. Only one of them has published findings. However, the foundations of their research are based in previous pre-clinical studies and in the findings of related studies like those for anxiety, depression, and palliative care.[56]

Anorexia and bulimia nervosa both are co-occurring with body dysmorphic disorder. Patients have visual distortions and see their bodies very differently from external views of their weight and appearance. Imaging studies reflect that the distortions in how patients see their bodies may be because of changes in cortical function especially of the hippocampus and a part of the brain called the anterior cingulate cortex.[57] Eating disorders also co-occur with depression and anxiety. Some researchers consider disordered eating to be a behavioral addiction. As a result, when looking at disordered eating, it is critical to look at the form and function of different parts of the brain that are associated with addictive behaviors, as well as looking at their associated neurotransmitters along with receptors like dopamine.

Psilocybin does affect the release of dopamine. However, it is important to note that many mushroom species have trace levels of additional tryptamines like baeocystin, which may affect dopamine receptors differently. Some other addiction disorders have different expressions of the reward circuitry. Dopamine and the associated reward system activation are often very different in behavioral addictions like gambling and trichotillomania (obsessive hair pulling/removal). In disordered eating it can be even more unusual, with revulsion and control providing reward in anorexia, and imagining food without consuming it bringing reward in bulimia.[58] Research comparing healthy subjects and patients who have recovered from anorexia and bulimia (especially those who were treated early) shows that the reward circuits return to normal after treatment for disordered eating.

Stephanie Knatz Peck and her team at the University of California San Diego Eating Disorders Center for Treatment and Research completed a clinical study evaluating the effects of a single dose of psilocybin delivered alongside psychological support, which was published in *Nature Medicine* in 2023.[59] The study administered a relatively high dose (25 mg) to adult volunteers who had a clinical diagnosis of anorexia nervosa or partial anorexia nervosa. The researchers were primarily interested in evaluating the safety and tolerability of psilocybin treatment for anorexia nervosa. They were secondarily interested in exploring whether or not a single dose of psilocybin administered in a therapeutic environment and paired with psychotherapeutic integration would make a difference in several areas where patients with anorexia typically struggle. This was a small phase 1 open-label study, so the results are preliminary and exploratory; however, the study helped pave the way for continued research of psilocybin and eating disorders.

Their preliminary findings are very compelling. There were no serious adverse events, and the majority of participants endorsed the psilocybin treatment as highly therapeutically meaningful. Participants reported significant clinical improvements in most of the indicators they examined. Knatz Peck's research team asked for feedback from participants using multiple instruments, which is more than most studies. They collected data on participants at baseline before any medical or psychological interventions, and then recorded treatment effects 1 day, 7 days, 28 days, and, for some indicators, again at 84 days after treatment. Integrative therapy was provided one day after the medicine experience and at day 7. The research team was available afterward for the participants should any adverse effects appear.

The team recorded clinically significant improvements in scores on the Eating Disorder Exam, the State-Trait Anxiety Inventory, the Quick Depression Inventory Scale, and the Changes in Clinical Impairment Assessment, among others. They also took data on important medically relevant tests, like electrocardiograms, all with clinically significant results. An important observation is the timing of clinical results. For almost all of these results, the most relief was reported at the seven-day mark, which coincides with the day that the participants had an integration therapy session. Some of these results may be due to a positive experience with the therapist following treatment; thus, they could be a reflection of high-quality therapeutic support. Another possibility is that these findings reflect the often-reported week or so of feelings of well-being after psilocybin treatment as the neurotransmitter load titrates down from the initial flood associated with the dosing day. Kaye and Knatz Peck reported that it is still far too early for us to know all the possible ways psilocybin can be used or the required safety protocols for distinct populations. Despite their appropriate scientific conservatism, it is encouraging to see new protocols and medications being developed to treat patients for whom pharmacological treatments have often been spare and ineffective.

Obsessive-Compulsive Disorder

People who struggle with obsessive-compulsive disorder (OCD) exist in a world that is filled outside and in with fear, frustration, and persistent negative affect. What most people know about OCD is the stuff that turns up in movies. A man has to count the number of times that he locks the door, or a woman has to wash her hands repeatedly to avoid contamination. What the layperson may not know is that those behaviors are the *result* of internal thoughts that overwhelm the person suffering from OCD. These repetitive or ritualistic behaviors are an attempt to quiet internal critical thoughts or feelings. The real culprit in OCD is the client's persistent, unconscious negative thoughts and rumination that are then compounded by the added fear of how awful they feel in those states. When I explain OCD to therapists in training, I describe having the sense that someone is pouring mud and old food scraps all over you all the time and also describing it to you in detail as they continue to pour. Your attempt to wash everything off or to ritualize it is an effort to have some control in the deluge.

In a study early in the current psychedelic renaissance by Francisco Moreno et al., which was published in the *Journal of Clinical Psychiatry*, nine subjects who had been diagnosed with OCD were given either 100 mg, 300 mg, or a microdose of 25 mg of psilocybin. All of the participants were given multiple doses over the study period of four weeks. Researchers reported that all of the participants displayed significant reductions in OCD symptoms during the study period.[60] Moreno's research team at the University of Arizona has a follow-up study listed on ClinicalTrials.gov.[61]

They have not posted any results as of this writing; the study is set to conclude in December 2023.

Yale University's psychedelic research program is also investigating psilocybin and OCD, with a specific look at the neural correlates of OCD in the brain and how psilocybin may work directly on the neurobiology of OCD. Only the study plan is available as of this writing. Researchers plan to measure the presence, prevalence, and intensity of OCD symptoms before and after psilocybin treatment. In their study they plan to administer the medication in the hospital and have the participants stay for a few days in order to fully monitor their symptoms. This way the clinical staff's observations can also be part of the data collection. This study proposes to study several different outcome measures, from symptom severity to mind-body dualism. I'm very much looking forward to following the Yale group's research as it progresses.[62]

An interesting aspect of Yale's research project is that they published a case report regarding one of their participants in the study.[63] The case report of this singular patient is very moving, and the importance the subject gave to the study conditions and the therapeutic aspect of the treatment was very telling. In the Yale study, psilocybin is not being considered a stand-alone pharmacological treatment. This is not unusual, and in almost every study the use of psilocybin is paired with psychotherapeutic preparation sessions to help patients address the possibility of difficult experiences. The studies also provide at least one integration therapy session to help participants make sense of material that arises in their journeys after they've been completed. Over and over again, it is the combination of preparation, medication, and integration that seems to create lasting positive outcomes.

The Yale case study reported on the experience of a man, given the pseudonym Daniel, who had struggled with the symptoms of OCD for more than two-thirds of his life, starting at the age of 10. When he started with the Yale group, he had already been through multiple types of medical treatment. Daniel had tried several medications and therapies to assist with the symptoms of OCD. While some of the interventions had been helpful, none had provided the kind of relief that his experience in the psilocybin trial produced. Daniel's story reads like a modern medical miracle.

Daniel reported that he had tried psychedelics recreationally a handful of times in his life, with no durable results. The Yale study offered him preparation sessions and integration sessions in addition to the "journey" of taking psilocybin in their clinical setting. The experience of working with trained therapists who prepared him to approach the images and feelings he would confront in his journey was a critical component of his positive experience, according to the case report. Daniel described experiences that align with many of the ideal goals of therapy. He gained a new perspective, partly by having the experience of "being" a tree. Far from being a laughable experience, this shift in perspective helped Daniel to see from a completely different perspective that life and all of its experiences are beautiful and necessary. This and other emotional explorations contributed to him feeling that it was safe for him to feel his feelings, which is another goal of psychotherapy. As mentioned in earlier chapters, in one of the kinds of therapy I practice (acceptance and commitment therapy), radical acceptance is a tenet of a healthy psyche. Learning how and when to let go of emotional resistance is an ideal outcome of therapy. That's not to say that a patient should seek out or welcome negative or unpleasant experiences, but rather that they should learn to tolerate discomfort without resistance.

When Daniel found himself dealing with some significant stressors more than a year after his participation in the Yale study, he was very afraid that he would slip back into old patterns. However, he reported to the researchers that he found himself returning to the tools of the therapeutic preparation and to the content of his psychedelic journey. The combination of the two helped him to traverse the complex ground of trauma and notice his psyche's predisposition toward returning to an old pattern. He acknowledged that to do things differently took effort, skill, and emotional regulation. But because he had both the therapeutic training and the psychedelic experience, he felt well equipped to proceed. Daniel reported that before psilocybin treatment, he would have returned to an old pattern and felt like a failure because of it, thereby reinvigorating the old pattern of internal criticism, bad feeling, and resistance to bad feeling. The meaning made in his original psychedelic journey and the toolbox that resulted from the journey not only changed Daniel's momentary outcome, but also created the potential for future healing.[64]

All of these disorders have similar dependencies and deficiencies. They are addressed by activating the serotonergic pathways of the affected brain structures, and in doing so they activate those and other downstream pathways like GABA and dopamine receptors. In addition, all have highly self-referential elements

(rumination, fear, concerns about others' opinions, internal negative feedback) that keep the DMN and amygdala active. Psilocybin's ability to reset the DMN, reduce activation of the amygdala, and increase activation of serotonergic and other neural pathways appears to be the critical role in calming the background noise so that a different option can be made available to the person experiencing the journey.

Finally, the experience of ego dissolution appears to give the sojourner the necessary psychological distance from their pain to help them make sense of it and help them not to identify with it in the same way as before their psychedelic experience. This combination of actions explains why Indigenous healers have always considered these fungi and other psychoactive components sacred. In what other context could any of us do years' worth of spiritual and psychological work in a matter of hours or days? Under what other conditions would our ancestors have believed it was possible? We have new names and new tools, but only recently have we started the challenging work of reconnecting an older form of knowledge to modern science. The work of healing is certainly worth the effort.

Addictions

Because of the association psychedelics have with the counterculture movements of the 1960s and 1970s, psilocybin, LSD, and many other substances like cannabis have been made illegal in many parts of the world. Despite more than a decade of successful research in using psychedelics to help patients with substance addictions prior to the creation of the current drug schedule system, psyche-delics were listed as Schedule I substances. The critical distinction of a Schedule I substance is that the drug is seen as having zero medicinal benefit. Medications that are highly addictive, like opioids, are Schedule II because they provide a benefit, despite their high potential for abuse.

In the 1950s and '60s there were more than 1,000 studies of psychedelics. Many of these were focused on the utility of these substances in treating alcoholism and other addictions. While we have far more rigor in our scientific studies today than we did in those earlier decades, their findings were mostly ignored in scientific and pharmacological research until the early 2000s. Researchers like Roland Griffiths, Franz Vollenweider, and Michael Bogenshutz revisited the early research done on addictions and psychedelics, and independently of one another began quiet and disciplined reexaminations of the possibility of using these substances to help patients with challenging problems like addiction.

Since the beginning of the 21st century there has been an explosion in research of psychedelics. One of the most active of these areas is the research into using psychedelics to treat addictions. With applications as diverse as alcoholism, opiate addiction, and smoking, the results continue to find that there is a potential benefit to exploring a psychedelic state to deal with addiction. From a psychological perspective, this may look absurd on its face to most people: *You're going to use a drug to stop your addiction to another drug?* If it were that simple, it would be preposterous. But why are most people abusing opioids, alcohol, nicotine, or street drugs like methamphetamine? As my favorite clinical supervisor

used to say, "Why do people use drugs? Because they work!" People who use these substances are doing so because they long for pain relief—the high is the only thing that can divert the psyche from their pain. Whether we are discussing the pain of trauma, abuse, combat, disease, or other physical suffering, people take drugs to diminish or treat their very real pain. It is true that there are some people for whom drugs or alcohol become a physical necessity; their bodies adapt to the substances in a way that they cannot safely quit by going cold turkey. These patients must be medically treated, and even if psychedelics were offered to them in treatment facilities, they must be carefully monitored for safety and any potential health complications.

People are taking nonpsychedelic substances in order to avoid, mask, or manage the challenges they face. They do this because they lack the capacity to tolerate the larger-than-life feelings that their traumas and pain generate in their bodies and psyches. People can't tolerate the high highs and low lows of these experiences. Research into depression and psilocybin that I've already discussed in these pages has demonstrated that after taking psychedelics, patients often describe being able to tolerate a greater breadth and depth of feeling. When administered properly, psychedelics help people expand their tolerance for joy and sorrow, pleasure and pain, elation and grief. People with substance addictions are most often using drugs and alcohol in order not to feel the waves and depths of their feelings. Psilocybin can make those peaks and troughs tolerable.

The results of scientific studies into the efficacy of psilocybin continue to be published and almost always with encouraging results.

A 2022 study led by Michael Bogenshutz at the NYU Medical School Langone Center for Psychedelic Medicine tested 93 participants who had been diagnosed with alcohol use disorder.[65] In this double-blind study, all the participants were given psychotherapy for 12 weeks and were administered either psilocybin or a placebo at weeks 4 and 8. The researchers examined how many "heavy" drinking days the participants reported over a 32-week period during the study period. As a back-up measure the researchers gathered hair or nail clipping samples from participants to confirm self-reports of abstinence from alcohol.

The researchers investigated patients' number of heavy drinking days during the study and asked patients to fill out questionnaires that measured complications from drinking. This study instrument is called the Alcohol Problems Questionnaire (APQ); it measures the relationship between alcohol use and personal and interpersonal problems that arise as a consequence of alcohol use. There are 44 questions on this scale. A higher score indicates more problems in the patient's life because of their alcohol use; a lower score means a decrease in social and interpersonal problems.

In the Bogenshutz team's study, respondents in the control group had an overall higher percentage of heavy drinking days during the study. Those who were part of the psilocybin group had 41% fewer heavy drinking days than their counterparts in the control group. In addition, the scores on the APQ for each group showed a clear treatment effect of psilocybin on drinking. The control group had a mean score of 13.00 on the APQ while the mean data for the psilocybin group was 6.59. Researchers pointed out that these scores

were already fairly low compared to other populations and may be the result of having had significant psychotherapy as part of the study. But looking at the comparisons to the baseline measures was particularly powerful. The control group's mean score on the APQ at baseline was 21.60, compared to the psilocybin group average of 20.26. The control group's mean score at the end of the study was 13.00, a reduction of 8.6 points. The psilocybin group's APQ average was 6.59 at the end of the study, a reduction of 13.67 points. In other words, those who had been administered psilocybin had a 67.5% drop in alcohol-related personal problems compared to 39.8% for their counterparts in the control group. It's critical to point out that in this study the participants had more than six months of therapy in addition to their psilocybin experience. The results of the placebo group show that there was a treatment effect from the therapy alone. That effect was much greater when paired with psilocybin.[66]

Several trials in the US and in Europe in the last several years have used psilocybin in an effort to treat alcoholism. There have also been several analyses of the historical data from the 1960s and '70s. The data are compelling. Psilocybin is helpful in reducing alcohol dependence when paired with therapy. Some researchers have speculated that the ego dissolution facilitates a mystical sensation or awareness that is analogous to the "higher power" that is central to the culture of Alcoholics Anonymous and other 12-step programs. Regardless of the belief system that is invoked by the patient's psyche in the psilocybin experience, it is clear that the effects of the journey last well beyond the initial treatment.

Smoking Cessation

Several trials have been done to see if psilocybin can have a positive effect on people wishing to quit smoking. One of the highlights of my time at Pacifica Graduate Institute was the amazing cohort of colleagues I got to study with as we learned the foundations of psychology necessary to become a psychotherapist. One of my closest colleagues in that program had already completed a doctorate in neuroscience. Her specialty was examining the toll that nicotine addiction took on the brain. In our first year spent learning about addictions she would wow me with her understanding of neuroscience as side commentary explaining the underlying neurological mechanisms during our lectures.

Though the reality of nicotine addiction and the havoc it can wreak terrified me, my colleague's experience in neuroscience inspired me, and it was likely the seed of my current fascination . . . some might say obsession. The brain was so much more than I had ever understood before meeting her. The door into my understanding was her description of the effect that nicotine has on the brain. She explained that almost every type of neuron had receptors for nicotine, and that it took only seconds for those receptors to stimulate the release of dopamine, serotonin, and GABA in the brain. This flood of neurotransmitters explains why, when people smoke cigarettes or vape pens, they immediately feel both more alert and also a little more at ease. Nicotine gives you focus, a surge in positive mood, and a reduction in anxiety. And the neurotransmitter cascade begins almost as soon as the nicotine hits your system, because it is inhaled

and travels to the brain without having to be translated through the digestive system.[67]

As most of us know by now, the dangers of smoking aren't limited to the brain. Nicotine causes stress on the heart, and it can contribute to making the arteries more inflexible. It also promotes cell growth in inconvenient or dangerous ways, including helping to vascularize tumors. The ways we get nicotine also mean that we ingest other chemical additives. Research over the last several decades has shown that some of these additives are carcinogenic, like the tar found in commercially produced cigarettes. We know less about the additives in vape cartridges, but there have been enough illnesses and deaths to let us know that there are safety issues with those products as well.

Nicotine is one of the most addictive substances in the world. Could a course of psilocybin therapy make that big of an impact? One of the first trials of psilocybin in this new era was a pilot study conducted by Matthew Johnson at Johns Hopkins University School of Medicine, the results of which were published in 2017.[68] Since then, teams at Johns Hopkins, NYU, the University of Alabama, and many others have initiated or published studies on the efficacy of psilocybin therapy in assisting clients to quit nicotine.

In every study using psychedelics there is a clear protocol that fuses psychotherapy and psychedelics. Most of the studies have at least two psilocybin sessions in combination with therapy. The overwhelming reporting shows that people quit smoking with greater ease after a course of psilocybin therapy. In one of the first pilot studies run by Johnson et al., there was a success rate of 80%, with only

3 people out of 15 resuming smoking after six months.[69]

Most people who attempt to quit smoking have multiple failed attempts. In another study looking at the reasons people gave for their ability to maintain their abstinence, participants reported that the psilocybin journey provided them with deep insights into the reasons why they smoked.[70] The journey helped them more carefully examine the ways in which they had crafted their identities to include smoking and provided them with a sense of interconnectedness and awe. As seen in similar studies, participants reported that the therapeutic support provided in this study was a critical feature of their journey. Support and meaning making were necessary to the positive outcomes that were reported.

The researchers in the smoking cessation study were often surprised by their findings, and they pointed out that the outcomes resulted from the combination of therapy and psychedelics. In almost every article that was published, they promoted the combination of the two because they did not want to endorse psilocybin use as a self-help tool to stop smoking. A Harvard study published in 2022 examined a group of people who regularly used psychedelics to determine if there was a connection that would imply causation between psychedelic use and a lower dependence on nicotine.[71] Grant Jones and his team found that there was overall lower use of nicotine by people who were regular users of psychedelics with one exception: those who primarily used LSD.

Opioid Addiction

Opioids the world over are a major public health concern, but in the US they have been at a crisis point for over a decade. In 2017 there were approximately 70,000 deaths from opioid overdose.[72] The ubiquity and ease with which opioids were made legally available created an addiction problem that devastated whole communities, especially in areas with already depressed employment and income. Opioid addiction is particularly pernicious because opiates are the first line of treatment for addressing serious physical pain. Opioids do not work on the same pathways as psychedelics. They act to reduce the pain signal at the neuronal level. They bind to a different receptor on the neuron in parts of the brain that slow things down, from heart rate to thought. They can induce a sense of euphoria, which makes them easy candidates for abuse. They are receptor agonists, which means that they assist with binding at the neuron's receptor site. Lifesaving drugs like Narcan work as a very fast-acting receptor antagonist, blocking the neuron from using opiate molecules that may be floating around the intrasynaptic space.

In a study led by Vincent Pisano published in the *Journal of Psychopharmacology*, an interdisciplinary research team looked at data from the National Survey on Drug Use and Health from 2008 to 2013 to determine if there was a relationship between opioid and psychedelic use.[73] The researchers discovered that there was a different use pattern for those who used both opioids and psychedelics recreationally: they were found to have a 27% reduced risk of opioid dependence and a 40% reduced risk of opioid abuse.

The team from Harvard led by Grant Jones, who conducted the nicotine research, engaged in a study replicating and building on the Pisano team's project.[74] In their 2022 study, the Jones team examined the National Survey on Drug Use and Health from 2015 to 2019 and came to similar conclusions. The use of psilocybin lowers the incidence of harm from opioid use. The team reported that in their study, lifetime psilocybin use was associated with lower incidence of opioid harm and abuse. The team found that there was no other drug, including other classic psychedelics like LSD or peyote, whose use acted as a mediating factor to opioid addiction. Both research teams offer that it is likely that psilocybin's primary action on the serotonin system may act as a moderating force. Jones and his team speculated that psilocybin may be supportive in treating opioid addiction, because opioids disrupt the serotonin patterns in the brain. They propose that the combination of serotonin activation and dopamine release in psilocybin use may act as a powerful tool to assist people struggling with the effects of opioid use disorder. They acknowledge that their theories are speculative and concede that more research is needed to help understand the possible mechanisms, effects, and outcomes.

As of this writing there are at least four studies listed on ClinicalTrials.gov that plan to examine whether psilocybin can be useful in helping address the nation's opioid crisis. The studies use a range of approaches. They look at everything from adding psilocybin as an adjunct to assist with tapering off opioid

dosage under medical supervision to using psilocybin as a complement to methadone for heroin addiction. The researchers report a desire to understand the quality of the psychedelic experience and the impact that psilocybin may have on chronic pain and withdrawal as areas of interest. These and future studies are necessary to help us learn how psilocybin can be used to help address the devastating cost of opiate addiction.

Psilocybin and other classic psychedelics are being studied for their potential to bring a new dimension of healing to intractable social problems like addiction that have devastating effects not just on individuals but on whole communities. While psilocybin can't cure everything, it is clear that the mystical experiences and neurological impacts combined create a transformative experience for those seeking healing from addiction.

Neurodegenerative Disorders

Research into the application of psilocybin for psychiatric and psychological problems like addiction, depression, and other disorders has generated results that are currently inspiring scientists to look at adjacent applications. Neurogenerative disorders like Alzheimer's disease and frontotemporal dementia are categorized by cortical atrophy. The cortex is the most easily recognizable area of brain anatomy: it is the folded, layered gray and white matter that makes up the bulk of the organ. Cortical atrophy on the gross level consists of reduction in the overall body of the cortex. As you look more closely at the structures of the brain, cortical atrophy can look like a loss of synapses and death of neuronal axons and dendrites. As these structures die, the result is less volume, fewer neurons, fewer connections, and less surface area that can potentiate and execute neuronal activity. If you likened it to a cellphone network, it would be like the ends of the networks being destroyed and only the central towers remaining. It would make it more challenging to connect, and you'd have to work much harder for those connections to be maintained.

Another hallmark of these and related neurogenerative disorders is neuroinflammation. When neurons are inflamed, they produce chemicals called cytokines (and other related compounds). When the neuron is in a perpetual state of inflammation it is at risk of neuronal atrophy and death. When there is neuroinflammation in the central nervous system the cells mediating the immune response will activate the immune system as the central nervous system thinks that it is under attack. In doing so the surface of these neurons shifts to a more protective mode, activating the different receptors to focus on protection.[75] In diseases like Alzheimer's, the activation goes a little haywire. The inflammation becomes chronic, and the more the brain thinks it's under attack because of inflammation, the more the inflammatory response ramps up to protect the brain in an ever-growing cascade of neural effects that eventually lead to cell death and cortical loss.

Researchers believe that psilocybin and other classic psychedelics may be candidate substances to address some of these issues. Psilocybin is capable of initiating neurogeneration, and in some laboratory models this happens at the level of generating whole new neurons from adult stem cells. In other instances, psilocybin assists in the generation

of additional synapses, dendritic spines, or axons. Neurogenesis is one of the most powerful reasons to experiment with psilocybin as a treatment for neurogenerative disorders. Another is the release of brain-derived neurotropic factor, which has a primarily anti-inflammatory effect on the brain and is a necessary precursor for the expression of some genes and proteins in the central nervous system.

While multiple review articles and speculative papers written by neuroscientists endorse the potential of psilocybin and other classic psychedelics for the treatment of neurogenerative disorders like Alzheimer's disease, traumatic brain injury, and temporal-parietal dementia, there are no current clinical trials listed in the US clearinghouse ClinicalTrials.gov. As of this writing, a single study was recruiting with the intention of testing psilocybin for mild dementia of early Alzheimer's. If psilocybin has the ability to catalyze neurogenesis in a more directed way, or if the tryptamines in mushrooms can be harnessed to decrease cortical inflammation, our understanding of their potential is just beginning.

New Research Areas

It's been 20 years since a handful of scientists decided to reengage the scientific and medical communities into the research of psychedelics. The primary focus of their research has been on the ways that psilocybin and other classic psychedelics affect the serotonergic pathways in the brain. As the research has progressed, we have seen that there are secondary pathways or unexpected downstream activities like the release of brain-derived neurotropic factor (BDNF), which initiates neurogenesis and can interrupt neuroinflammation. These recent discoveries have encouraged research into areas beyond the psychiatric and neuropsychological domains. They cover multiple areas of medical research and interest, they share features that involve neuroimmunological, neurogenerative, and neuroinflammatory systems. We don't yet know how the research will impact most of these disorders or what changes will come as a result, but we can be sure that the research into new ways of using psilocybin will have a lasting impact across multiple domains in health and pharmacology.

LYME DISEASE

Though most of us have heard of Lyme disease or have done the obligatory tick checks after a hike in the woods, few people have experienced the disease at the level of severity that is currently being considered for treatment with psilocybin. This tick-borne illness—a bacterial infection spread via tick bite—can be very dangerous. Lyme disease can begin with a rash that looks like a bull's-eye and then spread to different systems in the body, ranging from the heart muscle to the joints. Some people may experience a long-term Lyme disease infection or a subsequent autoimmune response to the *Borrelia burgdorferi* bacterium that causes the disease. Once someone has the disease at this level, it can be very challenging to treat.

There have been some limited exploratory studies, and a clinical trial is underway that is treating people who are suffering from neuropsychiatric symptoms of Lyme disease with psilocybin.[76] The theory of using psilocybin either as a microdosing option or in a psychedelic therapy intervention is that the anti-inflammatory properties of the drug may have an impact on the autoimmune response common to those suffering with Lyme disease. The activation of serotonergic pathways may also assist patients by helping to boost the thalamus and immune system responses, while also assisting in addressing depression brought on by the complications and fatigue that occur with chronic Lyme disease.[77]

PHANTOM LIMB PAIN

It is not uncommon for someone who has had an amputation to experience the sensation that their severed limb is still attached to their body. For a long time, the medical establishment believed that phantom limb sensations and pain were psychological problems with no correlation to actual neurology. In the last several years, this thinking has been revised. While we don't fully understand the neuroscience behind phantom limb pain, scientists no longer believe that the experience is an illusion that is held in the mind alone.[78] I am careful not to call this pain psychosomatic, not because this is not a good descriptor, but because the word has become synonymous in recent years with being imaginary. Somatic psychology is reclaiming that word, but it has not fully succeeded as yet.

Somatic psychology is the study of a unified mind-body. As such, somatic psychologists use the same techniques as talk therapists, but they add to them. In somatic therapy the body is seen as also holding information about trauma, pain, love, and connection. This relates back to the discussion in chapter 2 about the mind-body problem, and how since the days of Rene Descartes we have separated the mind from the body. New research tells us that there is far more integration between brain and body than we have considered in the last 100 or so years of medicine and psychology.

One of the leading theories of phantom limb phenomena is that the brain needs to reorganize its own internal map of the body following an amputation, and that this takes time and neurological resources.[79] Treatment with psilocybin may assist in reducing inflammation and provide stimulation of neurogenesis at the level of the neuron, axon, dendrite, and synapse. This expanded capacity may assist the central (brain and spinal cord) and peripheral (extremities radiating off the spinal cord) nervous systems in reorganizing a cortical map of the body, thereby assisting the brain as it reorganizes its sense of the embodied self.[80]

MIGRAINE HEADACHE

People who suffer from migraine headaches and migraine-related disorders often have great difficulty once symptoms begin. A migraine disorder can make someone nauseated, sensitive to light and sound, and fatigued, and it can cause significant pain. Recently there have been some novel treatments for migraine including botulinum toxin, otherwise known as Botox.

A study by Emmanuelle Schindler and her research team at Yale University investigated the efficacy of psilocybin for people who suffer from chronic migraine.[81] Anecdotally, chronic migraine sufferers have experimented with psilocybin to relieve their pain and other symptoms for more than a decade. Because psilocybin is a Schedule I drug, physicians have been unable to recommend or prescribe it. In the Yale study, subjects were asked to

keep a journal describing their headaches and symptoms for two weeks before they were offered psilocybin, and then again for two weeks after the trial ended. The exploratory study was highly successful. There was a much greater reduction in weekly migraines after administering psilocybin when compared to those who received a placebo.

A review article published in the journal *Neuropharmacology* by Schindler examined several studies done on atypical treatments for migraine disorders. The overall evidence suggests that psychedelics generally are beneficial, even preventative for people with migraine disorders. Psilocybin in particular was reported in more than one study to prevent migraine pain for up to six weeks. In another study attacks for those who took psilocybin were diminished in 56% of patients who took psilocybin. Schindler reported that across the studies, the reduction from the patients' baseline migraine conditions was significant after psilocybin. As with other areas of inquiry with psilocybin, scientists aren't sure why psilocybin is successful in treating this disorder.[82] It is likely related to the action on the serotonergic pathways in the brain.

AUTISM SPECTRUM DISORDER

There is broad speculation that the condition we call autism spectrum disorder (ASD) is not a simple disease with a singular origin but a result of multiple possible variations of several systems in the brain. The serotonin system seems to be implicated in ASD, though whether this is because of different genes or environmental concerns is unclear. Researchers think that several proposed pathways may be involved in creating the conditions that might cause ASD. That being said, findings are primarily based on deductive reasoning and correlation studies. Researchers look at the brains of autistic people postmortem, compare them with those of laboratory animals who have similar traits, and look at neuropsychiatric and pharmacological research to make inferences about chemical signaling in the brain.

We don't know what causes autism. We do know that it has a complex origin, not a simple one. Researchers at the Institute of Psychiatry, Psychology, and Neuroscience at King's College London have proposed using psilocybin to test changes in the serotonin system in neurotypical and autistic individuals.[83] The hope is that by examining the ways that serotonin behaves in its various individual forms, in both neurotypical and neurodivergent individuals, perhaps scientists could get a little bit closer to understanding the serotonin mechanisms at work in ASD.

The research team spans several neurology-centered research groups at King's College. They hope to capture what they call serotonin shift in both populations, and then compare via functional MRIs, EEGs, questionnaires, behavioral observation, and other measures. The team published their proposed protocol in May 2023.[84] In it, they explain that they believe using psilocybin to help demonstrate how serotonin pathways vary and are activated in these two different populations (ASD and neurotypical controls) may be the key to understanding the role serotonin plays in ASD.

There have been other studies and case reports made of people who have self-medicated with psilocybin and who also have ASD. This self-selected group is clearly a group that, while neurodivergent, is not gravely impaired by their diagnosis. Their anecdotal reports are interesting, and they support similar findings to those reported in using psilocybin for other conditions. The results are positive. Those who have self-medicated with psilocybin report that they were able to feel empathy and develop an awareness of other people that is usually outside of their capacity.[85] This may be because the 5-HT2A receptors in the parts of the brain that affect empathy are more active, or it may be because the DMN is quieter. Either way, the data continues to trend toward positive outcomes.

CHRONIC PAIN

In a case review article published in April 2023 in the journal *Pain*, Matthew Lyes and his collaborators at the University of California San Diego Medical Center report on the cases of three patients who took pain management into their own hands when traditional treatments failed to provide relief.[86] Despite very different conditions and presentations of pain and very different therapeutic protocols of psilocybin, all three patients reported positive outcomes. One patient (known only by his initials, DC) found that daily microdosing at 250 mg of dried mushrooms gave him 8 to 10 hours per day of total relief from pain, despite eight prior years of constant pain following a vehicular accident. As a result of microdosing psilocybin, this patient discontinued cannabis and opioid use because he found their effects negligible in comparison. He reported that the relief he experienced from psilocybin was total. Prior to taking psilocybin, his baseline pain was self-reported as usually between 5 and 8 out of 10. When taking daily microdoses of psilocybin, his pain was reported as zero in the 8 to 10 hours immediately after ingestion.

The second patient (initials ES) was seeing the San Diego team for complex regional pain syndrome. She reported a significant drop in pain while taking a daily 500 mg dose of dried mushroom powder (not pure psilocybin), and she would take occasional days off of her psilocybin schedule. She would also occasionally increase her dose by approximately 50% to get greater relief when her pain was worse. This patient reported that she had gained functional mobility over time and greatly improved her pain management. She reported an approximately 80% reduction in pain about three hours or so after taking psilocybin. She experimented at higher doses but found the psychedelic effects unpleasant and unnecessary to her relief. She reportedly achieved 80–90% reduction in pain by taking a microdose as mentioned earlier without any psychedelic effects or alterations in mood.

Patient 3 (initials JP) decided to experiment with psilocybin to reduce her use of opioids for intense lower back pain brought on by degenerative disc disease. Despite having surgery and multiple epidural steroid injections, this third patient experienced no pain relief from traditional therapies. She reported that microdosing with approximately 1,000 mg of ground mushroom powder mixed into a chocolate bar alleviated her pain significantly. This patient reported that within one hour of taking psilocybin, her pain score went from a baseline of 8 out of 10 to zero. She also reported improved flexibility and relaxation in her muscles, which were usually uncomfortable due to muscle spasms and stiffness. When this patient took psilocybin, she adapted by doing stretches and exercises that helped with flexibility. When she was in acute pain, these exercises were not tolerable. The results reported by JP were some of the most compelling in the study. She was able to describe for the researchers how there were two types of pain that she was experiencing. One type was primarily musculoskeletal, and psilocybin was able to significantly reduce that pain for months at a time, after only a single dose. The patient described the other type of pain as neurological and reported that after her third session taking psilocybin, she experienced complete relief from that pain, and that her results were durable for more than six months following her last dose.

The authors of this study report that these results are clinically compelling and thus warrant investigation into the ways that psilocybin could be used to help treat chronic pain. In two of the three cases (DC and JP), the researchers report that the effects seemed additive over time. They point to the possibility of neurogenic effects as a possible explanation. These reports are unusual in that, unlike other research in this area, they reflect the effects of microdosing on its own and do not include any psychotherapy to produce a treatment effect.

In an article published in the journal *Nature*, Joel Castellanos, one of the authors on the UCSD case study just discussed, was interviewed along with several other leading scientists who are researching psilocybin as a potential treatment.[87] Castellanos is a pain medicine and rehabilitation physician. His patients' pain and their desperate desire for relief are a daily area of confrontation. He is quick to point out that some people's pain is made worse by psilocybin, so it is not a panacea. While there is a great deal of hope, Castellanos is wary of too much hype. He points to the need for more rigorous clinical trials and for more research into the neuropsychopharmacological mechanisms of psilocybin and other psychedelics.

The most exciting opportunity pointed to by the multiple researchers who administered these studies seems to be the possibility of pain relief that does not include the use of opiates. They were stoic about the toll the opioid crisis has taken on individuals and communities, and they expressed reservations about repeating those mistakes, saying that the medical community should move slowly as research deepens in the field of pain management and psychopharmacology. After all, pain is a unique application for this kind of research. The more distress one has about their pain or about the conditions that cause that pain, the more intense the patient's experience of the pain itself will be.[88] Learning to appropriately anticipate the experience of pain is a critical feature of pain management. The more someone who suffers with chronic pain has a negative anticipation of said pain, the worse their pain will feel.

To manage the anticipation of pain, patients need to be able to relax their minds and bodies. Resistance is a feature of both physical and psychological pain, as I have written in other chapters in this book. Furthermore, discussing the research in areas where psilocybin is clinically useful—like depression and anxiety—is important in this context because chronic pain doesn't only affect the pain receptors in the brain. Depression, anxiety, suicidality, and other psychological conditions accompany chronic pain, adding to the suffering of already beleaguered patients. A substance that can have an effect on both the neurological and psychological components of pain is a win for patients and doctors alike.

FIBROMYALGIA

Chronic, widespread pain in the muscles, bones, and joints with chronic fatigue, sleep difficulty, and a history of trauma are the hallmarks of fibromyalgia (FM). Diagnosing FM can be difficult, as the most consistent symptom reported by patients is pain—diffuse, shifting, and constant.[89] In the last 10 years doctors have accepted that FM is a real disorder, but there are still physicians who may not recognize it or who downright dismiss the symptoms. FM was, up until recently, often differentially diagnosed with hysteria, hypochondria, and conversion disorder. It should also be mentioned that this disorder has a tendency to be experienced by more female than male patients, which has added to the travesty of dismissing the symptoms as something more psychological than physical.[90]

A handful of studies examining the effects of psilocybin on FM are either recruiting or about to begin as of this writing. As with some of the other studies I've covered in this book, this disorder often co-occurs with significant neuroinflammation. Researchers also have deduced that autoimmunity plays a role in and correlates to trauma that is nearly always a prominent feature of the FM patient's history. Sleep disturbances, fatigue, brain fog, and cognitive concerns are common in patients as well. The proposed studies describe treating the pain associated with FM as well as the psychological effects. Unlike other chronic pain studies, anecdotal reports on the efficacy of psilocybin are more mixed than conclusive. Researchers report that this may point to a very different pain signal. This difference could be in the approach to pain experienced by those with the diagnosis, or more likely it is because there is a different neural signal in

FM pain compared to the origins of pain in other disorders. Despite this anecdotal concern, researchers are optimistic that psilocybin may bring relief to those suffering from FM.[91] This disorder continues to challenge providers and patients because of its complex etiology and presentation.

In some studies, patients who have been diagnosed with FM have had a primarily neutral response to psilocybin. In a journal article by Nicolas Glynos and his team at the University of Michigan,[92] researchers found that of 354 FM patients asked to participate in a survey about treatment interest, 29.9% reported having self-medicated using psilocybin or LSD for pain management. Their reports were mixed, with 59.4% reporting a neutral response and 36.8% reporting a positive one. Approximately 3% reported negative experiences, either to their overall health or their pain. Twelve of the participants who had tried a psychedelic reported improvement in their FM pain. While this study is encouraging, it also reminds us that research into the ways that psilocybin works is still in its early stages. The future is very promising but not yet defined.

SLEEP DISTURBANCES

One of the biggest surprises I had in becoming a psychotherapist was learning about sleep. While we all know how important sleep is, it is generally thought of as something pleasant, necessary, and sometimes annoying. We often treat sleep as an afterthought. We believe that we can "catch up" on the weekend, or that sleeping (what scientists consider) a healthy amount (seven to nine hours per night) is an indulgence. Americans in particular pride themselves on the amount of sleep deprivation they can tolerate. Research into mood and psychosis shows that sleep is a critically important regulator in mental health.

When I was training to be a therapist one of my psychopharmacology professors taught us that before you refer a patient to a psychiatrist for medication, you should first see if you could encourage the patient to regulate their sleep. Exercise and the occasional over-the-counter sleep aid were usually enough to encourage the body to sleep deeper and for a longer period of time. I have tried this with my clients over the years and have found it to be true—helping someone sleep better is an important tool in improving mental health.

Research into sleep has shown that there is a common theme between sleep regulation and traditional antidepressants like SSRIs. This similar pattern has led to some speculation that one of the actions of antidepressants is actually the improvement of sleep, and that this might be part of why SSRIs are effective treatments. Depression is also associated with sleep disturbances, with patients who suffer from depression reporting disrupted sleep schedules and poor-quality sleep.[93]

Sleep research shows that sleep is necessary for memory consolidation and for cleaning up the cellular structure of the brain. Researchers have investigated psilocybin's effect on sleep and have come to some interesting conclusions. Sleep is broken down into stages, the most well-known of which is rapid eye movement (REM) sleep. But there are three non-REM stages of sleep that are just as important. We may go through multiples of each stage over the course of a night. In the first stage our body is falling asleep, meaning that your brain and body are switching from wakefulness to sleep. Your body may have a few muscle spasms as the muscles relax and your brain slows down. In the second stage you will experience a light sleep; your muscles will relax more, and your heart rate will slow down. Your brain may have a few random electrical signals as it quiets down. Stage 2 is the most common form of sleep you will experience, and you may go through this stage several times in a single night. Stage 3 is often called slow-wave sleep to distinguish it from the other two non-REM stages. This stage of sleep often occurs in longer stretches. Your brain, heart rate, and body temperature are all at their lowest levels during this stage of sleep. It is in slow-wave sleep that we get most of the benefits of sleep. This stage is necessary for the consolidation of memory. Finally, after slow-wave sleep comes REM sleep. We used to think that this was when most dreaming occurred because of the brain's activity, but we now know that dreaming also occurs in other sleep stages.

Research into psilocybin's effect on sleep has reported that it doesn't change the overall quality of sleep, though sleep patterns immediately following a psychedelic experience may be altered. People will sometimes have a more difficult time falling asleep after taking psilocybin. Researchers have found that in laboratory experiments done with animals and also in sleep studies done with human subjects, psilocybin is often associated with a delay in the onset—and a shorter duration of—slow-wave sleep. However, researchers have also noted that these changes did not appear to affect mood or later sleep quality. They speculate that a psychedelic experience may augment sleep and that some of the work done during sleep, like memory consolidation or emotional homeostatic resetting, is actually being achieved during the psychedelic experience.[94]

Other psychedelics have similar effects on sleep. Researchers have investigated the effects of ketamine and ayahuasca on sleep patterns. Ketamine seems to bring about a more immediate and restorative sleep, while ayahuasca may create a sleep pattern similar to psilocybin—less sleep required with more activation—but that it may be doing the consolidation work of sleep, thus requiring less sleep of the person immediately following administration.[95]

Another core component of these findings is the relationship between depression and sleep. If the mechanisms underlying depression and insomnia are connected, the activation of these mechanisms via psilocybin administration may help address insomnia in some patients. In short, psilocybin will not help someone with insomnia sleep better on the next sleep cycle or the day after psilocybin, but it may help overall by addressing depressive symptoms, by helping to consolidate memory, or through neurogenerative effects.

Contraindications: Who Shouldn't Take Psilocybin or Other Psychedelics?

In most of the studies that have been conducted, there is a pretty long list of people who have been excluded. This isn't necessarily because psilocybin is inherently dangerous, but because there are other factors to consider that would limit the efficacy of the study. Additionally, there are some concerns about how psilocybin could affect people with certain conditions. Because the scientific community is still in the early stages of research, we cannot say for certain what the impact of psilocybin will be on someone who suffers from one of these disorders. Almost all the contraindications I'm about to list have to do with the action of neurotransmitters. We can infer from what we know about the mechanisms of action of a given disorder and that of psilocybin what we might expect and why it would be better to not combine them.

PERSONALITY DISORDERS

Some personality disorders, like borderline personality disorder and narcissistic personality disorder, are marked by an overly grandiose or negative affect. We have limited data on the neural processes that take place in these disorders, but we know that there is less inhibition, which is governed by the medial prefrontal cortex. While psilocybin has demonstrated increased activity in this area of the brain, these disorders have been shown to have other activation patterns in the brain, such as in the amygdala and the temporal lobe, and these could be aggravated by serotonergic action. There is one proposed study on using psilocybin to treat patients with co-occurring borderline personality disorder and major depressive disorder; as of this writing, the investigatory phase for this study should be concluded in 2024.[96] Because narcissistic and borderline personality disorders tend to include at least some delusional thought processes, these may be exacerbated in the psilocybin experience. In other words, it is more likely that a person with these personality structures might have a "bad trip." That doesn't mean that the overall healing would be difficult, or that there wouldn't be meaning and growth from the experience. But if someone has been diagnosed with one of these disorders, their experience with psilocybin could cause a substantial

negative episode that would then need to be worked through, or it could contribute to feelings of grandiosity in either a positive or negative way. For example, a borderline patient who has a bad journey might fixate on the idea that they can never get any relief and that they'll never get better. This would stand in the way of any actual healing that could take place by examining the images, sensations, and experiences that they had during their journey.

Some journal articles have been written about people who have bipolar disorder and have taken psilocybin, but these studies have primarily examined the use of recreational psychedelics by people diagnosed with bipolar disorder.[97] There are two primary types of bipolar disorder: I and II. In addition, there is a subclinical presentation that used to be referred to as cyclothymia; this diagnosis is no longer included in the *Diagnostic and Statistical Manual of Psychological Disorders*. The research into the mechanisms of all the different forms of bipolar disorder shows a significant contribution of serotonin pathway activation.

In a study published in the *Journal of Psychopharmacology* in January 2023, researchers asked more than 500 people in countries around the world to participate in an online survey about psilocybin and bipolar disorder.[98] Approximately one-third of the respondents reported challenging experiences in the journey followed by an increase in negative symptoms like mania, difficulty falling or staying asleep, and increased anxiety. The researchers were quick to add that even though these participants reported negative experiences, they said that the overall experience was still positive and described having received benefits in mood and understanding from their journeys.

PSYCHOSIS AND PSYCHOTIC DISORDERS

In the earliest research into psychedelics, scientists believed that psychedelics like LSD and psilocybin could create a psychotic state that mimicked the psychosis of illnesses like schizophrenia.[99] While hallucinations are hallmarks of both psychedelic and psychotic states, the reasons for their occurrence appear to be different. Psychosis is marked by an increase in dopamine, which could be a result of downstream serotonin signaling. The psychedelic state has a very different activation pattern. Importantly, when the neurotransmitter load begins to return to normal, any hallucinogenic effects also begin to subside.

New research comparing the neural correlates of psychedelics and psychosis found similar structural activation but different patterns and frequencies that appear to be differentiated by the neural structures of the patient. In psychosis there are disruptions in the connectivity of the basal ganglia with the thalamus that result in disruptions in neurotransmitter release. In both psychedelic states and psychotic states, the thalamus's connections to different parts of the brain are hyperactivated. Researchers believe that the difference between the two is that the activation pattern in psychosis is actually caused by the structure underlying the connections, which is different, and that allows only the psychotic pattern to be experienced.[100] In psychedelic states, the hyperconnection of the thalamus with other areas of the brain is part of a psychedelic activation pattern, not a structural difference. When the psychedelic

begins to break down in the body, the hyperconnection ceases, and the person returns to a normal state.

One of the differences in experience of psychosis versus a psychedelic trip is that the person in a psychotic state struggles with reality testing. In other words, they may have great difficulty assessing their inner world and differentiating it from the outer one. A person who experiences a schizophrenic state may hear voices and believe wholeheartedly that those voices are giving them very real, externally generated information. A person having a psychedelic experience will know that any incoming information is related to their use of a psychedelic, and they will usually assign meaning to a psychological or spiritual insight.

Because of the structural differences implied in people who experience psychosis (schizophrenia, bipolar disorder with psychosis), it is not recommended that these patients use any psychedelic substance. It may be that one day we will come to understand the underlying mechanisms of psilocybin and other psychedelics enough to allow us to create new classes of drugs that may be beneficial to people who struggle with psychotic disorders. But at this time, it is too early to tell, and there is a higher likelihood that a person who is already prone to psychosis would have a negative experience with the hallucinations and disruptions of psilocybin or other psychedelics.

SEROTONIN SYNDROME

If you have ever been on a psychedelic retreat, a responsible organizer will have asked if you regularly take selective serotonin reuptake inhibitors (SSRIs), serotonin and norepinephrine reuptake inhibitors (SNRIs), or monoamine oxidase inhibitors (MAOIs). This class of drugs is designed to increase the overall available serotonin in your system. Having too much serotonin in your body can lead to a condition called serotonin syndrome. This is a dangerous adverse reaction that needs to be treated in a hospital if you should suspect it is happening to you. It is most often found when people mix medications, like taking ayahuasca and an MAOI at the same time, or take too much of a very strong SSRI.

It is good to know the symptoms of serotonin syndrome, sometimes called serotonin toxicity. While it is rarely fatal, it is still very dangerous, and if left untreated it can lead to death. Some of the symptoms include myoclonus (jerking and twitching in specific muscle groups, similar to what sometimes happens when you're falling asleep), extreme and fluctuating vital signs, cognitive disturbances, unconsciousness, fever, seizures, and muscle rigidity. Any of these symptoms, either alone or in combination, require immediate medical attention. People with bipolar disorder or other serotonin system disorders should always check with a health care provider before using any psychedelic to make sure that they are tapered off of their serotonin medications.

CARDIAC CONCERNS

If you have any heart problems, you should get clearance from your cardiologist before trying any psychedelic medicine. While we have just started to understand the important role that psychedelics can play in mental health, we do not yet know the impact that these medicines may have on other biological systems, especially those that have serotonin receptor involvement. Physicians have been quick to point out in the literature that one of the necessary areas of study in the exposure of

patients to psychedelics is the affinity for the 5-HTA2A and 2B receptors. The 5-HTA2A receptor plays a significant role in the blood stream, especially in serum blood platelet function.[101] Increases in 5-HTA2A expression may be responsible for increases in vasoconstriction and coronary arterial spasms. There is also a link between 5-HTA2B receptors and problems with the valves in the heart. These receptors are activated to repair the valves in the heart, and some cardiologists have raised concerns that we need additional testing to make sure that the expression of this receptor doesn't lead to a thickening of heart valves.[102] If you have high blood pressure or cardiovascular disease, please talk to your physician before taking any psychedelics.

Reflections on the Research

Overwhelming evidence shows that there is a great potential benefit in developing medicines and practices around the use of psilocybin. Still, these are not without risks, and we are very early in our understanding of the effects this powerful tryptamine has on human biology. Moving forward in a clear-eyed fashion will be the key to a better future that includes psychedelic and nonpsychedelic medicines and treatments (like microdosing) derived from these exceptional organisms. Whether you are curious about treating your own conditions or doing research to assist someone you love, please do so with great caution. The research exists to support your efforts, but you should always work with a medical professional. Physicians, nurse practitioners, psychologists, and psychotherapists would prefer to know about your use of these substances. Understanding what you are experiencing and the effects—both positive and negative—is critical for a healthy body and mind. If you're concerned that your medical provider will judge you, then perhaps choose a new provider. Medical providers aren't bound by law to tell anyone about what substances you use. Most of them are less interested in moralizing and more concerned with doing right by their patients. So be candid with your health care provider and ask for their guidance whenever possible. They are unlikely to endorse a course of treatment that is currently illegal, so don't ask for their medical advice specifically. Legally, they cannot endorse any treatment that is prohibited by law, or they risk losing their medical license. Instead, ask them about possible drug-to-drug interactions that might occur, relate any concerns you have about the effects of psilocybin on your current condition, and ask if there is anything you should know so that you can make your own decisions. The laws may soon change, and it could soon be that you'll have a psilocybin option from your psychiatrist, but until then, be prudent, be careful, and stay informed.

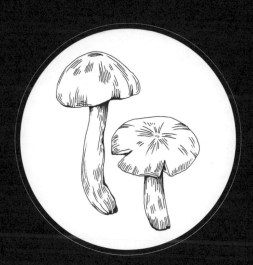

BOTTLE CAPS

Fight for the things that you care about but do it in a way that will lead others to join you.

—RUTH BADER GINSBURG

CHAPTER 8

Mushrooms, Psychedelics, and the Law

Hunting Unicorns

A unicorn is a mythical animal that represents something pure, wonderful, magical, and rare. The mythology of unicorns is invoked in everything from medieval courtly poetry to 21st-century venture capitalism. When hunting a unicorn, you're looking for something that shouldn't exist. In 13th-century courtly love, the unicorn was a metaphor for pure love that existed of and for itself, with no expectation of physicality or return of affection. Today a unicorn could be the perfect tryptamine-based medication that can deliver on the promise of psychedelics without the side effects and possibly without the psychedelic experience.

In the last several years several organizations have begun to invest significant resources into the future of psilocybin and other psychedelics. Some of these are nonprofit organizations like the Multidisciplinary Association for Psychedelic Studies (MAPS), whose phase 3 trial of MDMA may soon change how PTSD is treated in the United States. The drug is usually referred to as ecstasy or molly, but its official name is 3,4-methylenedioxymethamphetamine (you can see why it has enjoyed multiple nicknames). The drug that we would eventually come to call ecstasy started as a medicine for couples therapy, became a party drug, and is now finishing up a huge clinical trial for PTSD, with the possibility of being approved for treatment of PTSD in 2024 or 2025. Other unicorn hunters are more futuristic, like the New York firm Gilgamesh Pharmaceuticals, which has raised more than $30 million and uses artificial intelligence to help isolate novel compounds based on classic psychedelics.

Drugs and treatments based on psychedelics are on the horizon; we just aren't sure yet what the final presentation will look like. In the last several years it's been a little bit like the Wild West as companies try to become the first to decide the future of psychedelics. Some companies are isolating compounds; others are developing clinical protocols.

Recently, a company called Field Trip Health became a cautionary tale on moving too quickly in the psychedelic space. Field Trip Health raised more than $100 million in venture capital investments. Its premise seemed to be that the company could begin work using the only currently legal psychedelic in the United States, ketamine, and from there build a practice that would be ready when other psychedelics like psilocybin and MDMA were legalized. The company was founded by Canadian cannabis investors Hannan Fleiman, Ryan Yermus, Joseph del Moral, and Ronan Levy and by solar industry management professional Mujeeb Jafferi. Field Trip was headquartered in Toronto, Canada, and had an original and—one would think—winning approach. Field Trip Health invested in clinics meant to provide services to patients and in research and development to create its own psychedelic medicines. Its first product was based on psilocybin, and these efforts were intended to create a psychedelic experience that would be consistent, predictable, and about three hours in duration—half of the time of the psilocybin experience typically felt from using mushrooms. As of this writing, Field Trip Health has filed for creditor protection, sold off a number of its clinics to other providers, and spun off its research and development arm and its first psilocybin-based compound into a new company called Reunion Neuroscience.[1]

I attended a Field Trip training in late 2021. It proved to be a little disorganized, but the training, information, and overall environment were spectacular. Full disclosure: I was so inspired I bought a tiny bit of stock in the company as well, but in the end its reach was far beyond what it could sustain. Field Trip is an appropriate footnote as we examine the promise of psychedelics in this closing chapter.

The promise, potential, and possibility of Field Trip's ultimate goal—to "heal the sick, and better the well through psychedelic therapies"—is admirable and something everyone operating in the psychedelic space can get behind. Nevertheless, Field Trip went too far too fast, and it is an excellent reminder of how easy it is to trip (pun intended) while trying to fulfill the promise of psychedelics.

Schedules and Expectations

The way that psychedelics are currently organized in the US and in many other parts of the world is the result of the terror that psychedelics generated in the culture in the 1960s. In the 1950s, prior to the "Turn on, tune in, drop out" message promoted by former Harvard psychology professor Timothy Leary, research using psychedelics had been seen as avant garde. By the late 1960s psychedelics had escaped the laboratory and accompanied the first generation of the post–World War II boom (also known as boomers). The search for meaning drove many people to look beyond the nuclear family and buying a home in the suburbs. Young adults coming of age needed an alternative road to travel. If the traditional view was taking the I-10 to the burbs, psychedelics provided the yellow brick road to Oz. For many, the Vietnam War and growing instability in the world coalesced to act as deterrents from pursuing a "traditional" life, and young people by the millions tried to remake the world into something new. But there was no blueprint to follow, and many of them relied on psychedelics to help them make sense of their anxiety, frustration, and desire for something different, something better.

This rejection of social norms terrified parents and communities. During the 1960s, when psilocybin, LSD, and other psychedelics were being shared at parties and experimented with in college psychology labs, the upheaval being felt around social issues easily caught the psychedelic cause in its crosshairs. Richard Nixon was elected to the presidency in 1968, and the "war on drugs" would be one of his most enduring legacies. In 1970 Nixon signed into law the Controlled Substances Act. It basically codified our entire approach to medication and drugs in this and other countries. If a drug can be abused, it is studied, deliberated on, and placed on a list of controlled substances, which is broken down into five "schedules" based on the potential for harm. Which schedule it lands on is wholly dependent on its medical value and its potential for abuse or addiction. The highest level, Schedule I, is the most restrictive. Substances on this list are considered to have high abuse potential and no known medical value. These drugs are basically illegal substances and cannot even be prescribed by a doctor. Permits are not allowed for manufacturing, though occasionally a substance can be studied in a research environment.

The schedule system was created at a time when people weren't solely concerned with a drug's or substance's potential to create opportunities for addiction or contrarily individual relief. They were also concerned about the public cost of the substance and included the perception of social harm that the drug could do. This is why the drugs that are part of the most restrictive Schedule I category are substances that have a moral and a physical effect.

The Schedule I list includes marijuana, heroin, LSD, and psilocybin. MDMA was added later once it became a party drug. Schedule II includes drugs like cocaine, methamphetamine, oxycodone, Adderall, and other opiates and stimulants. As the schedule gets more relaxed, you are basically left with cold medicine and antipsychotics.

For psilocybin and other psychedelics to lose their Schedule I status they must demonstrate that they have medical value. More than 20 years into the psychedelic renaissance, that point has been proven. The US Food and Drug Administration has changed the status of psilocybin and MDMA to "breakthrough." This designation allows the FDA to reconsider the status of a medication and to fast-track its approval. With the wealth of research outcomes in the last decade, it is hard to believe that there won't be an approval in the next few years. Indeed, corporations, universities, and Silicon Valley are all poised to be the first at the psychedelic table.

The Future of Pharmaceutical Psilocybin

As of this writing there are at least 10 companies engaged in research that attempts to isolate the active components in psilocybin for the express pharmacological use of these compounds. There are some companies trying to do away with the psychedelic "trip" aspect all together, and others that are trying to control its effects so that it can be used predictably with clear timing, like surgical anesthesia. These companies are all playing their cards close to the vest, awaiting the moment when the breakthrough status is dropped and the schedule for psilocybin is lowered to something that can be prescribed by a medical doctor. When that happens, a new wave of psychedelic medicines will flood the experimental waters.

There are two probable first options, which I've already mentioned. It is likely that the first psilocybin pill made available will be one that provides a predictable, timetable-focused psychedelic experience. Most of the research into psychotropic uses of psilocybin have demonstrated that one of the healing aspects is the deep insight that comes from the psychedelic experience and the integration of that material into the patient's own personal understanding of their psychological and emotional life. The second likely candidate will be a low-dose psychedelic-inspired antidepressant/analgesic that works in a similar fashion to microdosing. Companies are researching these compounds now, and some are already providing the medications for clinical trials in big research programs. In some places, though, states and local governments aren't waiting for the schedules to change; they are allowing shared use of psilocybin in its natural form: the mushroom.

Decriminalization versus Legalization

For anyone who has followed the changes in cannabis legislation, decriminalization versus legalization is a basic concept. There is a difference between the legalization of something (i.e., making it legal to own, share, or sell) and the choice to decriminalize something. If a substance, activity, or product is legal, that doesn't mean it isn't regulated. Soup, spray paint, and unleaded gasoline are regulated. To decriminalize something generally means that

despite other laws that may prohibit that substance or product, the authoritative powers of the state—the police and the court system—are not going to spend their resources or time to enforce the laws that spell out the prohibition.

If, for example, I breed poodles, and suddenly poodles were described as Schedule I canines and could not legally be owned, then my dog would be illegal, and I would either have to hide her and face legal repercussions or give her up. If, however, the government decided that poodles were going to be decriminalized, I wouldn't have to worry as much, as it would mean that they wouldn't come after me for owning a poodle. It still wouldn't be legal for me to breed her, sell her, or share her with anyone, but I could relax because I wouldn't go to prison for owning my little fluff ball.

Decriminalization has created a host of problems in the cannabis industry. Cannabis, while decriminalized and legal in many US states, has not had its schedule changed at the federal level. This middle ground between legal and illegal has created problems that no one expected, like making banking and lending to cannabis-based businesses problematic at best and impossible at worst. Other problems have developed that were also unforeseen, like human trafficking for farm labor and the monopolizing of permits. The goal for psilocybin is to avoid some of the pitfalls while waiting for the schedules to change. These new laws could remain in place after the schedule eventually changes, provided that the proposed systems are respected, making it easier to use psilocybin therapeutically rather than just profiting from it. This is especially important in places where native fungi could be at risk of overharvesting without a plan in place for maintaining their natural habitats.

Legalization of psilocybin could be ideal, but it would come with its own range of complexities. Who gets to decide how these substances are used? How will dosing be defined? At what age will it be legal to use these substances, and in what context? Oregon and Colorado are coming to terms with these questions now, since passing laws to legalize and regulate psilocybin. Proposed legislation in California is similar to the legislation that passed in Colorado, where something defined as "shared use" went into effect in 2023.

The shared use model allows people to grow and consume psychedelic mushrooms for personal use, and it allows mushrooms to be shared for therapeutic or spiritual purposes. The shared use law does not allow personal, unlicensed growers to profit from the sale of psilocybin mushrooms. As community programs are developed, tested, and rolled out, the system will add regulations for greater commercialization. Oregon's original legislation was similar to Colorado's, and to what has recently been proposed in California. Despite Oregon being the first state to embrace psilocybin for its citizens, the state has lately changed course as it struggles under the history of cannabis industrialization. Currently, the requirements in Oregon are much more stringent than what was originally proposed.

Where Psilocybin Mushrooms Are Legal

ARGENTINA
In Argentina, the possession of psychedelics has been decriminalized, yet a tangled web of conflicting legislation persists. In the landmark 2009 *Arriola* decision, the nation's Supreme Court unanimously declared that the criminalization of personal possession of drugs (in the *Arriola* decision it was cannabis) was unconstitutional.[2] Despite this ruling, the framework for drug criminalization remains intact in the country's legal statutes, leaving enforcement to the discretion of individual judges.

AUSTRALIA
Australia recently passed legislation rescheduling MDMA and psilocybin. As of right now the country has yet to fully implement the changes that would allow psychiatrists to prescribe psilocybin. Under the changed law, psilocybin can be prescribed for depression and MDMA for PTSD.

AUSTRIA
Austria takes a relatively progressive stance on psilocybin. In 2016, Austria decriminalized the possession of psilocybin mushrooms for personal use. Austria also had changes in overall drug laws that prioritize treatment over punishment. The sale and distribution of controlled substances remain illegal. Nonprofit organizations such as the Vienna Psychedelic Society are working to destigmatize psilocybin and other psychedelics.

BAHAMAS
In the Bahamas, psilocybin-containing mushrooms are legal. The Bahamian government does not classify magic mushrooms as "dangerous drugs." This results in the legal possession, sale, distribution, and cultivation of psilocybin mushrooms within the Bahamas. Several all-inclusive luxury psychedelic retreats operate legally there.

BOLIVIA

Psilocybin is not mentioned by name in Bolivia's drug laws, but the Bolivian government exercises strict control around most drugs. A local judge or magistrate could determine that using psilocybin falls under the restrictive drug laws, so approach psilocybin use carefully. Bolivia recognizes ayahuasca as an integral part of Indigenous traditions. Ingredients required for preparing ayahuasca can be freely obtained from local markets. Nevertheless, it's crucial to note that other psychedelics and psychoactive substances remain illegal in the country.

BRAZIL

Brazil navigates a unique legal landscape regarding psychedelics, with some notable distinctions. Psilocybin and psilocin as individual compounds are illegal under Brazilian law, but having the mushrooms themselves is not.

BRITISH VIRGIN ISLANDS

The British Virgin Islands exercises autonomy in its laws, operating independently of the British Crown. Psilocybin mushrooms are illegal in Britain but they are legal both for personal use and possession in the British Virgin Islands, though selling them is prohibited.

CANADA

Psilocybin, psilocin, and magic mushrooms are illegal in Canada under the Controlled Drugs and Substances Act. Under this law psilocybin and psilocin are illegal unless authorized by Health Canada, which can issue a license or exemption. The government accepts applications for the special access program, and if approved, a health care provider will receive a letter of authorization that allows them to legally conduct their treatment. Several clinical trials are underway in Canada that might be options for those seeking treatment; a database is available through Health Canada, or individuals can write to the Office of Clinical Trials. Health Canada also permits health care providers to apply for permits to administer special treatments when a patient has a life-threatening illness, or when a treatment has been successfully researched elsewhere. In May 2023, Prime Minister Justin Trudeau announced that the enforcement of laws prohibiting psychedelic mushrooms would be left to individual provinces. British Columbia has decriminalized drug use, with the federal government granting an exception through 2026. Similar exemptions have been explored in Toronto and Hamilton, Ontario.[3]

COLOMBIA

Drug possession for personal consumption has been decriminalized in Colombia since a landmark 1994 Constitutional Court decision that deemed laws prohibiting such possession unconstitutional.[4] Ayahuasca retreats are common in Colombia, and psilocybin mushrooms grow natively.

DENMARK

The Danish government has strict drug laws, but it acknowledges psilocybin's therapeutic potential, especially in treating substance abuse. Pharmacies, including hospital pharmacies, are authorized to dispense psychedelics. Ketamine is also available for medical use in Denmark.

JAMAICA

Psilocybin mushrooms are legal in Jamaica and have never been prohibited there. They are not considered controlled substances. This has led to a burgeoning psilocybin industry, with legal retreats and companies operating on the island.

NETHERLANDS

In the Netherlands, there's a unique legal landscape regarding psychedelic substances. While psilocybin mushrooms are technically illegal, several products exploit legal loopholes. Possession of small amounts of fresh or dried psychoactive mushrooms has been decriminalized, with quantity limits.

PORTUGAL

Small quantities of psychedelic substances have been decriminalized since 2001, setting a precedent for drug policy reform.

SPAIN

Small quantities of psychedelic substances are legal for personal use in Spain, although selling or distributing them remains illegal.

THAILAND

Thailand has started adopting a new approach to psychedelics and illegal substances since 2017, reducing penalties for possession, cultivation, and sale of substances like MDMA, LSD, and psychoactive mushrooms. Thailand has considered relaxing its drug laws, and recent articles by travel writers describe eating meals prepared with or finding that their morning smoothies were prepared with psilocybin mushrooms.[5]

UNITED STATES: STATES WHERE MUSHROOMS ARE LEGAL OR DECRIMINALIZED

Oregon

The Pacific Northwest state that also led the way in the cannabis industry made history in November 2020 by becoming the first state to legalize psilocybin-assisted therapy and to decriminalize personal drug possession. Measure 109, known as the Oregon Psilocybin Services Act, tasked the Oregon Health Authority (OHA) with the responsibility of licensing and regulating aspects of psilocybin products and services. These include manufacturing, transportation, delivery, sale, and purchase of psilocybin products, as well as the provision of psilocybin services like psychotherapy and retreats. The OHA collaborated with the Oregon Psilocybin Advisory Board to establish comprehensive rules and regulations governing Measure 109 and the utilization of psilocybin products and services.

Beginning January 2, 2023, the OHA started accepting applications related to the manufacture, sale, and purchase of psilocybin products, as well as the provision of psilocybin services. As of this writing, the Oregon Psilocybin Services Section has received thousands of inquiries from all over the world. Individuals who aren't based in Oregon and retreat centers looking for a place to establish themselves have spooked the regulators. They do not want a repeat of the cannabis industry's problems in Oregon. As of this writing, there are 10 licensed service centers in Oregon. It is now notoriously difficult for someone to create a facility in Oregon if they aren't already a resident there. Therapists must be trained and certified. In addition, after the difficulties that some communities have had with cannabis farming, state legislators included a provision that allows local communities to ban psilocybin facilities.[6]

Colorado

In a groundbreaking decision, Colorado made history by passing Proposition 122, becoming the second US state to legalize psychedelics and establish treatment centers for their supervised use. The journey toward this milestone began in 2019 when Denver became the first city in the United States to deprioritize law enforcement against individuals possessing psilocybin mushrooms. This groundbreaking shift came with the passing of Initiative 301, which explicitly declared personal possession of mushrooms as the city's "lowest law enforcement priority." The initiative effectively barred the allocation of city funds for criminal enforcement related to the personal use and possession of psilocybin mushrooms among adults.[7]

Building upon this initial progress, Colorado activists introduced two closely related ballot measures, Initiative 49 and Initiative 50, in December 2021. These initiatives aimed to establish psychedelic treatment centers. Later efforts, in the form of Proposition 122, garnered enough signatures to secure a place on the 2022 general election ballot. The Decriminalization and Regulated Access Program for Certain Psychedelic Plants and Fungi Initiative went on to achieve approval in November 2022, with 54% of the vote, marking the state as the second in the nation to establish a regulated access program for psychedelics.

This proposition paves the way for the creation of the Natural Medicine Advisory Board, which will advise Colorado regulators in establishing state-sanctioned "healing centers." These centers will provide adults over the age of 21 access to "natural medicines," including psilocybin. Initially, the term *natural medicine* covered only psilocybin and psilocin, but it currently is expected to expand on June 1, 2026, to encompass dimethyltryptamine

(DMT), ibogaine, and mescaline (but not peyote, as this is a protected class).[8]

The Colorado Department of Regulatory Agencies had until January 1, 2024, to establish the qualifications, education, and training requirements for facilitators providing natural medicine services. Additionally, by September 30, 2024, the department must adopt the necessary rules to implement the regulated natural medicine access program and begin accepting licensure applications, with decisions on all applications made within 60 days of receipt. The specific administrative rules developed in the coming years will play a pivotal role in shaping the landscape of regulated access to psychedelics in Colorado and elsewhere.[9]

Proposition 122 also decriminalizes "possessing, storing, using, processing, transporting, purchasing, obtaining, and ingesting natural medicine for personal use" for adults. It also extends decriminalization to the cultivation and processing of plants or fungi capable of producing natural medicine for personal use, as long as these activities occur within a "private home or residence" and are protected from access by anyone under the age of 21.

Nevada
A bill to decriminalize the possession, use, and manufacturing of psilocybin for adults and create a research program passed the state senate and the assembly in June 2023.

Washington, DC
The residents of Washington, DC, passed a resolution in November 2020 lowering the enforcement priority to the lowest possible level for naturally occurring psychedelics.

In other states and cities in the US, there is a checkerboard of decriminalization, legalization, proposed research, and enabling legislation to study the effects of changing the law.

Depending on where you live, there may be a city or state where the law is about to change, or a small jurisdiction where there have been quiet decriminalization efforts. This list is not exhaustive, but it hopefully shows that psychedelics are broadly more accepted than in years past. For the most up-to-date information, check local and state ballot measures, talk to your state representatives, and learn about local efforts in your community through nonprofits, mycology clubs, or lobbying efforts.

WHO'S NEXT

California

Several cities in California have championed resolutions that prioritize personal use and possession of specific psychedelics as the lowest law enforcement priority. The cities of Oakland, Santa Cruz, Arcata, Berkeley, and San Francisco unanimously passed resolutions that redirected city resources away from enforcing laws penalizing the use and possession of naturally occurring psychedelics.

In February 2021 Senator Scott Wiener introduced Senate Bill 519. This bill sought to remove criminal penalties for personal possession and social sharing of various psychedelics, including psilocybin, psilocin, MDMA, LSD, DMT, ibogaine, and mescaline (excluding peyote). The law failed for several reasons; one was the inclusion of MDMA and LSD. Law enforcement strongly advocated to eliminate laboratory-created compounds at this stage, saying that it would make enforcement much more difficult. The bill failed in the state assembly.[10]

In December 2022, Wiener reintroduced the bill under a new number, SB 58, described as allowing the legal possession, transportation, transfer, and preparation of psilocybin and other naturally occurring psychedelics. The assembly bill also allowed psychedelics for personal use by individuals 21 years and older and eliminated the prior inclusion of MDMA and LSD. In September 2023, the California state senate finalized the bill. It was vetoed by Governor Gavin Newsom. If he had signed the bill, it would have gone into effect in the beginning of 2025. The governor signed an executive order that if the schedule changes for psilocybin, MDMA, and other psychedelics, they would immediately be decriminalized in all of California. While there was a great deal of criticism immediately following the announcement of the veto, the governor's office offered that it is working to understand the complex regulatory changes that will be necessary when the schedules change. California wants to be ready to be a leader in this space, not follow Oregon and Colorado and run the risk of repeating the complex problems those states have been struggling with.[11]

Illinois

Illinois is poised to be the first Midwestern state to legalize psilocybin for medicinal use under the Compassionate Use and Research of Entheogens (CURE) Act. This law would also create an advisory board similar to those in Colorado and Oregon to help guide the development of psilocybin-related services. As of this writing, the CURE Act is still pending.[12]

Iowa

Legislation has been proposed to legalize psilocybin and decriminalize certain psychedelics for patients with life-threatening illnesses.

Kansas

A bill was introduced to legalize "homegrown mushrooms" and would decriminalize the cultivation and use of less than 50 g of psilocybin mushrooms. The bill was forwarded to the Committee on Assessment and Taxation as of March 2023.[13]

Maryland

In April 2022 Maryland lawmakers presented a bill aimed at establishing a state fund designed to grant "cost-free" access to psychedelic substances such as psilocybin, MDMA, and ketamine. This initiative primarily targeted military veterans grappling with PTSD and traumatic brain injury, with the goal of providing them with potential therapeutic relief.

In May 2022, Maryland's then governor, Larry Hogan, announced that he would permit SB0709 to become law without affixing his signature to it. Another bill, HB 0927, was introduced proposing a reduction in penalties for de minimis possession of small, specific quantities of controlled substances. If this bill wins approval, it will create a significant shift in the legal landscape of the state.[14]

Massachusetts

Massachusetts has seen several developments regarding the legalization of psilocybin and other naturally occurring psychedelics. These include the introduction of two state bills that shared the objective of removing penalties for individuals over 18 years old who possess, ingest, obtain, grow, or share limited quantities of psilocybin, psilocin, and DMT. In addition, several cities have decriminalized psilocybin, including Somerville, Cambridge, Northampton, Easthampton, and Salem.

Michigan

Detroit, Hazel Park City, Ann Arbor, and Washtenaw County decriminalized entheogenic plants in 2021. A ballot initiative is underway to decriminalize psilocybin mushrooms and other plants and fungi. It is proposed to go before the voters on November 5, 2024.

Montana

In March 2023, a final bill was delivered for review that would legalize psilocybin for psychiatric care. The bill establishes guidelines for the administration, cultivation, and distribution of psilocybin.

New York

Two bills have been advanced through the state assembly and state senate. Assembly bill A00114 was referred to the health committee and would legalize possession of naturally occurring psychedelics and allow for the development of psychological and spiritual services for psychedelic therapy or support. Senate bill S3520 seeks to create a psilocybin-assisted therapy grant fund and was referred to the finance committee. As of this writing there are no updates.[15]

NOT QUITE THERE YET . . .

Several states have established exploratory groups or enacted legislation to study psychedelics and the benefits that they may convey. Depending on where these states are in their research, they might be some of the next to allow psilocybin use. Here's a list of states that have created task forces or enacted enabling legislation to study these substances:

- Arizona
- Connecticut
- Georgia
- Hawaii
- Minnesota
- Missouri (this state is trying very hard to legalize psilocybin for veterans and those suffering from life-threatening illness; they aren't looking to decriminalize or legalize in general)
- New Mexico
- North Carolina
- Oklahoma
- Pennsylvania
- Rhode Island
- Texas
- Utah
- Vermont
- Virginia
- Washington

Retreats and More

Several retreat centers around the world promise a unique and healing experience for people using psychedelics. Some of these are expensive, all-inclusive resort-style options, and others are simply huts where you stay with a shaman and his family as you work through your trauma. The most challenging aspect of these varying retreat options is that they are absolutely caveat emptor, or buyer beware. There are very few guidelines, and some stories have emerged in the last several years about psychedelic practitioners taking

advantage of their clients and preying on people when they are in a vulnerable state. Some of these stories have been disturbing and describe rape and sexually inappropriate behavior on the part of teachers and workshop leaders.

If you are considering attending a psychedelic retreat, it is best to do so with a group or company that is established in this space. Working with psychotherapists and medical professionals is advised, not only because you'll have confidence that the person you're working with has the knowledge required to help you with any psychological, emotional, or medical issues, but also because people who have licenses and practices are much more careful with their professional credentials and therefore are more likely to provide good service.

There are websites where you can learn more about psychedelic retreat options. Some of these are backed by scientific research like those with the Beckley Retreats or my own therapy practice at Hope Therapy Center. You can also find options on Retreat.guru, which is sort of like a clearinghouse for psychedelic retreats. Practitioners and facilities are listed, and you can search profiles and locations and read reviews.

Be sure to ask questions about the experience of the staff, what training they've had, and how they came to this work. Ask about their safety protocols. Don't be afraid to ask about how they handle negative situations or "challenging experiences." You'll soon learn that retreat leaders and psychedelic practitioners avoid the language of the "bad trip." But it's important to pay attention to how they respond to your questions. Most practitioners will answer with something that may sound a little "woo" but is symbolic of the nonresistant approach: "it's all welcome." This means that the practitioners are ready to manage whatever shows up and to be with you through the experience. Beware of anyone who promises you that everything is wonderful and beautiful. Anyone who is trying to sell you solely on the positive and blissful either has not done their own work or is not equipped to manage the depths of your experience. Better to move on and interview someone else.

A word of caution about retreats and group experiences: there are many underground practitioners in this space right now. Many of them are well trained, and some have spent time working closely with Indigenous shamans. Some in the underground psychedelic world are psychotherapists or physicians. If you live in a place where psychedelics are illegal and are working with a medical professional, you want to make sure that they are licensed. A medical doctor or psychotherapist who has lost their license is a danger to patients—not because they don't know their science, but because their livelihood now depends on underground work. I have more faith in people who are risking their license than those who have lost one. This is not because I don't have compassion for their circumstances, but because I fear the desperation of someone who has lost something critical to their identity and livelihood. If you can afford it, spring for a retreat in a beautiful location where the psychedelic experience is legal. You'll be surrounded by practitioners who don't feel constrained, and if something goes wrong, you'll be in a community that likely has medical facilities or practitioners that have experienced it in the past and therefore know what to do without fear for their livelihood or reputation.

Ayahuasca and Other Medicines

In the development of practices and efforts to legalize psilocybin there is a great deal of interest in other naturally occurring psychedelics. Sometimes these will be available in retreat settings along with psilocybin. Over the last decade it has become trendy for people who can afford it to travel outside of the US to experience ayahuasca ceremonies. In these ritualized experiences participants are given a substance or drink made by combining multiple plant species into a decoction or concentrated liquid including the caapi (*Banisteriopsis caapi*) vine, and the leaves of the chacruna (*Psychotria viridis*) shrub. The drink is said to help the person drinking it purge their sorrows and confront meaning in a new way.

The substance that brings this mystical experience to fruition is N,N-dimethyltryptamine (DMT). Ayahuasca ceremonies have become something of a destination in the last two decades. People who have been trained in the proper creation of this elixir are far outnumbered by people who haven't been properly trained. In many parts of the world, this psychedelic brew is a secret handed down from shaman to shaman. When done properly, ayahuasca can facilitate profound healing. When taken too lightly or treated disrespectfully, ayahuasca can be dangerous. Taking ayahuasca is considered a sacrament in the Indigenous cultures that practice it. Sometimes the journey is taken to help find someone a spouse or to heal them of a profound illness or psychological condition like grief. Treating ayahuasca as though it is nothing more than a drug is a misunderstanding of its utility as an agent of Indigenous psychiatry or psychotherapy.

In many Indigenous cultures, sacraments that help a person see a forward path or make amends with their ancestors are central to their worldview. It is a relatively new idea that human beings are autonomous individuals with no ties through space and time to their ancestors or descendants. If you are invited or wish to take part in an ayahuasca ceremony, please find someone qualified who is trained in the making of the brew. Also interview the shaman or guide to learn where they learned, how they learned, and how they approach their practice. A dedicated person isn't looking for a quick payday and will have invested their own time and money to learn these Indigenous practices. Their education will likely also include other psychoactive substances and spiritual practices.

BUFO

DMT can be found in multiple species of plants and in the glands of some animals. The most well known (and easily accessible) of these is in the skin of toads of the Bufonidae family, the most common of which is the Sonoran Desert toad (*Bufo alvarius*). The toad can be quite large, about three to five pounds. Some people will lick these amphibians, which can be very dangerous as this can cause muscle weakness, rapid heart rate, and vomiting. Dogs sometimes catch them, and they should be rushed to the veterinarian if this happens.

If you encounter this substance on a retreat, it may simply be called bufo, toad, or sapo (the Spanish word for toad). The toad excretes a form of DMT called 5-methoxy-N, N-dimethyltryptamine (5-MeO-DMT).

Some people have taken to harvesting the venom ducts from the toads, drying them, and then smoking them. Kinder practices involve people holding the toads gently while encouraging them to salivate onto a glass tile. A member of the Comcáac (aka Seri) tribe in Northern Mexico told me they tickle the toads, though I think he may have been joking with me. The venom on the tile is dried and then later scraped off and smoked. This preserves the life of the toad, which is a critical aspect of many Indigenous practices. While either method sounds disgusting, there is new research that indicates this version of DMT might become a useful future medication.

Most psychedelic sessions last a long time in comparison to traditional therapy; this makes it complex to try to offer these treatments in a medical or therapeutic setting. Most of the substances being investigated for their therapeutic benefits have fairly long effect windows. A psilocybin experience often lasts three to six hours. An MDMA experience can last five to eight hours. Ketamine, depending on its administration (oral, nasal, intramuscular injection, or IV), can last anywhere from two to four hours, and it could require multiple administrations. The 5-MeO-DMT or bufo experience is much shorter than that of psilocybin: the active period is less than an hour.

In an article in *Mexico News Daily*, Comcáac shaman Octavio Rettig Hinojosa, who practices traditional shamanism, described the experience of taking bufo as "anti-hallucinogenic." He declared that "it removes the madness from your mind, everything that removes you from the here and now, everything that is not real."[16] While it is possible to get bufo venom for sale, it is most effectively used in a ceremonial fashion. The Comcáac have been working with this medicine for a long time. They consider the toad a sacred partner, one they must protect. I had the privilege of participating in a bufo ceremony at the Comcáac reservation in Sonora, Mexico, in 2023. It was a deeply meaningful experience, and the feelings of overwhelming love and care I felt afterward have stayed with me to this day.

CHANGA

Changa is another form of DMT that is a combination of *Banisteriopsis caapi* leaves and other plants, which may or may not contain tryptamines or other psychoactive substances. It is sometimes mixed with tobacco. Changa was created through the inspiration of an Australian man named Julian Palmer, who asked for a vision during an ayahuasca ceremony in the early 2000s. Changa is smoked, and the psychedelic experience lasts less than an hour. It is very popular in modern shamanic practices, having been introduced to Western pilgrims who wanted to have a psychedelic experience. This is a related use of the *Banisteriopsis caapi* plant, one of the primary ingredients in ayahuasca. Changa is considered gentle when compared to some other versions of DMT.[17]

MESCALINE (SAN PEDRO)

Mescaline, also known as San Pedro, was once relatively well received in the psychology circles of the 19th and early 20th centuries. It quickly became popular with poets and artists. As a result, it didn't take too long for psychologists to reject it. The San Pedro cactus is the source of mescaline and should not be confused with peyote. However, its origins are similar, and there is evidence that mescaline has been used for more than 1,000 years by Indigenous peoples in Mexico and the southwestern United States.[18]

Mescaline is a naturally occurring alkaloid (3,4,5-trimethoxyphenethylamine). Some anthropologists date its use back more than 5,000 years. Mescaline is legal in some places, as it has been associated with the Native American Church since 1920. Its use has spread among different Indigenous groups over the last 100 years, with some reports of people indigenous to Canada adopting it for spiritual use. It has a similar mechanism of action to psilocybin, working on the serotonergic system in the brain. In a psychedelic ritual setting, mescaline causes a voyage that lasts between six and eight hours. Sojourners report seeing fractal patterns and changes in the perception of time. Mescaline is traditionally used in a ceremonial way similar to ayahuasca. A petitioner and other members of the community will partake of the parts of the cactus together and journey together. There is usually drumming and chanting throughout the time of the journey. Participants in these rituals report improvements in well-being and symptoms of depression and, in some instances, healing from addiction and resolution of grief.[19]

PEYOTE

Similar to mescaline, peyote is extracted from a cactus. While the San Pedro cactus is relatively robust and widely distributed, the peyote cactus is endangered and takes many years to cultivate. It is a relatively flat cactus with no spiny protections. The body of the cactus resembles a pumpkin or squat green gourd.

The flowering part of the peyote cactus grows where a pumpkin's stem would be.

Indigenous people from southern Texas and northern Mexico, where the peyote cactus grows natively, have been on a mission in recent years to protect it from Western psychedelic interests. It is a potent psychedelic whose use should be reserved for the people to whom it is sacred, especially given its endangered status.[20]

IBOGAINE

A psychedelic plant from Africa, ibogaine has become very popular in recent years due to the popularized idea that it provides a cure for addiction. Ibogaine can have many interactions that are unpleasant, including cardiac arrhythmias, nausea, and vomiting. It is currently being investigated in a handful of laboratories. Scientists in these labs have been working with the drug to isolate the active compounds. The experience of an ibogaine journey is almost never pleasant, unlike other psychedelics, which bring about an equal number of both challenging and positive experiences.[21]

Ibogaine experiences often share a theme of a life review. The person taking the journey has the experience of reviewing the hardest parts of their lives and making peace with trauma, illness, violence, and grief. One of the most inspiring effects of the ibogaine journey is that people who are in active addiction often describe their life before and after ibogaine. Before ibogaine, a drug like heroin is something that the patient craves and needs; it makes them feel better. After ibogaine, heroin feels different, and most patients report few to no withdrawal symptoms. Ibogaine is illegal in most countries, but it is a psychedelic of interest in many of the research proposals being brought before state governments.[22] A psychedelic that has a high rate of reliably treating and curing addiction is a rare unicorn indeed, one that we should dedicate our time to luring out of the shadows.

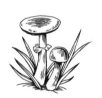

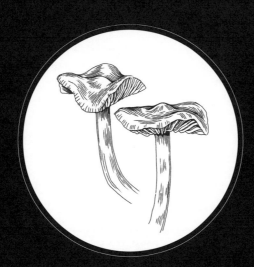

WAVY CAPS

CONCLUSION

THE FIELDS OF psychology, psychiatry, and psychopharmacology are all experiencing a radical shift in how they think about treating mental illness. The work of scientists, politicians, volunteers, agriculturalists, preservationists, mycologists, physicians, and anthropologists has opened up new doors to psychoactive substances, especially fungi that have the power to change our experience of mental illness and that could greatly increase our ability to bring relief to those suffering. Further, these drugs don't create a dependent state in their users like opiates, nor do they trim the capacity for feeling emotion like some SSRIs. Instead, when coupled with therapy or meaningful spiritual guidance, these substances can make greater, deeper meaning easier to tolerate. The capacity for greater feeling rather than less is one of the aspects of working with psychedelics that brings me the most satisfaction. My primary goal as a therapist is to help my patients feel their feelings without being broken by them. If any substance assists in that goal, it will have aided the profession and assisted in providing healing not just to the person I'm treating but to the generations who follow them.

If you are considering learning more, or if you would like to become trained in psychedelic psychotherapy, please connect with me and my practice online (admin@hope-therapy-center.com). We are actively developing retreats, trainings, and new psychedelic protocols so that when the rules change, we are ready to bring these new modalities to patients who need healing.

Psychedelics have changed the world many times, and this may be one of the first times that we are documenting the changes in real time. Whether we are discussing the mysteries of Eleusis, the visions of Maria Sabina, or the healing of a soldier's PTSD, the world shifts with psilocybin. It is a new application for an old technology. Psilocybin has the power to change your world, and when your world changes, it will shift from the inside out. Your experience of the world you live in will more closely align with your inner world. Your pain and trauma will find relief, and your capacity for love and empathy will expand. Mushrooms and mycelial networks are a great example of how life actually works. We are all connected, even if the connections are underground, and those connections are feeding us and making us stronger. We can't always see it clearly, but there is a great network that supports us all, and it is . . . us.

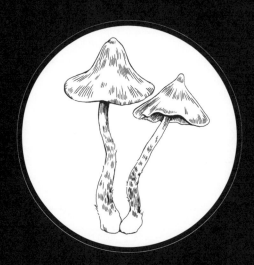

BADO

acknowledgments

ANY BOOK IS a labor of love, and this one is no different. My life has always been one of seeking, but psychedelics wasn't a topic I was interested in until becoming fascinated with neuroscience. Since going on the journey of depth psychotherapy over the last decade, psychedelics and altered states of consciousness have become central to my understanding of the psyche and the unconscious. This book would not have been possible without the love and support of my husband, Ched Hover; my dear friends Laura Voglesong, Patricia McGrath, Jane Henricksen, and Samuel C. Spitale; and my friend and colleague Jennie Marie Battistin. My writers group was instrumental in giving me the confidence to move forward—thank you Selene Castrovilla and all the members of the Writer's Pinnacle. I am deeply grateful to my agent, Mark Gottlieb, who encouraged me that a book on psychedelics was needed—you were right! A huge expression of gratitude to my editor, Joe Davidson, who read every word and made thoughtful edits and raised valuable questions, turning around big chunks of often very nerdy material in short order. Deep gratitude as well to my editorial assistant, Zoe Simmons-Mills, who helped me stay on top of the research and citations and advised me on the glossary contents. A deep debt of gratitude to the work of all the researchers who responded to questions and to those who opened the door to this new era, especially Kelly O'Donnell, Franz Vollenweider, Robin Carhart-Harris, the late Roland Griffiths, and my friend Will Van Deveer, who read the first draft and wrote the foreword. Words are not enough, and yet, somehow, words are everything. Thank you all!

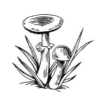

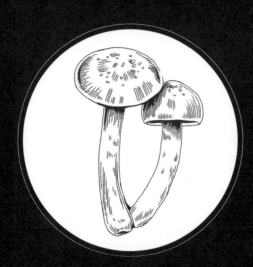

DR. WEIL'S

GLOSSARY

Acetylcholine: Acetylcholine is the primary neurotransmitter associated with activating neurons in the autonomic and peripheral nervous system.

Adrenaline (epinephrine): A hormone produced primarily in the adrenal glands (sometimes called epinephrine), adrenaline plays a critical impact in the regulation of the body and nervous system. It helps to prepare the body for dangerous or stressful situations. Some of the ways it does this are by signaling increases in heart rate, activating the stomach and intestines, and preparing muscles to contract. In addition, when adrenaline is active in the system, attention is increased, and the perception of pain is reduced. All of these activities assist in survival in dangerous situations.

Aeruginascin: This tryptamine is also known as N,N,N-trimethyl-4-phosphoryloxy-tryptamine. It naturally occurs in some mushroom species and produces effects similar to psilocin or psilocybin.

Agonist molecules: In a biological context an agonist facilitates the action of a neuron by activating the process of a neurotransmitter creating a bond at the synapse of a neuron. This process tells the neuron what to do.

Amatoxins: Amatoxins are a family of toxic chemicals that primarily target the liver. These compounds naturally occur in some mushroom species and can be fatal if ingested. They are commonly found in *Amanita phalloides* (Death Cap) and some species of *Galerina* mushrooms.

Amygdala: This almond-shaped structure in the brain is associated with emotional processing. The amygdalae (plural because it has two "halves" on either side of the corpus callosum in the brain) process emotional stimuli and communicate with other parts of the brain to help those signals make sense.

Amyloid tryptamine: These naturally occurring compounds are aggregates of alkaloid proteins with an indol core structure. In animals, the original source of the tryptamine comes from tryptophans found in the diet. Serotonin and melatonin are two essential tryptamines found in animals. There are more than 1,500 natural varieties of tryptamines, including psilocin, dimethyltryptamine, psilocybin, mescalin, and lysergic acid.

Anhedonia/anhedonic mood: The word *anhedonia* translates to "absent pleasure" and refers in psychology and psychiatry to the inability of someone to experience pleasure or happiness.

Antagonist molecules: In a biological context, an antagonist blocks the action of a neuron by inhibiting the process of activation. This process tells the neuron to stop.

Atropine: This naturally occurring compound is found in some plants like belladonna. Atropine is primarily used to counter anticholinergic poisoning and bradycardia and acts as antagonist for muscarine receptors, blocking the effects of acetylcholine.

Axon: The longest part of a nerve cell or neuron, the axon conducts the electrical signal from the neuronal cell body to the end of the nerve, called the axon terminal.

Ayahuasca: A concoction (tea-like drink) created by traditional healers in South America as a traditional psychiatric treatment for spiritual and psychological problems. The concoction is made with several plants known by native shamans, the most potent of which are the *Psychotria viridis* and the *Banisteriopsis caapi* plants.

Baeocystin: An amyloid tryptamine found in some psychedelic mushrooms, baeocystin is similar in structure to psilocin, though there has not been as much detailed research on this compound.

Basal ganglia: A part of the brain comprised of several structures that interconnect and communicate with each other and with other parts of your brain. They are deeply connected to movement and emotional control, especially with regard to inhibitory signals. Studies in recent years have revealed that the basal ganglia are much more complex than previously believed.

Body high: Traditionally associated with cannabis use, a body high refers to physical sensations that are usually relaxing and euphoric. However, with psilocybin, sometimes there can be an activation of all types of body sensations; these can feel tingly and energizing or calming and expansive, depending on the strain of mushrooms being consumed.

Brain-derived neurotropic factor (BDNF): This molecule found primarily in the brain is critical for memory and learning. Increased BDNF is also associated with reductions in inflammation and improved neuroplasticity and neurogenesis.

Central executive network (CEN): One of the key hubs of brain activity, the CEN is made up of parts of the prefrontal cortex and the parietal cortex. It is necessary for decision-making and goal-directed behavior. Decreased interaction between this hub and others is implicated in several psychiatric conditions, including schizophrenia, depression, and PTSD, to name a few. The CEN and default mode network (DMN) appear to have an inverse relationship; as one is activated, the other is reduced, and vice versa.

Cerebral cortex: This area is the outermost layer of the brain. It is responsible for activities like memory, learning, emotions, and sensory functions. Layers of the cortex are made of neurons and are frequently referred to as "gray matter" because of the color of the neurons. The folds of the cortex allow greater complexity in the connectivity and organization of the brain. The frontal lobe, parietal lobes, temporal lobes, and occipital lobes are all part of the cortex.

Cognitive behavioral therapy (CBT): This type of therapy is one of the most well-studied forms of psychotherapy in the world. The premise of CBT is that there is a dynamic relationship between thoughts, feelings, and behavior. The premise is that by changing one of these, a person can impact the other two. One of the hallmarks of CBT is learning to observe thoughts so that a person can have an influence on their feelings, behaviors, and beliefs. By making decisions about a thought or feeling, the person observing the thought has greater control.

Coprophilic: This means liking poop or feces. In discussing mushrooms, coprophilic species often grow in or around feces dropped by animals.

Corpus callosum: A thick, subcortical bundle of nerve fibers that connects the two hemispheres of the brain. The corpus callosum helps the brain to communicate more efficiently. A strong corpus callosum helps to provide greater neuroplasticity to the brain; for example, people with a robust corpus callosum have better recovery from some kinds of brain injuries. Damage to the corpus callosum can create many problems, including visual disturbances, speech problems, and difficulty retrieving memories.

Cortical hierarchies: The brain appears to work by organizing its functions according to hierarchies that prioritize its functions based on need, sequence, memory, threat, and action. Processing of stimuli and other forms of information are determined by these hierarchies. There are also developmental hierarchies that continue to be studied in an effort to determine the ways that these change over the lifespan.

Corticotropin releasing hormone: The primary regulating hormone of the hypothalmus-pituitary-adrenal axis. This hormone is key in regulating the body's response to stress.

Cortisol: This hormone is the body's primary stress hormone. It is secreted by the adrenal glands. Long-term, chronic cortisol release is often seen in PTSD. Research has shown that prolonged exposure to cortisol may increase inflammation in several parts of the body, including the brain, reducing the efficacy of the hormone and negatively impacting neurogenesis and neuroplasticity.

Cyclothymia: Cyclothymia is a milder presentation of bipolar disorder marked by mild, hypomanic symptoms and milder depressive episodes. Some people with this disorder don't even know that they have any psychiatric issues.

Default mode network (DMN): A hub of activity that is activated when the brain lacks a cognitive task. It is implicated in rumination and in disorders characterized by negative self-talk. Parts of the DMN include the medial prefrontal cortex (mPFC), the posterior cingulate cortex (PCC), and the middle temporal lobe.

Dendrite: These tiny projections off the cell body of a neuron receive the signal from the axons of other neurons.

Diploid: A diploid cell has two complete sets of chromosomes, with each set being contributed by one parent.

Dopamine: This critical neurotransmitter is implicated when something feels good, rewarding, or pleasurable. Sometimes called "the molecule of more," dopamine regulation is critical to the brain functioning properly. Scientists have known for many years that excess dopamine is found in certain disorders like schizophrenia. Too little dopamine is associated with some disorders like attention deficit hyperactivity disorder (ADHD) and depression.

Dorsal attention network (DAN): This network hub in the brain is associated with visual attention and goal-directed behavior. Reductions in connectivity with the DAN are implicated in disorders like ADHD and depression.

Downregulation: The process by which the body normalizes its relationship with a substance or chemical by reducing its natural production of or affinity for those compounds is called downregulation.

Entheogens: Literally translated as "bringing the God within," the term has come to describe psychedelic medicines generally and usually refers to naturally occurring substances like mushrooms or DMT rather than laboratory-generated compounds like LSD or MDMA.

Entropic brain theory: This theory, originated by neuroscientist Robin Carhart-Harris, says that the brain will seek a higher state of entropy when it is in the presence of psychedelics. This is achieved by a reduction in orchestration of the brain's networks, most clearly achieved by reducing the impact of the default mode network.

Epinephrine: See *adrenaline*.

Ethnomycologist: An ethnomycologist is a scientist who studies mushrooms in the context of cultural use, significance, and intergenerational knowledge and transmission.

Flush: A crop of mushrooms is called a flush.

Fluvoxamine: See *selective serotonin reuptake inhibitors*.

Frontal cortex: This part of the brain in the front of the skull is one of the most highly developed areas of the brain in humans, who have a higher concentration of neurons in this part of the brain than most other mammals. The frontal cortex is responsible for orchestrating thought, memory, logic, and other complex cognitive processes. It is associated with personality traits. Damage to the frontal cortex often results in significant changes to personality, memory, and the ability to remember, reason, and make decisions.

GABA: This inhibitory neurotransmitter blocks impulses in the neurons of the brain. Most often GABA inhibits neurons that had been activated with the agonist glutamate.

Genus (plural: genera): Genus is a taxonomic category that falls between species and family. Members of a genus share common characteristics or genetics.

Glutamate: This neurotransmitter is the most widely distributed and used in the brain. It is the primary excitatory neurotransmitter in the nervous system.

Gut-brain axis: This complex system consists of the microbiome of bacteria in the gut/enteric system and the serotonergic connections in the brain. These two systems appear to communicate bidirectionally via serotonin pathways activated in the gut that then provide feedback to the serotonin systems in the brain.

Haploid: A haploid cell has only one set of chromosomes contributed by one parent. These are typically the reproductive cells that will eventually combine to become a new organism.

Heterogeneous: Heterogeneous means having very different constituent parts or having different consistencies.

Hippocampus: The hippocampus is a subcortical part of the brain necessary for the formation and retrieval of memory. It gets its name from its shape, which looks like a seahorse.

Hymenium: The layer of a mushroom structure that holds the reproductive spores.

Hyphae: These are the nutrient-seeking and reproductive structures of the mushroom.

The hyphae expand from the spores during the reproductive phase, each hypha seeking a partner to fuse with. Once the hyphae expand, they will fuse and form mycelia that will feed the overall mushroom structure.

Hyphal knot: Once two hyphae fuse, the mushroom reproductive process begins. A hyphal knot is the first aspect of the reproductive cycle where the mushroom begins to take form.

Hypothalamic-pituitary-adrenal (HPA) axis: The hypothalamus, pituitary gland, and adrenal glands work together in coordination in the regulation of the body's response to stress. When the HPA axis is not functioning properly, or when it has been in a state of chronic activation, the body may demonstrate problems like loss of cortical volume in the brain.

Ibogaine: This psychedelic is one of the only ones found natively in Africa. Ibogaine is made from the roots of the *Tabernanthe iboga* shrub. It has been widely hailed as very helpful in treating addiction.

Inner healing intelligence (IHI): Psychedelic psychotherapists coined this term to discuss the unconscious direction of healing processes of the psyche. In the same way that the body's defenses unconsciously direct physical healing processes when there is an injury to the body, so too the body appears to direct healing of the mind/psyche/psychological self in the presence of psychedelics.

Integration process: In psychotherapy and other transformative processes, integration is a critical component. Integration takes the content and insights gained in the medicine session or other transformative process and works through them, helping the person to make sense of the insights and connecting them to meaningful events and feelings. Integration is similar to learning a new vocabulary word. Once learned, integration is the experience of using the new word in day-to-day language.

Interleukin: Interleukins are one type of a group of proteins known as cytokines that are expressed as part of immune response. Interleukin is an indicator of the expression of white blood cells and is often present when there is significant inflammation.

Intrasynaptic space: The space in between the synapses of the neuronal architecture is called the intrasynaptic space.

Lateral temporal cortex: The lateral temporal cortex is the upper part of the cortex associated with the temporal lobe. There is one on each side (hemisphere) of the brain. Many important functions are coordinated in this part of the brain, from emotions to social cognition.

Limbic system: This is a subcortical network hub in the brain that connects several parts of the brain focused on defenses and drives, from food to sex to the ability to defend against threats. Some of the parts that make up the limbic system are the amygdala, the hippocampus, and the hypothalamus.

Mass spectrometry: This analytical technique is used to identify chemical compounds. The process measures the weight and speed of ions to identify the chemical constituents.

Medial prefrontal cortex (mPFC): This hub in the brain sits at the most distal part of the prefrontal cortex. New research identifies it as coordinating a great deal of our behavior and thought processes. It is implicated primarily in self-referential thought, helping us to integrate ourselves into experiences with others and consider the connection of our individual selves with the social world.

Memory consolidation: This neuropsychological process translates experience into stable memory. Certain brain structures like the hippocampus are necessary for this process. In addition, there are time and process dependencies that are necessary for this set of tasks. Sleep is considered necessary for proper memory consolidation. There are some hypothetical possibilities that a psychedelic experience could also assist in memory consolidation in a manner similar to sleep.

Mendelian inheritance: This was one of the first theories of how traits are passed from parents to their offspring. Gregor Mendel was a monk who learned about inheritance by examining the flowers of pea plants in his garden. He first wrote about his findings in 1865. His discoveries were the precursor to modern genetics.

Metabolites: A metabolite is any compound, molecule, or substance that is a product of or results from the digestive/metabolic process.

Microdosing: The practice of using a very low dose of a substance for a mild or nominal clinical effect is called microdosing. In psychedelics, a microdose refers to a small dose that produces no psychedelic effect but may have an effect that improves mood.

Monoamine: A monoamine is a chemical compound that has only one amino acid group, a carbon chain, and an aromatic group. Typically in animals these are neurotransmitters (serotonin, adrenaline, etc.) or analogs of neurotransmitters (psilocybin, psilocin).

Muscimol: The primary psychoactive compound in the classic psychedelic mushroom *Amanita muscaria*. This compound is a powerful GABA agonist. It can produce hallucinations but also can make people sleepy.

Mycelium: The mycelium is the branching part of the mushroom that resembles a root system but acts like an external digestive system, breaking down nutrients and connecting species. Mycelial networks are necessary for life on earth, as they break down other organisms so that the molecular components can be recycled in nature.

Neural correlates: In research studies on the brain, the neural correlates are those parts of the brain that can be associated with either a functional behavior or a structural component. In looking for a neural correlate of emotions for example, a functional MRI image might show a higher concentration of activity in the amygdala or temporal lobes. These areas would be considered the neural correlates of the emotional state being studied.

Neurochemical: Processes that influence the chemistry of the brain and/or nervous system generally are called neurochemical.

Neurogenesis: The process of developing new neurons or neural parts is called neurogenesis. Neurogenesis can be as comprehensive as the growth of an entirely new neuron or can be concentrated in certain neuronal structures like axons, dendrites, and synapses.

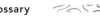

Neuromodulating compounds: These chemicals are important to the proper functioning of neurons and receptors but may not act on the activation or deactivation process.

Neuropeptide: A neuropeptide is a molecule of small-chain amino acids. They can act as signaling molecules in the central nervous system, meaning that they can behave similarly to neurotransmitters.

Neuroplasticity: This term refers to the brain's ability to reconfigure network connections, grow new neurons, and reorganize or reprioritize connections across the cortex and subcortical brain structures.

Neurotransmitter: These molecules act as chemical messengers between neurons. They initiate the nerve impulses and help direct the task of the neuron based on the signal.

Nondirective therapy: This model of therapy keeps the focus on the client's process without guiding the client in a particular direction or toward a specific goal. This is especially important in working with psychedelics, as the direction of the therapy and integration should be orchestrated by the client's inner healing intelligence.

Norepinephrine: Also called noradrenaline, norepinephrine is a hormone that can also act as a neurotransmitter. It is released in the body in response to stress.

Norpsilocin: Norpsilocin is a recently discovered tryptamine that is more potent than psilocin. This compound is an analog of serotonin that has a much stronger effect on neurons in the nervous system.

Nucleus accumbens: This subcortical structure in the brain is part of the basal ganglia and helps to regulate attention, motivation, and reward.

Papillate: Papillate means similar to the shape of a nipple.

Pellicle: A thin film or membrane found on the exterior cap of some mushrooms is called a pellicle.

Peripheral nervous system: The peripheral nervous system consists of the nerves that extend from the brain and spinal cord and connect to all of the other enervated structures in the body.

Phallotoxins: Phallotoxins are a type of toxic molecules found in some mushrooms of the *Amanita* and *Galerina* species.

Phylogenetic: This means relating to the study of evolution, nomenclature, and organization of different species.

Posterior cingulate cortex (PCC): This part of the brain is considered a central part of the default mode network (DMN) and is connected to multiple other hubs in the brain.

Prefrontal cortex (PFC): This part of the brain most distinguishes humans from other animals. The PFC is responsible for cognitive thought, planning, logic, and some aspects of personality, especially those regulated by inhibition and moderating behavior.

Primordial: Primordial means the beginning of a phase or era, a time of newness.

Prodrug: A prodrug is a substance that is inert before it is metabolized but transitions to an active compound once it goes through a metabolic change.

Pseudorhiza: An extension from the base of a mushroom's stipe that resembles, but has a different function from the roots of, a plant. The pseudorhiza helps to ground the stipe and may aid in conducting water.

Psilocin: The active tryptamine that is metabolized in the human body from psilocybin, and which appears in its pure form in some mushroom species. Psilocin is not as stable a molecule as psilocybin.

Psilocybin: A prodrug tryptamine found in psychedelic mushrooms. The body metabolizes psilocybin into psilocin.

Psychedelic-assisted psychotherapy: The process of using a psychedelic substance as a catalyst for the therapeutic process. Psychedelic-assisted psychotherapy sessions usually include preparation, medicine, and integration sessions as part of the overall process.

Psychedelic tourism: Tourist experiences based on the ability to engage in (usually legal) psychedelic experiences as part of their appeal are called psychedelic tourism. In recent years this has mostly been built on ayahuasca experiences but has grown to include other psychedelics.

Psychodynamic orientation: This theoretical perspective in psychology and psychiatry is concerned with the interplay between the conscious and the unconscious. It highlights ways of engaging with the unconscious that often extend beyond talk therapy, such as through art, creativity, symbolism, and dreams.

Psychonaut: A psychonaut is a person who is going on the inner journey of the psyche. This often refers to someone who is engaging in a psychedelic practice, but it isn't limited to psychedelics. It can be true of people engaged in other forms of inducing an altered state of consciousness, such as breath work or trance.

Psychosomatic: In recent years this term has come to mean far deeper things than it has in years previous. Prior to the development of somatic psychology, a psychosomatic symptom or illness was often synonymous with imaginary. Recent work has shifted this perspective to mean that something happening on the soma (body) level is being activated by or in response to the psyche or mind.

Psychotropic: Usually, this term is used in describing medication. A psychotropic medication typically is a drug that has an effect on the brain, or behavior.

Recreational use: When a medication is used occasionally for fun or diversion, it is often described as "recreational" use. This differs from medical treatment, self-medication, or abuse.

Salience network: This brain hub is believed to be primarily focused on integrating internal and external stimuli, and managing the switching between the DMN and the CEN. Research into this area is in the early stages.

Selective serotonin reuptake inhibitor (SSRI): SSRIs are a class of drugs used to treat depression and anxiety. Their primary mechanism of action is in slowing down the serotonin reuptake cycle in the synaptic area of neurons.

Sensorimotor system: This network is responsible for both the motor functions and sensory functions of an organism. It relies on a hierarchy of neuronal networks in the central and peripheral nervous systems to help make sense of information and give it meaning so that the organism knows how to initiate, move through, and respond to stimuli.

Serotonergic: Serotonergic means relating to the serotonin production and receptors of the nervous system.

Serotonin: Also called 5-hydroxytryptamine (5-HT), this neurotransmitter is one of the most important in the nervous system. Multiple subtypes of serotonin and serotonin receptors are used in the nervous system. Serotonin is used most frequently in the brain, the gut, and the heart.

Shaman: This word has roots in anthropology and was originally used to describe the role of a mystical practitioner among Indigenous Siberians. However, the word has become synonymous with a person in almost any Indigenous culture who interacts with the spirit world. Controversially, in the last several years, many Westerners have begun adopting the term to describe anyone who is skilled or educated in how to use and guide others in the use of psychedelics.

Sojourner: A sojourner is a person on a voyage, a seeker. See also *psychonaut*.

Spore print: A critical part of mushroom identification, spore prints are used to identify and differentiate species of mushrooms. Once made, they can be used to grow mushrooms from the spores.

Subclinical presentation: When a symptom, illness, or disorder doesn't cause sufficient impairment to register in a clinical examination or test, it is called subclinical presentation.

Substrate: The element or environment where an organism lives and feeds itself is a substrate. For mushrooms, this is the environment where the mycelia grows as it seeks nutrients.

Synapse: The gaps between neurons where the chemical signals pass via neurotransmitters are called synapses. The full area of the synapse is made up of the synaptic cleft, the presynaptic terminal, and the receiving dendrite of the next cell.

Synaptic cleft: This is a small area between the presynaptic and postsynaptic areas where neurotransmitters concentrate so that they can be used by the neuron.

Synthesis: The production of complex molecular compounds from simpler substances or chemicals is called synthesis.

Temporal lobe(s): There is one temporal lobe on each side (hemisphere) of the brain, located near the temples and ears. It is primarily associated with auditory and emotional processing.

Temporal-parietal junction (TPJ): This part of the brain is where the temporal and parietal lobes meet. Language, social learning, and a sense of self are associated with this part of the brain.

Thalamus: This subcortical part of the brain regulates and coordinates numerous relationships in the brain and plays a central role in consciousness, immune system regulation, motor functions, and more.

Titration: The process by which concentrations of chemicals are changed and regulated in any system is called titration.

Translational research: This form of research is dedicated to taking basic science (referring to science purely for the sake of discovery) and translating it into forms with real-world applications.

Underground therapist/practitioner: This is someone who may be a trained therapist or a lay practitioner who is working outside of the legal structures that regulate medical and psychological practice. For the most part this refers to practitioners who are working with psychedelics in places where those substances are not (yet) legal.

Valvulopathy: Valvulopathy refers to diseases that affect the valves of the heart. This can reflect the valves not working properly due to a mechanical problem or disease process.

Ventral tegmental area (VTA): This area of the brain is implicated in the development of the dopamine system; as such, it is connected to the reward system in the brain.

Vermiculite: Vermiculite is a substance used in some fertilizers and substrates to assist in the retention of moisture.

Whole self/deep self: In some forms of psychological theory or practice, the whole or deep self is considered a fundamental aspect of the psyche or mind. It is considered a higher form of the self that is affected by and has an effect on the conscious and the unconscious. It is separate from the persona, or the aspect of self that is presented in the day-to-day experience of life. It is also separate from the ego structures that help the person identify and differentiate from others. It is often considered the goal of psychotherapy to make a more clear path between the whole or deep self and the persona and/or ego.

NOTES

INTRODUCTION

1 Hofmann et al. (1958), 107–109.
2 Wasson (1957, May 13).
3 Bragagnolo (2023, March 8).

1. A BRIEF HISTORY OF MUSHROOMS AND PSYCHEDELICS

1 Calder & Hasler (2023); Calder et al. (2013).
2 Graves (1960); Samorini & Camilla (1995).
3 Martin (2004, February 22).
4 Martin (2004, February 22).
5 Miller, G. (n.d.).
6 Roberts (1997).
7 Shipley (2014).
8 Doblin et al. (2019).
9 Doblin et al. (2019).
10 Mitchell et al. (2023).
11 Strassman (1996).
12 Vollenweider et al. (1998).
13 Griffiths, Johnson, et al. (2016).
14 Johnson, Garcia-Romeu, Cosimano & Griffiths (2014).
15 Griffiths, Hurwitz, et al. (2019).

2. MUSHROOMS AS MEDICINE

1 American Psychiatric Association (2022).
2 Jones & Graff-Radford (2021).
3 Twomey (2010).
4 Haber & Robbins (2022).
5 Preuss & Wise (2022).
6 Raichle et al. (2001, January 16).
7 Shulman et al. (1997).
8 Foster, B. L., et al. (2023).
9 Leech & Sharp (2014).
10 Domínguez-Borràs & Vuilleumier (2022).

11 Domínguez-Borràs & Vuilleumier (2022).
12 Anand & Dhikav (2012).
13 Kiernan (2012).
14 Carhart-Harris, Leech, Hellyer, et al. (2014).
15 Carhart-Harris, Leech, Hellyer, et al. (2014); Carhart-Harris (2018); Carhart-Harris & Friston (2019).
16 Carhart-Harris, Leech, Hellyer, et al. (2014).
17 Daws et al. (2022).
18 Carhart-Harris (2018).
19 Daws et al. (2022).
20 DiSabato et al. (2016).
21 National Institute of Mental Health (n.d.-b).
22 American Psychiatric Association (2022).
23 Akil et al. (2018).
24 Goodwin et al. (2022).
25 Goodwin et al. (2022).
26 Gukasyan et al. (2022).
27 Carhart-Harris, Giribaldi, et al. (2021).
28 Carhart-Harris, Giribaldi, et al. (2021).
29 Carhart-Harris, Giribaldi, et al. (2021).
30 Wall et al. (2023).
31 Wall et al. (2023).
32 Korr & Schmitz (1999).
33 Toda et al. (2019).
34 Toda et al. (2019); Aimone et al. (2010).
35 Aimone et al. (2010); Leschik et al. (2021).
36 De Gregorio et al. (2021).
37 Hesselgrave et al. (2021).
38 Mason et al. (2020).
39 Calder & Hasler (2023).
40 *Psychology Today* (n.d.); Hayes et al. (1999).
41 Fernández-Rodríguez et al. (2018).

42 Zeifman et al. (2023).
43 Zeifman et al. (2023).
44 Zeifman et al. (2023).
45 van Elk & Snoek (2020); Monroy & Keltner (2023).
46 Griffiths, Richards, et al. (2006).
47 Zhang et al. (2022).
48 Mans et al. (2021).
49 Griffiths, Johnson, et al. (2016).
50 Nayak & Griffiths (2022).
51 Griffiths, Hurwitz, et al. (2019).

3. MUSHROOM ANATOMY
1 Stamets (2011).
2 Wu et al. (2019).
3 McKernan et al. (2021).

4. MUSHROOM ENVIRONMENTS
1 Haard & Haard (1977).
2 Haze & Mandrake (2016).
3 Stamets (2000).

5. WORKING WITH MUSHROOMS
1   Carey (2019, September 4).
2   Siebert (2021, February 25).
3   Garcia-Romeu et al. (2021).
4   Garcia-Romeu et al. (2021).
5   Fadiman (2011).
6   Lea et al. (2020).
7   Kuypers et al. (2019).
8   Johnstad (2018); Ross (2019).
9   Hasler et al. (2004).
10 Rootman, Kiraga, et al. (2022).
11 Hartong & van Emmerik (2023).
12 Grind & Bindley (2023, June 27).
13 Mikhail (2023, June 27).
14 Prochazkova et al. (2018).
15 Prochazkova et al. (2018).
16 Rootman, Kiraga, et al. (2022).

17 Yale Center for Clinical Investigation (n.d.).
18 Fadiman (2011).
19 McIntyre (2023).
20 McIntyre (2023); Thomas, K. (2022, April 13).
21 Surapaneni et al. (2011).
22 McIntyre (2023).

6. VARIETIES OF MUSHROOMS
1   Thomas, K. (2022, April 13); McIntyre (2023).
2   Holtzheimer & Mayberg (2011).
3   Mason et al. (2020).
4   Calder & Hasler (2023).
5   Mastinu et al. (2023).
6   Oughli et al. (2021).
7   Beug & Bigwood (1981).
8   Strauss et al. (2022).
9   Stamets (1996); Bauer (2018, December 21).
10 Cooke (2021, September 12).
11 Zoomies Canada (2023, July 31).
12 Beatrice Society (2022, December 22).
13 Perez (2022, June 12).
14 Perez (2022, June 12).
15 Cooke (2021, September 12).
16 Perez (2022, June 12).
17 Fun Guys (n.d.).
18 Micro Zoomers (n.d.-a).
19 Cooke (2021, September 12).
20 Guy (2021, June 29).
21 Cooke (2021, September 12).
22 Shāfaa (n.d.).
23 McElroy (2023, June 18).
24 Shāfaa (n.d.).
25 Simms (2022, July 9).
26 Cooke (2021, September 12).
27 Guy (2021, June 25).
28 Cooke (2021, September 12).

29 Cooke (2021, September 12).
30 Guy (2021, May 13).
31 Perez (2022, June 12).
32 Cooke (2022, March 10).
33 Perez (2022, June 12).
34 Guy (2021, June 11).
35 Guy (2021, June 11).
36 Cooke (2021, September 12).
37 Pallay (2022, March 7); Frshminds (2021, August 1).
38 Lubiano (2022, June 1).
39 Pilger (2023, August 28).
40 Lubiano (2022, June 1).
41 Lubiano (2022, June 1).
42 Stamets (2011).
43 Stamets (1996).
44 Stamets (1996).
45 Stamets (1996).
46 Strauss et al. (2022).
47 Merlin & Allen (1993).
48 Stamets (1996).
49 Perez (2022, June 12).
50 Alchimia (n.d.).
51 Stamets (1996).
52 Barlow (2021, August 17).
53 Leung & Paul (1968).
54 Glatfelter et al. (2022).
55 Barlow (2021, August 17).
56 Perez (2022, June 12).
57 Alchimia (n.d.).
58 Stamets (1996).
59 Mandrake (2023, April 20).
60 Cooke (2021, September 12); Leung & Paul (1968).
61 Stamets (1996).
62 Stamets (1996).
63 See https://doubleblindmag.com/psilocybe-cyanescens/.
64 Beck (2021).
65 McElroy (2023, June 20).
66 Stamets (1996).
67 Omissi (2016).
68 Stamets & Gartz (1995).
69 McElroy (2023, January 24).
70 Barlow (2020, July 30).
71 Cooke (2021, September 12).
72 Cooke (2021, September 12).
73 Stamets (1996).
74 Borovička, Oborník, et al. (2015); Mandrake (2023, April 13).
75 Cooke (2021, September 12).
76 Stamets (1996).
77 Cooke (2021, September 12).
78 Stamets (1996).
79 Heim & Hofmann (1958); Stamets (1996).
80 McKenna (1992).
81 Diaz (1977).
82 Cooke (2021, September 12).
83 Stamets (1996).
84 Stamets (1996).
85 Barlow (2021, August 31).
86 Cooke (2021, September 12).
87 Guy (2023, August 7).
88 Diaz (1977).
89 Mérida Ponce et al. (2019).
90 Cooke (2021, September 12).
91 Stamets (1996).
92 Stamets (1996).
93 Cooke (2021, September 12).
94 Guy (2021, September 7).
95 Stamets (1996).
96 Musha et al. (1988).
97 Matsushima et al. (2009).
98 Matsushima et al. (2009).
99 Guzmán et al. (1991).
100 Stamets (1996).
101 Cooke (2021, September 12).
102 Stamets (1996).
103 The Global Fungal Red List Initiative (n.d.).

104 Diaz (1977).
105 Stamets (1996).
106 Guzmán, Allen & Gartz (1998).
107 Stamets (1996).
108 Cooke (2021, September 12).
109 Shroomery (n.d.-b).
110 Stamets (1996).
111 Stamets (1996).
112 Guzman (1978a).
113 van de Peppel et al. (2022).
114 Cooke (2021, September 12); Stamets (1996).
115 Guzmán & Bas (1977).
116 Stamets (1996).
117 Stamets (1996).
118 Bastos et al. (2023).
119 McKenna (1992).
120 Stamets (1996).
121 Mandrake (2023, April 13).
122 Stamets (1996).
123 Mandrake (2023, April 13).
124 Moser & Horak (1968).
125 Stamets (1996).
126 Guzmán, Ott, et al. (1976).
127 Strauss et al. (2022).
128 Borovička, Oborník, et al. (2015).
129 Stamets (1996).
130 Chang & Mills (1992).
131 Puls (n.d.).
132 Barlow (2021, November 4).
133 Singer & Smith (1958a).
134 Stamets (1996).
135 Stamets (1996).
136 Rockefeller (2013).
137 Stamets (1996).
138 Hausknecht et al. (2004).
139 Cooke (2021, September 12).
140 Stamets (1996).
141 Stamets (1996).
142 Dias (2023, August 14).

143 Kendrick (2000).
144 Jo et al. (2014).
145 National Audubon Society (2023); Dickinson & Lucas (1979).
146 First Nature (n.d.).
147 National Audubon Society (2023).
148 Wieczorek et al. (2015).
149 McKnight et al. (2021).
150 Kendrick (2000).
151 Phillips (2005).
152 Stamets (1996).
153 Besl (1993).
154 Enjalbert et al. (2004).
155 *Galerina—The Genera and Species from A to Z* (n.d.).
156 Gulden, Dunham & Stockman (2001).
157 McKnight et al. (2021).
158 Stamets (1996).
159 Patocka et al. (2021).
160 Bresinsky & Besl (1989).
161 Raufman et al. (2008).
162 Hausknecht & Krisai-Greilhuber (2007).
163 Hausknecht, Krisai-Greilhuber & Voglmayr (2004).
164 Stamets (1996).

7. MEDICINAL USES FOR MUSHROOMS

1   Zhu et al. (2022).
2   Cuthbert (2022).
3   Nestler et al. (2002).
4   Köhler, S., et al. (2016).
5   de la Cruz et al. (2021).
6   Carhart-Harris, Leech, Hellyer, et al. (2014).
7   Nunez (2016).
8   Marstaller et al. (2020).
9   Carhart-Harris, Leech, Hellyer, et al. (2014).
10 Salvat-Pujol et al. (2017).
11 Smith & Vale (2006).

12 Dunlavey (2018).
13 Wang et al. (2021).
14 Catlow et al. (2013).
15 Banskota et al. (2019).
16 Banskota et al. (2019).
17 Dayabandara et al. (2017).
18 Berlucchi & Marzi (2019).
19 Cozolino (2017).
20 van der Kolk (2014).
21 Wall et al. (2023).
22 Radiolab (2022, June 30).
23 Mentlein & Kendall (2000).
24 Jairaj, Fitzsimons, et al. (2019).
25 Jairaj & Rucker (2022).
26 Cheng et al. (2022).
27 Jairaj & Rucker (2022).
28 Crocq & Crocq (2000).
29 Jones, E. (2023).
30 Krediet et al. (2020).
31 Fernández-Rodríguez et al. (2018).
32 Etkin & Wager (2007).
33 American Psychiatric Association (2022).
34 Krediet et al. (2020).
35 Smith & Vale (2006).
36 Lanius et al. (2006).
37 Van Overwalle (2009).
38 Krediet et al. (2020).
39 Carhart-Harris (2018).
40 National Institute of Mental Health (n.d.-a).
41 de la Mora et al. (2015).
42 American Psychiatric Association (2022).
43 Griffiths, Johnson, et al. (2016).
44 DeYoung (2010).
45 Goldstein et al. (2020).
46 MacLean et al. (2011).
47 Kiraga et al. (2022).
48 Felsch & Kuypers (2022).
49 Borasio (2011).
50 Agin-Liebes et al. (2020).
51 Griffiths, Johnson, et al. (2016).
52 Marchese (2023, April 7).
53 Moskowitz & Weiselberg (2017).
54 Via et al. (2018).
55 Ledwos et al. (2023).
56 Kaye (2022).
57 Lucherini Angeletti et al. (2022).
58 McAdams & Smith (2015).
59 Peck et al. (2023).
60 Moreno et al. (2006).
61 Moreno (2023).
62 Kelmendi (2023); Kelmendi et al. (2022).
63 Kelmendi et al. (2022).
64 Kelmendi et al. (2022).
65 Bogenschutz et al. (2022).
66 Bogenschutz et al. (2022).
67 Noorani et al. (2018).
68 Johnson, Garcia-Romeu & Griffiths (2017).
69 Johnson, Garcia-Romeu, Cosimano & Griffiths (2014).
70 Noorani et al. (2018).
71 Jones, G., et al. (2022).
72 Centers for Disease Control and Prevention (2023, August 8).
73 Pisano et al. (2017).
74 Jones, G., et al. (2022).
75 Oughli et al. (2021).
76 Johns Hopkins University (2023).
77 Kinderlehrer (2023).
78 Zeidan (2023).
79 Collins et al. (2018).
80 Zeidan (2023).
81 Schindler et al. (2021).
82 Schindler (2022).
83 McAlonan (2022).
84 McAlonan (2022).
85 Katsnelson (2022, May 31).
86 Lyes et al. (2023).
87 Watson (2022).

88 Goel et al. (2023).

89 Ablin et al. (2016).

90 Ablin et al. (2016).

91 Glynos et al. (2023).

92 Glynos et al. (2023).

93 Posada-Quintero et al. (2019).

94 Nikolič et al. (2023).

95 Froese, Leenen & Palenicek (2018).

96 University of Chicago (2023).

97 Morton et al. (2023).

98 Morton et al. (2023).

99 Vollenweider et al. (1998).

100 Carhart-Harris, Leech, Erritzoe, et al. (2013).

101 Nebigil et al. (2003).

102 Rothman et al. (2000).

8. MUSHROOMS, PSYCHEDELICS, AND THE LAW

1   Gunther (2023, June 1).

2   Blickman (n.d.).

3   Government of Canada (n.d.).

4   Treaster (1994, May 7).

5   Foster (2023, November 14).

6   Culver & Kravarik (2022, November 4).

7   Kenney (2023, July 4).

8   Kenney (2023, June 21a).

9   Kenney (2023, June 21b).

10 Zavala (2023, September 8).

11 Sosa (2023, October 7).

12 Illinois General Assembly (n.d.).

13 Kansas State Legislature (2022).

14 McLeod (2022, April 12).

15 Jacobs (2021, November 11).

16 MND Staff (2021, July 20).

17 Lewis-Healey (2021, May 25).

18 May (1999, October).

19 Abbott, A. (2019).

20 ScienceDirect (n.d.).

21 Oaklander (2021, April 5).

22 Rodríguez-Cano et al. (2023).

BIBLIOGRAPHY

Abbott, A. (2019). Altered minds: Mescaline's complicated history. *Nature, 569*(7757), 485–486. https://doi.org/10.1038/d41586-019-01571-2

Abbott, B., and Hernandez, D. (2023, June 27). As psychedelics become more mainstream, here's what you need to know. *Wall Street Journal*. https://www.wsj.com/articles/psychedelics-ketamine-lsd-drug-what-to-know-d552ee9c

Ablin, J. N., Zohar, A. H., Zaraya-Blum, R., and Buskila, D. (2016). Distinctive personality profiles of fibromyalgia and chronic fatigue syndrome patients. *PeerJ, 4*, e2421. https://doi.org/10.7717/peerj.2421

Academic Accelerator (n.d.). *Panaeolus Cambodginiensis:* Most Up-to-Date Encyclopedia, News & Reviews. Retrieved October 12, 2023, from https://academic-accelerator.com/encyclopedia/panaeolus-cambodginiensis

Agin-Liebes, G. I., Malone, T., Yalch, M. M., et al. (2020). Long-term follow-up of psilocybin-assisted psychotherapy for psychiatric and existential distress in patients with life-threatening cancer. *Journal of Psychopharmacology, 34*(2), 155–166. https://doi.org/10.1177/0269881119897615

Aimone, J. B., Deng, W., and Gage, F. H. (2010). Adult neurogenesis: Integrating theories and separating functions. *Trends in Cognitive Sciences, 14*(7), 325–337. https://doi.org/10.1016/j.tics.2010.04.003

Akil, H., Gordon, J., Hen, R., et al. (2018). Treatment resistant depression: A multi-scale, systems biology approach. *Neuroscience and Biobehavioral Reviews, 84*, 272–288. https://doi.org/10.1016/j.neubiorev.2017.08.019

Alchimia. (n.d.). Differences between *Panaeolus cyanescens* (Hawaiian *Copelandia*) and *Psilocybe cubensis*. Retrieved June 17, 2023, from https://www.alchimiaweb.com/blogen/differences-panaeolus-cyanescens-hawaiian-copelandia-psilocybe-cubensis/

Allen-Kiersons, C. (2022, September 7). *Psilocybe cyanescens* (the wavy cap) is one of the most potent psychedelic fungi. Beatrice Society. https://beatricesociety.com/psilocybe-cyanescens-the-wavy-cap-is-one-of-the-most-potent-psychedelic-fungi-2/

Allitt, M. (2023, January 16). 5 Best Strains of Magic Mushrooms. Third Wave. https://thethirdwave.co/top-five-strains-of-magic-mushrooms/

Amer, T., and Davachi, L. (2023). Extra-hippocampal contributions to pattern separation. *eLife, 12*, e82250. https://doi.org/10.7554/eLife.82250

American Psychiatric Association. (2022). *Diagnostic and statistical manual of mental disorders* (5th ed., text rev.). American Psychiatric Association.

Anand, K. S., and Dhikav, V. (2012). Hippocampus in health and disease: An overview. *Annals of Indian Academy of Neurology, 15*(4), 239–246. https://doi.org/10.4103/0972-2327.104323

Andersson, C., Kristinsson, J., and Gry, J. (2009). *Occurrence and Use of*

Hallucinogenic Mushrooms Containing Psilocybin Alkaloids. Copenhagen: Nordic Council of Ministers.

Angel, Sr. K., and Wicklow, D. T. (1975). Relationships between coprophilous fungi and fecal substrates in a Colorado grassland. *Mycologia, 67*(1), 63–74. https://doi.org/10.1080/00275514.1975.12019722

Aragaki, M., and Uchida, J. Y. (2001). Morphological distinctions between *Phytophthora capsici* and *P. tropicalis sp. nov. Mycologia, 93*(1), 137–145. https://doi.org/10.1080/00275514.2001.12061285

Atasoy, S., Roseman, L., Kaelen, M., et al. (2017). Connectome-harmonic decomposition of human brain activity reveals dynamical repertoire re-organization under LSD. *Scientific Reports, 7*(1), 1–18.

Atlas Obscura. (n.d.). Peyote. Retrieved September 18, 2023, from https://www.atlasobscura.com/foods/peyote-cactus-mexico

Austin, E., Myron, H. S., Summerbell, R. K., and Mackenzie, C. A. (2018). Acute renal injury cause by confirmed *Psilocybe cubensis* mushroom ingestion. *Medical Mycology Case Reports, 23*, 55–57. https://doi.org/10.1016/j.mmcr.2018.12.007

Badham, E. R. (1980). The effect of light upon basidiocarp initiation in *Psilocybe cubensis. Mycologia, 72*(1), 136–142. https://doi.org/10.1080/00275514.1980.12021162

Badham, E. R. (1982). Tropisms in the mushroom *Psilocybe cubensis. Mycologia, 74*(2), 275–279. https://doi.org/10.1080/00275514.1982.12021501

Badham, E. R. (1985). The influence of humidity upon transpiration and growth in *Psilocybe cubensis. Mycologia, 77*(6), 932–939. https://doi.org/10.1080/00275514.1985.12025182

Balconi, M., and Angioletti, L. (2023). Hemodynamic and electrophysiological biomarkers of interpersonal tuning during interoceptive synchronization. *Information, 14*(5), 289. https://www.mdpi.com/2078-2489/14/5/289

Banskota, S., Ghia, J.-E., and Khan, W. I. (2019). Serotonin in the gut: Blessing or a curse. *Biochimie, 161*, 56–64. https://doi.org/10.1016/j.biochi.2018.06.008

Barba, T., Buehler, S., Kettner, H., et al. (2022). Effects of psilocybin versus escitalopram on rumination and thought suppression in depression. *BJPsych Open, 8*(5), e163. https://doi.org/10.1192/bjo.2022.565

Barbanoj, M. J., Riba, J., Clos, S., et al. (2008). Daytime ayahuasca administration modulates REM and slow-wave sleep in healthy volunteers. *Psychopharmacology, 196*(2), 315–326. https://doi.org/10.1007/s00213-007-0963-0

Barlow, C. (2020, July 30). *Psilocybe azurescens*: This magic mushroom is stronger than what you're used to. *DoubleBlind Mag.* https://doubleblindmag.com/mushrooms/types/flying-saucer-shrooms/

Barlow, C. (2021, May 27). *Psilocybe cubensis* isn't the only magic mushroom—here's what to know about its cousin, Liberty Caps aka *Psilocybe semilanceata. Double Blind Mag.* https://doubleblindmag.com/mushrooms/types/liberty-caps/

Barlow, C. (2021, August 17). Blue Meanies mushrooms: Are they really that potent? *DoubleBlind Mag.* https://doubleblindmag.com/blue-meanies-mushrooms-panaeolus-cyanescens/

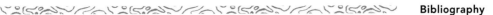

Barlow, C. (2021, August 31). The tragic story of magic truffles: The elusive wild *Psilocybe*. *DoubleBlind Mag*. https://doubleblindmag.com/magic-truffles-psilocybe-tampanensis/

Barlow, C. (2021, November 4). Meet the crazy strong Australian shroom we almost forgot. *DoubleBlind Mag*. https://doubleblindmag.com/psilocybe-subaeruginosa/

Barlow, C. (2022, June 23). 10 most potent magic mushrooms. *HealingMaps*. https://healingmaps.com/most-potent-magic-mushrooms-species/

Barlow, C. (2022, December 17). Psychedelic mushroom types; beyond *Psilocybe cubensis*. Third Wave. https://thethirdwave.co/psilocybe-cubensis/

Barsuglia, J., Davis, A. K., Palmer, R., et al. (2018). Intensity of mystical experiences occasioned by 5-MeO-DMT and comparison with a prior psilocybin study. *Frontiers in Psychology*, 9. https://doi.org/10.3389/fpsyg.2018.02459

Bastos, C., Liberal, Â., Moldão, M., et al. (2023). Ethnomycological prospect of wild edible and medicinal mushrooms from Central and Southern Africa—A review. *Food Frontiers*, 4(2), 549–575. https://doi.org/10.1002/fft2.215

Bates, S. T., Miller, A. N., and the Macrofungi Collections and Microfungi Collections Consortia. (2018). The protochecklist of North American nonlichenized fungi. *Mycologia*, 110(6), 1222–1348. https://doi.org/10.1080/00275514.2018.1515410

Bauer, B. E. (2018, December 21). Wood lover paralysis: An unsolved mystery. *Psychedelic Science Review*. https://psychedelicreview.com/wood-lover-paralysis-unsolved-mystery/

Bauer, B. E. (2020, November 13). Aeruginascin identified in *Psilocybe cubensis* magic mushrooms. *Psychedelic Science Review*. https://psychedelicreview.com/aeruginascin-identified-in-psilocybe-cubensis-magic-mushrooms/

Baumeister, D., Barnes, G., Giaroli, G., and Tracy, D. (2014, March 17). Classical hallucinogens as antidepressants? A review of pharmacodynamics and putative clinical roles. *Therapeutic Advances in Psychopharmacology*, 4(4), 156–169. https://journals.sagepub.com/doi/full/10.1177/2045125314527985

Bayer, E. (n.d.). The mycelium revolution is upon us. Scientific American Blog Network. Retrieved June 12, 2023, from https://blogs.scientificamerican.com/observations/the-mycelium-revolution-is-upon-us/

Beadle, A. (2021, October 25). Medicinal genomics publishes genome of *Psilocybe cubensis*. (n.d.). Analytical Cannabis. https://www.analyticalcannabis.com/news/medicinal-genomics-publishes-genome-of-psilocybe-cubensis-313459

Beatrice Society. (2022, December 22). Psilocybin mushroom strains to know about, from Wavy Caps to Golden Teacher. https://beatricesociety.com/5-psilocybin-mushroom-strains-to-know-about-from-wavy-caps-to-golden-teacher/

Beaty Biodiversity Museum. (n.d.). *Psilocybe pelliculosa*. Retrieved June 24, 2023, from https://explore.beatymuseum.ubc.ca/mushroomsup/P_pelliculosa.html

Beck, M. (2021). *Psilocybin Mushrooms of the United States: A Visual Guide*. Mockingbird Press.

Becker, A. M., Holze, F., Grandinetti, T., et al. (2022). Acute effects of psilocybin after escitalopram or placebo pretreatment in a randomized, double-blind, placebo-controlled, crossover study in healthy subjects. *Clinical Pharmacology and Therapeutics*, 111(4), 886–895. https://doi.org/10.1002/cpt.2487

Bedry, R., Baudrimont, I., Deffieux, G., et al. (2001). Wild-mushroom intoxication as a cause of rhabdomyolysis. *New England Journal of Medicine*, 345(11), 798–802. https://doi.org/10.1056/NEJMoa010581

Benedict, R., Brady, L. R., and Tyler, V. E. (1962). Occurrence of psilocin in *Psilocybe baeocystis. J Pharm Sci*, 51(4), 393–394. https://doi.org/10.1002/jps.2600510428

Berger, M., Gray, J. A., and Roth, B. L. (2009). The expanded biology of serotonin. *Annual Review of Medicine*, 60, 355–366. https://doi.org/10.1146/annurev.med.60.042307.110802

Berlucchi, G., and Marzi, C. A. (2019). Neuropsychology of consciousness: Some history and a few new trends. *Frontiers in Psychology*, 10, 50.

Bermejo, D. (2022, December 2). A list of the strongest *Psilocybe cubensis* strains. *Psychedelic Spotlight*. https://psychedelicspotlight.com/a-list-of-the-strongest-psilocybe-cubensis-strains/

Besl, H. (1993). "Galerina steglichii" spec. Nov, ein halluzinogener Haeubling. *Zeitschrift Für Mykologie*, 59, 215–218.

Beug, M. W. (2011). The Genus Psilocybe in North America. *Fungi Magazine*, 4(3), 6–17.

Beug, M. W., and Bigwood, J. (1981). Quantitative analysis of psilocybin and psilocin in *Psilocybe baeocystis* (Singer and Smith) by high-performance liquid chromatography and by thin-layer chromatography. *J. Chromatogr.*, 207(3), 379–385. https://doi.org/10.1016/S0021-9673(00)88741-5

Beug, M. W., and Bigwood, J. (1982). Psilocybin and psilocin levels in twenty species from seven genera of wild mushrooms in the Pacific Northwest, U.S.A. *Journal of Ethnopharmacology*, 5(3), 271–285. https://doi.org/10.1016/0378-8741(82)90013-7

Bionity. (n.d.). *Gymnopilus*. Retrieved June 26, 2023, from https://www.bionity.com/en/encyclopedia/Gymnopilus.html

Bird, C. I. V., Modlin, N. L., and Rucker, J. J. H. (2021). Psilocybin and MDMA for the treatment of trauma-related psychopathology. *International Review of Psychiatry*, 33(3), 229–249. https://doi.org/10.1080/09540261.2021.1919062

Blei, F., Dörner, S., Fricke, J., et al. (2020). Simultaneous production of psilocybin and a cocktail of β-carboline monoamine oxidase inhibitors in "magic" mushrooms. *Chemistry – A European Journal*, 26(3), 729–734. https://doi.org/10.1002/chem.201904363

Blickman, T. (n.d.). The "Arriola" ruling of the supreme court of Argentina on the possession of drugs for personal consumption. TNI Drugs and Democracy Programme. Retrieved October 25, 2023, from https://www.druglawreform.info/en/country-information/latin-america/argentina/item/235-the-arriola-ruling-of-the-supreme-court-of-argentina

Bogadi, M., and Kaštelan, S. (2021). A potential effect of psilocybin on anxiety in neurotic personality structures in adolescents. *Croatian Medical Journal*, 62(5), 528–530.

https://doi.org/10.3325/cmj.2021.62.528

Bogenschutz, M. P., Ross, S., Bhatt, S., et al. (2022). Percentage of heavy drinking days following psilocybin-assisted psychotherapy vs placebo in the treatment of adult patients with alcohol use disorder: A randomized clinical trial. *JAMA Psychiatry*, 79(10), 953–962. https://doi.org/10.1001/jamapsychiatry.2022.2096

Bononi, V. L. R., Oliveira, A. K. M. de, Gugliotta, A. de M., and Quevedo, J. R. de. (2017). Agaricomycetes (basidiomycota, fungi) diversity in a protected area in the Maracaju Mountains, in the Brazilian central region. *Hoehnea*, *44*, 361–377. https://doi.org/10.1590/2236-8906-70/2016

Borasio, G. D. (2011). Translating the World Health Organization definition of palliative care into scientific practice. *Palliative & Supportive Care*, 9(1), 1–2. https://doi.org/10.1017/S1478951510000489

Borgford, G. (2023, May 5). The Wonderful and Diverse World of Psilocybin Mushroom Strains. Pychedelic Support. https://psychedelic.support/resources/psilocybin-mushroom-strains/

Borgford, G. (2023, June 12). How to Get Legal Psychedelics in Colorado. PsychedelicSupport. https://psychedelic.support/resources/how-to-get-legal-psychedelics-in-colorado/

Borovička, J. (2003). The bluing *Psilocybe* species of the Czech Republic III. *Psilocybe moravica* sp. *Nova*, the Moravian *Psilocybe*. *Mykologický Sborník*, 80(4), 126–141.

Borovička, J., and Hlaváček, J. (2001). The bluing *Psilocybe* species of the Czech Republic I. *Psilocybe arcana* Borovička et Hlaváček, the mysterious *Psilocybe*. *Mykologický Sborník*, 78(1), 2–7.

Borovička, J., Noordeloos, M. E., Gryndler, M., and Oborník, M. (2010). Molecular phylogeny of *Psilocybe cyanescens* complex in Europe, with reference to the position of the secotioid *Weraroa novae-zelandiae*. *Mycological Progress*, 10(2), 149–155. https://doi.org/10.1007/s11557-010-0684-3

Borovička, J., Oborník, M., Stříbrný, J., et al. (2015). Phylogenetic and chemical studies in the potential psychotropic species complex of *Psilocybe atrobrunnea* with taxonomic and nomenclatural notes. *Persoonia—Molecular Phylogeny and Evolution of Fungi*, 34(1), 1–9. https://doi.org/10.3767/003158515X685283

Bradshaw, A. J., Dentinger, B., Backman, T., et al. (2022). DNA authentication and chemical analysis of *Psilocybe* mushrooms reveal widespread taxonomic misdeterminations and inconsistencies in metabolites. SSRN Scholarly Paper 4038523. https://doi.org/10.2139/ssrn.4038523

Bragagnolo, C. (2023, March 8). Maria Sabina—the story of the priestess of mushrooms. Women on Psychedelics. https://www.womenonpsychedelics.org/post/maria-sabina-the-story-of-the-priestess-of-mushrooms

Bresinsky, A., and Besl, H. (1989). *A Colour Atlas of Poisonous Fungi: A Handbook for Pharmacists, Doctors, and Biologists*. Manson Publishing Ltd.

Cahn, B. R., and Polich, J. (2006). Meditation states and traits: EEG, ERP, and neuroimaging studies. *Psychological Bulletin*, 132(2), 180.

Calder, A. E., and Hasler, G. (2023). Towards an understanding of psychedelic-induced neuroplasticity. *Neuropsychopharmacology*, 48(1), 104–112. https://doi.org/10.1038/s41386-022-01389-z

Carey, B. (2019, September 4). Johns Hopkins opens new Center for Psychedelic Research. *New York Times*. https://www.nytimes.com/2019/09/04/science/psychedelic-drugs-hopkins-depression.html

Carhart-Harris, R. L. (2018). The entropic brain—revisited. *Neuropharmacology*, 142, 167–178.

Carhart-Harris, R. L. (2019). How do psychedelics work? *Current Opinion in Psychiatry*, 32(1), 16–21.

Carhart-Harris, R. L., Erritzoe, D., Williams, T., et al. (2012). Neural correlates of the psychedelic state as determined by fMRI studies with psilocybin. *Proceedings of the National Academy of Sciences*, 109(6), 2138–2143.

Carhart-Harris, R. L., and Friston, K. J. (2019). REBUS and the anarchic brain: Toward a unified model of the brain action of psychedelics. *Pharmacological Reviews*, 71(3), 316–344.

Carhart-Harris, R. L., Giribaldi, B., Watts, R., et al. (2021). Trial of *Psilocybin* versus escitalopram for depression. *New England Journal of Medicine*, 384(15), 1402–1411. https://doi.org/10.1056/NEJMoa2032994

Carhart-Harris, R. L., Leech, R., Erritzoe, D., et al. (2013). Functional connectivity measures after psilocybin inform a novel hypothesis of early psychosis. *Schizophrenia Bulletin*, 39(6), 1343–1351. https://doi.org/10.1093/schbul/sbs117

Carhart-Harris, R. L., Leech, R., Hellyer, P. J., et al. (2014). The entropic brain: A theory of conscious states informed by neuroimaging research with psychedelic drugs. *Frontiers in Human Neuroscience*, 8, 20.

Cassol, H., Pétré, B., Degrange, S., et al. (2018). Qualitative thematic analysis of the phenomenology of near-death experiences. *PLOS ONE*, 13(2), e0193001.

Castelhano, J., Lima, G., Teixeira, M., et al. (2021). The effects of tryptamine psychedelics in the brain: A meta-analysis of functional and review of molecular imaging studies. *Frontiers in Pharmacology*, 12. https://www.frontiersin.org/articles/10.3389/fphar.2021.739053

Castellano, M., and Cázares, E. (n.d.). *Handbook to additional fungal species of special concern in the Northwest Forest Plan (General Technical Report PNW-GTR-572)*. USDA, Forest Service, Pacific Northwest Research Station. http://www.fs.fed.us/pnw/pubs/gtr572/gtr572.pdf

Catlow B. J., Song S., Paredes D. A., et al. (2013). Effects of psilocybin on hippocampal neurogenesis and extinction of trace fear conditioning. *Experimental Brain Research*, 228(4), 481–491. https://doi.org/10.1007/s00221-013-3579-0

Centers for Disease Control and Prevention. (2023, August 8). Understanding the opioid overdose epidemic. https://www.cdc.gov/opioids/basics/epidemic.html

Chang, Y. S., and Mills, A. K. (1992). Re-examination of *Psilocybe subaeruginosa* and related species with comparative morphology, isozymes and mating compatibility studies. *Mycological Research*, 96(6), 429–441. https://doi.org/10.1016/S0953-7562(09)81087-3

Charnay, Y., and Leger, L. (2010). Brain serotonergic circuitries. *Dialogues in Clinical Neuroscience, 12*(4), 471–487.

Chatelle, C., Lesenfants, D., and Noirhomme, Q. (2018). Electrophysiology in disorders of consciousness: From conventional EEG visual analysis to brain-computer interfaces. In C. Schnakers and S. Laureys (Eds.), *Coma and Disorders of Consciousness* (pp. 51–75). Springer International Publishing. https://doi.org/10.1007/978-3-319-55964-3_4

Cheng, B., Roberts, N., Zhou, Y., et al. (2022). Social support mediates the influence of cerebellum functional connectivity strength on postpartum depression and postpartum depression with anxiety. *Translational Psychiatry, 12*(1), 54. https://doi.org/10.1038/s41398-022-01781-9

Chiesa, A., and Serretti, A. (2010). A systematic review of neurobiological and clinical features of mindfulness meditations. *Psychological Medicine, 40*(8), 1239–1252.

Ching, S., Chen, S., Glasauer, S., et al. (n.d.). Neural mechanisms of sequential dependence in time perception: The impact of prior task and memory processing. *bioRXIV: The Preprint Server for Biology*. https://doi.org/10.1101/2023.05.07.538104

Coleman, P. (2020, May 21). The psychedelic science of pain. *UC San Diego Today*. https://today.ucsd.edu/story/the-psychedelic-science-of-pain

Collins, K. L., Russell, H. G., Schumacher, P. J., et al. (2018). A review of current theories and treatments for phantom limb pain. *Journal of Clinical Investigation, 128*(6), 2168–2176. https://doi.org/10.1172/JCI94003

Cooke, J. (2021, September 11). Magic mushroom strain guide (100+ strains explained). Tripsitter. https://tripsitter.com/magic-mushrooms/strains/

Cooke, J. (2021, September 12). List of psilocybin mushroom species (and other psychoactive fungi). Tripsitter. https://tripsitter.com/magic-mushrooms/species/

Cooke, J. (2022, March 10). Penis Envy: The World's Trippiest Mushroom. Tripsitter. https://tripsitter.com/magic-mushrooms/strains/penis-envy/

Cornell Small Farms Program. (n.d.). Harvest to Market Guide, Section 2: Enterprise Planning. https://smallfarms.cornell.edu/projects/mushrooms/harvest-to-market-guide/section-2-enterprise-planning/

Cortés-Pérez, A. (2013a). *Psilocybe yungensis Singer & A.H. Sm*. https://commons.wikimedia.org/wiki/File:Psilocybe_yungensis_Singer_%26_A.H._Sm_368727.jpg

Cortés-Pérez, A. (2013b). *Psilocybe yungensis Singer & A.H. Sm*. https://commons.wikimedia.org/wiki/File:Psilocybe_yungensis_Singer_%26_A.H._Sm_368728.jpg

Cozolino, L. (2017). *The Neuroscience of Psychotherapy: Healing the Social Brain* (3rd ed.). Norton Series on Interpersonal Neurobiology. W. W. Norton & Company.

Crocq, M.-A., and Crocq, L. (2000). From shell shock and war neurosis to posttraumatic stress disorder: A history of psychotraumatology. *Dialogues in Clinical Neuroscience, 2*(1), 47–55. https://doi.org/10.31887/DCNS.2000.2.1/macrocq

Cuijpers, P., Reynolds, C. F. I., Donker, T., et al. (2012). Personalized treatment of adult depression: Medication, psychotherapy, or both? A systematic review. *Depression and Anxiety*, 29(10), 855–864. psyh. https://doi.org/10.1002/da.21985

Culver, D., and Kravarik, J. (2022, November 4). It's legal to use psilocybin, or "magic mushrooms," in Oregon. But that could soon change. CNN. https://www.cnn.com/2022/11/04/us/oregon-psilocybin-voter-pushback-ctrp/index.html

Curran, M., and Kobos, J. (1980). Therapeutic engagement with a dying person: Stimulus for therapist training and growth. *Psychotherapy: Theory, Research, and Practice*, 17(3), 343–351.

Cuthbert, B. N. (2022). Research domain criteria (RDoC): Progress and potential. *Current Directions in Psychological Science*, 31(2), 107–114. https://doi.org/10.1177/09637214211051363

Daniel, J., and Haberman, M. (2018). Clinical potential of psilocybin as a treatment for mental health conditions. *Mental Health Clinician*, 7(1), 24–28. https://doi.org/10.9740/mhc.2017.01.024

Davis, A. K., Barrett, F. S., May, D. G., et al. (2021). Effects of psilocybin-assisted therapy on major depressive disorder: A randomized clinical trial. *JAMA Psychiatry*, 78(5), 481–489. https://doi.org/10.1001/jamapsychiatry.2020.3285

Davis, A. K., So, S., Lancelotta, R., et al. (2019). 5-methoxy-N,N-dimethyltryptamine (5-MeO-DMT) used in a naturalistic group setting is associated with unintended improvements in depression and anxiety. *American Journal of Drug and Alcohol Abuse*, 45(2), 161–169. https://doi.org/10.1080/00952990.2018.1545024

Davis, A. K., Xin, Y., Sepeda, N. D., et al. (2021). Increases in psychological flexibility mediate relationship between acute psychedelic effects and decreases in racial trauma symptoms among people of color. *Chronic Stress*, 5. https://doi.org/10.1177/24705470211035607

Daws, R. E., Timmermann, C., Giribaldi, B., et al. (2022). Increased global integration in the brain after psilocybin therapy for depression. *Nature Medicine*, 28(4), article 4. https://doi.org/10.1038/s41591-022-01744-z

Dawson, B. (2022, April 21). How to identify the most common types of magic mushrooms. *MEL Magazine*. https://melmagazine.com/en-us/story/types-of-psychedelic-mushrooms

Dayabandara, M., Hanwella, R., Ratnatunga, S., et al. (2017). Antipsychotic-associated weight gain: Management strategies and impact on treatment adherence. *Neuropsychiatric Disease and Treatment*, 13, 2231–2241. https://doi.org/10.2147/NDT.S113099

De Gregorio, D., Aguilar-Valles, A., Preller, K. H., et al. (2021). Hallucinogens in mental health: Preclinical and clinical studies on LSD, psilocybin, MDMA, and ketamine. *Journal of Neuroscience* 41(5), 891–900. https://doi.org/10.1523/JNEUROSCI.1659-20.2020

de la Cruz, F., Wagner, G., Schumann, A., et al. (2021). Interrelations between dopamine and serotonin producing sites and regions of the default mode network. *Human Brain Mapping*, 42(3), 811–823. https://doi.org/10.1002/hbm.25264

de la Mora, M. P., Gallegos-Cari, A., Arizmendi-García, Y., et al. (2010).

Role of dopamine receptor mechanisms in the amygdaloid modulation of fear and anxiety: Structural and functional analysis. *Progress in Neurobiology, 90*(2), 198–216. https://doi.org/10.1016/j.pneurobio.2009.10.010

Dean, J., and Keshavan, M. (2017). The neurobiology of depression: An integrated view. *Asian Journal of Psychiatry, 27,* 101–111. https://doi.org/10.1016/j.ajp.2017.01.025

Denton, W. H., Carmody, T. J., Rush, A. J., et al. (2010). Dyadic discord at baseline is associated with lack of remission in the acute treatment of chronic depression. *Psychological Medicine, 40*(3), 415–424.

Denzin, N., and Lincoln, Y. (Eds.). (2013). *The Landscape of Qualitative Research* (4th ed.). Sage Publications.

DeYoung, C. G. (2010). Toward a theory of the big five. *Psychological Inquiry, 21*(1), 26–33. https://doi.org/10.1080/10478401003648674

Dias, D. (2023, August 14). New details emerge in lethal mushroom mystery gripping Australia. CBS News. https://www.cbsnews.com/news/lethal-mushroom-mystery-australia-new-details/

Diaz, J. L. (1977). Ethnopharmacology of sacred psychoactive plants used by the Indians of Mexico. *Annual Review of Pharmacology and Toxicology, 17,* 647–675. https://doi.org/10.1146/annurev.pa.17.040177.003243

DiBella, J. (2023, January 6). *Psilocybe cyanescens.* Sanctuary Wellness Institute. https://sanctuarywellnessinstitute.com/blog/psilocybe-cyanescens/

Dickinson, C., and Lucas, J. (Eds.). (1979). *The Encyclopedia of Mushrooms.* G.P. Putnam's Sons.

Dietrich, A. (2003). Functional neuroanatomy of altered states of consciousness: The transient hypofrontality hypothesis. *Consciousness and Cognition, 12*(2), 231–256.

DiSabato, D., Quan, N., and Godbout, J. P. (2016). Neuroinflammation: The devil is in the details. *Journal of Neurochemistry, 139*(Suppl 2), 136–153. https://doi.org/10.1111/jnc.13607

Doblin, R. E., Christiansen, M., Jerome, L., and Burge, B. (2019). The past and future of psychedelic science: An introduction to this issue. *Journal of Psychoactive Drugs, 51*(2), 93–97. https://doi.org/10.1080/02791072.2019.1606472

Domínguez-Borràs, J., and Vuilleumier, P. (2022). Amygdala function in emotion, cognition, and behavior. *Handbook of Clinical Neurology, 187,* 359–380. https://doi.org/10.1016/B978-0-12-823493-8.00015-8

Dumas, G., Fortier, M., and González, J. C. (2017). Les états modifiés de conscience en question, anciennes limites et nouvelles approches. *Intellectica, 67.*

Dunlavey, C. J. (2018). Introduction to the hypothalamic-pituitary-adrenal axis: Healthy and dysregulated stress responses, developmental stress, and neurodegeneration. *Journal of Undergraduate Neuroscience Education, 16*(2), R59–R60.

Eden Industries. (2023, May 10). B+ mushrooms (*P. Cubensis*) strain and cultivation guide. https://edenshrooms.com/collections/magic-mushroom-spores/

products/b-spore-syringe-kit-psilocybe-cubensis

Ehrmann, K., Allen, J. J. B., and Moreno, F. A. (2022). Psilocybin for the treatment of obsessive-compulsive disorders. *Current Topics in Behavioral Neurosciences*, 56, 247–259. https://doi.org/10.1007/7854_2021_279

Elsouri, K. N., Kalhori, S., Colunge, D., et al. (2022). Psychoactive drugs in the management of post traumatic stress disorder: A promising new horizon. *Cureus*, 14(5), e25235. https://doi.org/10.7759/cureus.25235

Emboden, W. A. (1979). *Narcotic plants* (rev. and enl.). Macmillan.

Emmons, C. W. (1961). Mycology and medicine. *Mycologia*, 53(1), 1–10. https://doi.org/10.1080/00275514.1961.12017928

Encyclopedia of Life. (n.d.). *Psilocybe liniformans Guzmán & Bas*. Retrieved June 24, 2023, from https://eol.org/pages/6688575/articles

Enjalbert, F., Cassanas, G., Rapior, S., et al. (2004). Amatoxins in wood-rotting *Galerina marginata*. *Mycologia*, 96(4), 720–729. https://doi.org/10.1080/15572536.2005.11832920

Epel E. S., Blackburn E. H., Jue, L., et al. (2004). Accelerated telomere shortening in response to life stress. *Proceedings of the National Academy of Sciences*, 101(49), 17312–17315. https://doi.org/10.1073/pnas.0407162101

Ermakova, A. O., Dunbar, F., Rucker, J., and Johnson, M. W. (2021). A narrative synthesis of research with 5-MeO-DMT. *Journal of Psychopharmacology*, 36(3), 273–294. https://doi.org/10.1177/02698811211050543

Erowid. (2002, November 29). Legality of psilocybin mushroom spores. http://www.erowid.org/plants/mushrooms/mushrooms_law8.shtml

Etkin, A., and Wager, T. D. (2007). Functional neuroimaging of anxiety: A meta-analysis of emotional processing in PTSD, social anxiety disorder, and specific phobia. *American Journal of Psychiatry*, 164(10), 1476–1488. https://doi.org/10.1176/appi.ajp.2007.07030504

Fadiman, J. (2011). *The Psychedelic Explorer's Guide: Safe, Therapeutic, and Sacred Journeys*. Inner Traditions/Bear and Company.

Fantastic Fungi. (2021, May 4). The R. Gordon Wasson trip that changed everything. https://fantasticfungi.com/the-r-gordon-wasson-trip-that-changed-everything/

Fayod, V. (1889). Prodrome d'une histoire naturelle des Agaricinés. *Annales Des Sciences Naturelles, Botanique, 9,* 181–411, 359.

Felsch, C. L., and Kuypers, K. P. C. (2022). Don't be afraid, try to meditate-potential effects on neural activity and connectivity of psilocybin-assisted mindfulness-based intervention for social anxiety disorder: A systematic review. *Neuroscience & Biobehavioral Reviews*, 139, 104724. https://doi.org/10.1016/j.neubiorev.2022.104724

Fernández-Rodríguez, C., Paz-Caballero, D., González-Fernández, S., and Pérez-Álvarez, M. (2018). Activation vs. experiential avoidance as a transdiagnostic condition of emotional distress: An empirical study. *Frontiers in Psychology*, 9. https://www.frontiersin.org/articles/10.3389/fpsyg.2018.01618

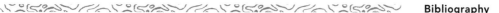

Fewster, E. (2022, January 21). *Panaeolus cyanescens*. Frshminds. https://frshminds.com/panaeolus-cyanescens/

First Nature. (n.d.). *Amanita muscaria*, Fly Agaric mushroom. Retrieved June 26, 2023, from https://www.first-nature.com/fungi/amanita-muscaria.php

First Nature. (n.d.). *Psilocybe semilanceata*, magic mushroom, Liberty Cap. Retrieved October 11, 2023, from https://www.first-nature.com/fungi/psilocybe-semilanceata.php

Fitzpatrick, S. M. (Ed.). (n.d.). *Ancient Psychoactive Substances*. University Press of Florida.

Food and Drug Administration. (2018). Questions and answers: Risk of next-morning impairment after use of insomnia drugs; FDA requires lower recommended doses for certain drugs containing zolpidem (Ambien, Ambien CR, Edluar, and Zolpimist). https://www.fda.gov/drugs/drug-safety-and-availability/questions-and-answers-risk-next-morning-impairment-after-use-insomnia-drugs-fda-requires-lower

Forrester-Jones, R., Dietzfelbinger, L., Stedman, D., and Richmond, P. (2018). Including the 'spiritual' within mental health care in the UK, from the experience of people with mental health problems. *Journal of Religion and Health*, 57(1), 384–407. https://doi.org/10.1007/s10943-017-0502-1

Foster, B. L., Koslov, S. R., Aponik-Gremillion, L., et al. (2023). A tripartite view of the posterior cingulate cortex. *Nature Reviews. Neuroscience*, 24(3), 173–189. https://doi.org/10.1038/s41583-022-00661-x

Foster, J. S. (2023, November 14). Drinking Mushroom Shakes in Thailand. TravelFreak. https://travelfreak.com/how-to-trip-on-mushrooms-in-thailand/

Fox, M. E., and Lobo, M. K. (2019). The molecular and cellular mechanisms of depression: A focus on reward circuitry. *Molecular Psychiatry*, 24(12), 1798–1815. https://doi.org/10.1038/s41380-019-0415-3

Freddy, F. (2021, April 22). Golden Teacher mushrooms strain review. https://fungushead.com/golden-teacher-mushrooms-strain-review/

Freddy, F. (2022, September 9). Golden Teacher mushroom effects of the brain and body. https://fungushead.com/golden-teacher-mushroom-effects-of-the-brain-and-body/

Fricke, J., Blei, F., and Hoffmeister, D. (2017). Enzymatic synthesis of psilocybin. *Angewandte Chemie International Edition*, 56(40), 12352–12355. https://doi.org/10.1002/anie.201705489

Froese, T., Guzmán, G., and Guzmán-Dávalos, L. (2016). On the origin of the genus *Psilocybe* and its potential ritual use in ancient Africa and Europe. *Economic Botany*, 70(2), 103–114. https://doi.org/10.1007/s12231-016-9342-2

Froese, T., Leenen, I., and Palenicek, T. (2018). A role for enhanced functions of sleep in psychedelic therapy? *Adaptive Behavior*, 26(3), 129–135. https://doi.org/10.1177/1059712318762735

Frshminds. (2021, August 1). Z strain magic mushroom species. https://frshminds.com/psilocybin-mushroom-species-guide/psilocybe-cubensis/z-strain/

Frshminds. (2021, October 14). *Panaeolus tropicalis* magic mushrooms. https://

frshminds.com/psilocybin-mushroom-species-guide/panaeolus/panaeolus-tropicalis-magic-mushrooms/

Frshminds. (2021, October 21). *Psilocybe fimetaria* magic mushrooms. https://frshminds.com/psilocybin-mushroom-species-guide/psilocybe/psilocybe-fimetaria-magic-mushrooms/

FunGuy Grow Supply. *Psilocybe cubensis*: Distribution, morphology, and strains. https://www.funguygrowsupply.com/the-black-truffle/psilocybe-cubensis-distribution-morphology-and-strains/

Fun Guys. (n.d.). Alacabenzi—dried mushroom. https://thefunguys.co/product/alacabenzi-dried-mushroom-premium/

Furst, P. T. (1976). *Hallucinogens and Culture*. Chandler and Sharp.

Furst, P. T., and Furst, P. E. (1986). *Mushrooms, Psychedelic Fungi*. Chelsea House Publishers.

Galerina—The Genera and Species from A to Z: The Encyclopedia of Psychoactive Plants: Ethnopharmacology and Its Applications. (n.d.). Retrieved June 27, 2023, from https://doctorlib.info/herbal/encyclopedia-psychoactive-plants-ethnopharmacology/120.html

Garcia-Romeu, A., Barrett, F. S., Carbonaro, T. M., et al. (2021). Optimal dosing for psilocybin pharmacotherapy: Considering weight-adjusted and fixed dosing approaches. *Journal of Psychopharmacology*, 35(4), 353–361. https://doi.org/10.1177/0269881121991822

Gartz, J. (1995). Cultivation and analysis of *Psilocybe* species and an investigation of *Galerina steglichi*. *Annali Museo Civico Di Rovereto*, 10, 297–306.

Gartz, J., and Wiedemann, G. (2015). Discovery of a new caerulescent *Psilocybe* mushroom in Germany: *Psilocybe germanica sp. nov. Drug Testing and Analysis*, 7(9), 853–857. https://doi.org/10.1002/dta.1795

Gattuso, J. J., Perkins, D., Ruffell, S., et al. (2022). Default mode network modulation by psychedelics: A systematic review. *International Journal of Neuropsychopharmacology*, 26(3), 155–188. https://doi.org/10.1093/ijnp/pyac074

Gavin, N. I., Gaynes, B. N., Lohr, K. N., et al. (2005). Perinatal depression: A systematic review of prevalence and incidence. *Obstetrics & Gynecology*, 106(5, Part 1), 1071–1083. https://doi.org/10.1097/01.AOG.0000183597.31630.db

Georgia Code, Crimes and Offenses, Title 16, Section 16-13-71. (n.d.). http://law.onecle.com/georgia/16/16-13-71.html

Gilbertson, R. L. (1980). Wood-rotting fungi of North America. *Mycologia*, 72(1), 1–49.

Glatfelter, G. C., Pottie, E., Partilla, J. S., et al. (2022). Structure–activity relationships for psilocybin, baeocystin, aeruginascin, and related analogues to produce pharmacological effects in mice. *ACS Pharmacology & Translational Science*, 5(11), 1181–1196. https://doi.org/10.1021/acsptsci.2c00177

Global Biodiversity Information Facility. (n.d.-a). *Psilocybe azurescens Stamets & Gartz*. Retrieved June 18, 2023, from https://www.gbif.org/species/5242469

Global Biodiversity Information Facility. (n.d.-b). *Psilocybe mairei Singer*. (n.d.). Retrieved June 24, 2023, from https://www.gbif.org/species/165555614/verbatim

Global Fungal Red List Initiative. (n.d.). Retrieved June 20, 2023, from https://redlist.info/iucn/about/

Glynos, N. G., Pierce, J., Davis, A. K., et al. (2023). Knowledge, perceptions, and use of psychedelics among individuals with fibromyalgia. *Journal of Psychoactive Drugs*, 55(1), 73–84. https://doi.org/10.1080/02791072.2021.2022817

Goel, A., Rai, Y., Sivadas, S., et al. (2023). Use of psychedelics for pain: A scoping review. *Anesthesiology*, 139(4), 523–536. https://doi.org/10.1097/ALN.0000000000004673

Goldberg, S. B., Pace, B. T., Nicholas, C. R., et al. (2020). The experimental effects of psilocybin on symptoms of anxiety and depression: A meta-analysis. *Psychiatry Research*, 284, 112749. https://doi.org/10.1016/j.psychres.2020.112749

Goldstein, B. L., Perlman, G., Eaton, N. R., et al. (2020). Testing explanatory models of the interplay between depression, neuroticism, and stressful life events: A dynamic trait-stress generation approach. *Psychological Medicine*, 50(16), 2780–2789. https://doi.org/10.1017/S0033291719002927

Goodwin, G. M., Aaronson, S. T., Alvarez, O., et al. (2022). Single-dose psilocybin for a treatment-resistant episode of major depression. *New England Journal of Medicine*, 387(18), 1637–1648. https://doi.org/10.1056/NEJMoa2206443

Gosseries, O., Fecchio, M., Wolff, A., et al. (n.d.). Letter to the editor: Behavioral and brain responses in cognitive trance: A TMS-EEG case study. *Clinical Neurophysiology*, 131(2020), 586–588.

Gotvaldová, K., Borovicka, J., Hajkova, K., et al. (2022). Extensive collection of psychotropic mushrooms with determination of their tryptamine alkaloids. *International Journal of Molecular Sciences*, 23(22), 14068. https://doi.org/10.3390/ijms232214068

Gotvaldová, K., Hájková, K., Borovička, J., et al. (2021). Stability of psilocybin and its four analogs in the biomass of the psychotropic mushroom *Psilocybe cubensis*. *Drug Testing and Analysis*, 13(2), 439–446. https://doi.org/10.1002/dta.2950

Government of Canada. (n.d.). Psilocybin and psilocin (magic mushrooms). https://www.canada.ca/en/health-canada/services/substance-use/controlled-illegal-drugs/magic-mushrooms.html

Grandjean, J., Buehlmann, D., Buerge, M., et al. (2021). Psilocybin exerts distinct effects on resting state networks associated with serotonin and dopamine in mice. *NeuroImage*, 225, 117456. https://doi.org/10.1016/j.neuroimage.2020.117456

Graves, R. (1960). *Food for Centaurs: A Collection of the Best of the Author's Short Stories, Essays, Poems*. Doubleday.

Greco, A., Gallitto, G., D'Alessandro, M., and Rastelli, C. (2021). Increased entropic brain dynamics during deep dream-induced altered perceptual phenomenology. *Entropy*, 23(7), 839.

Griffiths, R. R., Hurwitz, E. S., Davis, A. K., et al. (2019). Survey of subjective "God encounter experiences": Comparisons among naturally occurring experiences and those occasioned by the classic psychedelic psilocybin, LSD, ayahuasca, or DMT. *PLOS ONE*, 14(4), e0214377. https://doi.org/10.1371/journal.pone.0214377

Griffiths, R. R., Johnson, M. W., Carducci, M. A., et al. (2016). Psilocybin produces substantial and sustained decreases in depression and anxiety in patients with life-threatening cancer: A randomized double-blind trial. *Journal of Psychopharmacology (Oxford, England)*, 30(12), 1181–1197. https://doi. org/10.1177/0269881116675513

Griffiths, R. R., Richards, W. A., McCann, U., and Jesse, R. (2006). Psilocybin can occasion mystical-type experiences having substantial and sustained personal meaning and spiritual significance. *Psychopharmacology*, 187(3), 268–283; discussion 284–292. https://doi. org/10.1007/s00213-006-0457-5

Grind, K., and Bindley, K. (2023, June 27). Magic mushrooms. LSD. Ketamine. The drugs that power Silicon Valley. *Wall Street Journal*. https://www.wsj. com/articles/silicon-valley-microdosing-ketamine-lsd-magic-mushrooms-d381e214

Grob, C. S., and Grigsby, J. (Eds.). (2021). *Handbook of Medical Hallucinogens*. Guilford Press.

Guerrilla Mycology. (n.d.). Retrieved June 25, 2023, from https://www. guerrillamycology.com

Gukasyan, N., Davis, A. K., Barrett, F. S., et al. (2022). Efficacy and safety of psilocybin-assisted treatment for major depressive disorder: Prospective 12-month follow-up. *Journal of Psychopharmacology*, 36(2), 151–158. https://doi. org/10.1177/02698811211073759

Gulden, G., Dunham, S., and Stockman, J. (2001). DNA studies in the "Galerina marginata" complex. *Mycological Research*, 105, 432–440.

Gulden, G., Stensrud, O., Shalchian-Tabrizi, K., and Kauserud, H. (2005). *Galerina earle*: A polyphyletic genus in the consortium of dark-spored agarics. *Mycologia*, 97(4), 823–837.

Gunther, M. (2023, June 1). The collapse of field trip health. Lucid News. https:// www.lucid.news/the-collapse-of-field-trip-health/, https://www.lucid.news/the-collapse-of-field-trip-health/

Guy, T. M. (2020, July 14). *Psilocybe ovoideocystidiata*: The psychedelic ovoid mushroom. Healing Mushrooms. https:// healing-mushrooms.net/psilocybe-ovoideocystidiata/

Guy, T. M. (2021, May 13). Albino Penis Envy: APE mushroom effects, potency and more. Healing Mushrooms. https:// healing-mushrooms.net/albino-penis-envy-ape/

Guy, T. M. (2021, June 8). Best *Psilocybe cubensis* strains ranked by potency, visuals, and effects. Healing Mushrooms. https://healing-mushrooms.net/psilocybe-cubensis-strains/

Guy, T. M. (2021, June 11). Z-Strain *cubensis* mushrooms: Growing, effects, potency, and legality. Healing Mushrooms. https:// healing-mushrooms.net/z-strain/

Guy, T. M. (2021, June 25). Orissa India *cubensis*: Growing, effects, potency, and legality. Healing Mushrooms. https:// healing-mushrooms.net/orissa-india/

Guy, T. M. (2021, June 29). *Psilocybe Fanaticus*: Robert Mcpherson's PF Classic effects and potency. Healing Mushrooms. https://healing-mushrooms.net/pf-classic/

Guy, T. M. (2021, September 7). A comprehensive list of common wild mushrooms in Georgia. Healing

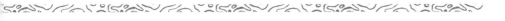

Mushrooms. https://healing-mushrooms. net/georgia/

Guy, T. M. (2023, August 7). *Psilocybe tampanensis*: Identification, look alikes, and safety. Healing Mushrooms. https:// healing-mushrooms.net/psilocybe- tampanensis/

Guzmán, G. (1973). Some distributional relationships between Mexican and United States mycofloras. *Mycologia*, 65(6), 1319–1330. https://doi.org/10.1080/ 00275514.1973.12019555

Guzmán, G. (1978a). *Psilocybe herrerae*. https://eol.org/pages/6688539/articles

Guzmán, G. (1978b). Variation, distribution, ethnomycological data and relationships of *Psilocybe aztecorum*, a Mexican hallucinogenic mushroom. *Mycologia*, 70(2), 385–396. https://doi.org/10.1080/00 275514.1978.12020239

Guzmán, G. (1983). *The Genus* Psilocybe: A *Systematic Revision of the Known Species Including the History, Distribution and Chemistry of the Hallucinogenic Species.* J. Cramer.

Guzmán, G. (2008). Hallucinogenic mushrooms in Mexico: An overview. *Economic Botany*, 62(3), 404–412. https:// doi.org/10.1007/s12231-008-9033-8

Guzmán, G., Allen, J. W., and Gartz, J. (1998). A worldwide geographical distribution of the neurotropic fungi, an analysis and discussion. *Annali Del Museo Civico Di Rovereto*, 14, 189–280. http://www.museocivico.rovereto.tn.it/ UploadDocs/104_art09-Guzman%20 &%20C.pdf

Guzmán, G., Bandala, V. M., and King, C. (1991). A new species of *Psilocybe* of section *Zapotecorum* from New

Zealand. *Mycological Research*, 95(4), 507–508. https://doi.org/10.1016/S0953- 7562(09)80856-3

Guzmán, G., and Bas, C. (1977). A new bluing species of *Psilocybe* from Europe. *Persoonia-Molecular Phylogeny and Evolution of Fungi*, 9(2), 233–238.

Guzmán, G., Jacobs, J. Q., Ramírez, and Murrieta-Hernández, D. M. (2005). The taxonomy of *Psilocybe fagicola*- complex. *Journal of Microbiology*, 43(2), 158–165. https://www.researchgate.net/ publication/7861094_The_taxonomy_of_ Psilocybe_fagicola-complex

Guzmán, G., Kroger, P., Ramirez-Guillen, F., and Castillo Del-Moral, R. (2006). *Psilocybe* (Basidiomycotina, Agaricales, Strophariaceae) in Canada, with a special review of species from British Columbia. *Mycotaxon*, 106, 179–193.

Guzmán, G., and Ott, J. (1976). Description and chemical analysis of a new species of hallucinogenic *Psilocybe* from the Pacific Northwest. *Mycologia*, 68(6), 1261–1267. https://doi.org/10.1080/00275514.1976.1 2020019

Guzmán, G., Ott, J., Boydston, J., and Pollock, S. H. (1976). Psychotropic mycoflora of Washington, Idaho, Oregon, California, and British Columbia. *Mycologia*, 68(6), 1267–1272. https://doi.org/10.1080/00275 514.1976.12020020

Guzmán, G., Tapia, F., Ramírez-Guillén, F., et al. (2003). New species of *Psilocybe* in the Caribbean, with an emendation of *P. guilartensis*. *Mycologia*, 95(6), 1171– 1180. https://doi.org/10.1080/15572536.20 04.11833026

Guzmán, G., Walstad, L., Gándara, E., and Ramírez-Guillén, F. (2007). A new bluing species of *Psilocybe*, section *Stuntzii*, from New Mexico, U.S.A. *Mycotaxon*, 99, 223–226. http://www.cybertruffle.org.uk/cyberliber/59575/0099/0223.htm

Haard, R., and Haard, K. (1977). *Poisonous and Hallucinogenic Mushrooms* (2nd ed.). Cloudburst Press.

Haber, S. N., and Robbins, T. (2022). The prefrontal cortex. *Neuropsycho-pharmacology*, 47(1), 1–2. https://doi.org/10.1038/s41386-021-01184-2

Halama, M., Poliwoda, A., Jasicka-Misiak, I., et al. (2014). *Pholiotina cyanopus*, a rare fungus producing psychoactive tryptamines. *Open Life Sciences*, 10(1). https://doi.org/10.1515/biol-2015-0005

Halpern, J., and Roth, B. L. (2004). Hallucinogens and dissociative agents naturally growing in the United States. *Pharmacology & Therapeutics*, 102(2), 131–138. https://doi.org/10.1016/j.pharmthera.2004.03.003

Haro-Luna, M. X., Ruan-Soto, F., Blancas, J., and Guzmán-Dávalos, L. (2022). The cultural role played by the ethnomyco-logical knowledge of wild mushrooms for the peoples of highlands and lowlands in Tlaltenango, Zacatecas, Mexico. *Mycologia*, 114(4), 645–660. https://doi.org/10.1080/00275514.2022.2068114

Hartney, E. (2023, August 8). What are shrooms (magic mushrooms)? Verywell Mind. https://www.verywellmind.com/what-are-magic-mushrooms-22085

Hartong, V., and van Emmerik, A. (2023). Psychedelic microdosing, mindfulness, and anxiety: A cross-sectional mediation study. *Journal of Psychoactive Drugs*, 55(3), 310–320. https://doi.org/10.1080/02791072.2022.2080616

Hasler, F., Grimberg, U., Benz, et al. (2004). Acute psychological and physiological effects of psilocybin in healthy humans: A double-blind, placebo-controlled dose-effect study. *Psychopharmacology*, 172(2), 145–156. https://doi.org/10.1007/s00213-003-1640-6

Hatfield, G. M., and Brady, L. R. (1969). Occurrence of bis-noryangonin in *Gymnopilus spectabilis*. *Journal of Pharmaceutical Sciences*, 58(10), 1298–1299.

Hausknecht, A., and Krisai-Greilhuber, I. (2007). Infrageneric division of the genus *Pholiotina*—a classical approach. *Österreichische Zeitschrift Für Pilzkunde*, 16(1), 133–145.

Hausknecht, A., Krisai-Greilhuber, I., and Voglmayr, H. (2004). Type studies in North American species of *Bolbitiaceae* belonging to the genera *Conocybe* and *Pholiotina*. *Österreichische Zeitschrift Für Pilzkunde*, 13, 153–235 (see pp. 180, 212).

Hayes, S. C., Strosahl, K. D., and Wilson, K. G. (1999). *Acceptance and Commitment Therapy: An Experiential Approach to Behavior Change*. Guilford Press.

Haze, V., and Mandrake, K. (2016). *The Psilocybin Mushroom Bible: The Definitive Guide to Growing and Using Magic Mushrooms*. Green Candy Press.

Healing Mushrooms. (n.d.). The ultimate guide to the PF Tek method: Recipe, yield, and more. Retrieved August 9, 2023, from https://healing-mushrooms.net/pf-tek

Heim, R., and Cailleux, R. (1959). Nouvelle contribution à la connaissance des *Psilocybes* hallucinogènes du Mexique. *Revue de Mycologie*, 24, 437–441.

Heim, R., and Hofmann, A. (1958). La Psilocybine et la psilocine chez les

Psilocybes et strophaires hallucinogenes. In *Les Champignons Hallucinogenes du Mexique* (Vol. 6, pp. 258–267).

Heim, R., and Wasson, G. (1956). Les champignons divinatoires recueillis par Mme Valentina Pavlovna Wasson et M. R. Gordon Wasson au cours de leurs missions de 1954 et 1955 dans les pays mije, mazateque, zapoteque et nahua du Mexique meridional et central. *Comptes Rendus de l'Académie Des Sciences, 242*, 1389–1395.

Heim, R., and Wasson, G. (1957). Les agarics hallucinogenes du genre *Psilocybe*. *Comptes Rendus de l'Académie Des Sciences, 244*, 659–700.

Herrington, A. J. (2023, October 9). California governor vetoes psychedelics legalization bill. *Forbes*. https://www.forbes.com/sites/ajherrington/2023/10/09/california-governor-vetoes-psychedelics-legalization-bill/

Hesselgrave, N., Troppoli, T. A., Wulff, A. B., et al. (2021). Harnessing psilocybin: Antidepressant-like behavioral and synaptic actions of psilocybin are independent of 5-HT2R activation in mice. *Proceedings of the National Academy of Sciences, 118*(17), e2022489118. https://doi.org/10.1073/pnas.2022489118

Hincks, S. W., Bratt, S., Poudel, S., et al. (2017). Entropic brain-computer interfaces: Using fNIRS and EEG to measure attentional states in a Bayesian framework. *PhyCS*, 23–34.

Hofmann, A., Heim, R., Brack, A., and Kobel, H. F. (1958). Psilocybin, ein psychotroper Wirkstoff aus mexikanischen Rauschpilz Psilocybe mexicana Heim. *Experientia, 14*(3), 107–112. https://doi.org/10.1007/BF02159243

Holtzheimer, P. E., and Mayberg, H. S. (2011). Stuck in a rut: Rethinking depression and its treatment. *Trends in Neurosciences, 34*(1), 1–9. https://doi.org/10.1016/j.tins.2010.10.004

Hove, M. J., Stelzer, J., Nierhaus, T., et al. (2015). Brain network reconfiguration and perceptual decoupling during an absorptive state of consciousness. *Cerebral Cortex, 26*(7), 3116–3124.

Huberman, A. (Director). (2023, May 22). Dr. Robin Carhart-Harris: The Science of Psychedelics for Mental Health, *Huberman Lab Podcast*. https://www.youtube.com/watch?v=fcxjwA4C4Cw

ICEERS. (n.d.). Psilocybin mushrooms: Basic info. https://www.iceers.org/psilocybin-mushrooms-basic-info/

Illinois General Assembly. (n.d.). Bill Status for HB0001. Retrieved September 18, 2023, from https://www.ilga.gov/legislation/BillStatus.asp?DocNum=1&GAID=17&DocTypeID=HB&SessionID=112&GA=103

iNaturalist. (n.d.-a). *Psilocybe* mushrooms (genus *Psilocybe*). Retrieved June 17, 2023, from https://www.inaturalist.org/taxa/54026-Psilocybe

iNaturalist. (n.d.-b). *Psilocybe silvatica*. Retrieved June 24, 2023, from https://www.inaturalist.org/guide_taxa/636084

iNaturalist. (n.d.-c). *Psilocybe yungensis*. Retrieved June 25, 2023, from https://www.inaturalist.org/taxa/206148-Psilocybe-yungensis

iNaturalist Canada. (n.d.). *Psilocybe quebecensis*. (n.d.). Retrieved June 24, 2023, from https://inaturalist.ca/taxa/511407-Psilocybe-quebecensis

iNaturalist Guatemala. (n.d.). *Psilocybe mescaleroensis*. Retrieved June 25, 2023, from https://guatemala.inaturalist.org/taxa/518961-Psilocybe-mescaleroensis

Irizarry, R., Winczura, A., Dimassi, O., et al. (2022). Psilocybin as a treatment for psychiatric illness: A meta-analysis. *Cureus, 14*(11), e31796. https://doi.org/10.7759/cureus.31796

Irwin, M. R., Olmstead, R., Carrillo, C., et al. (2014). Cognitive behavioral therapy vs. tai chi for late life insomnia and inflammatory risk: A randomized controlled comparative efficacy trial. *Sleep, 37*(9), 1543–1552. https://doi.org/10.5665/sleep.4008

IsHak, W. W., Garcia, P., Pearl, R., et al. (2023). The impact of psilocybin on patients experiencing psychiatric symptoms: A systematic review of randomized clinical trials. *Innovations in Clinical Neuroscience, 20*(4–6), 39–48.

IsHak, W. W., Greenberg, J. M., et al. (2011, September 15). Quality of life: The ultimate outcome measure of interventions in major depressive disorder. *Harvard Review of Psychiatry, 19*(5), 229–239. https://www.tandfonline.com/doi/abs/10.3109/10673229.2011.614099

Jacobs, A. (2021, May 9). The psychedelic revolution is coming. Psychiatry may never be the same. *New York Times*. https://www.nytimes.com/2021/05/09/health/psychedelics-mdma-psilocybin-molly-mental-health.html

Jacobs, A. (2021, November 11). Veterans have become unlikely lobbyists in push to legalize psychedelic drugs. *New York Times*. https://maps.org/news/media/the-new-york-times-veterans-have-become-unlikely-lobbyists-in-push-to-legalize-psychedelic-drugs/

Jairaj, C., Fitzsimons, C. M., McAuliffe, F. M., et al. (2019). A population survey of prevalence rates of antenatal depression in the Irish obstetric services using the Edinburgh Postnatal Depression Scale (EPDS). *Archives of Women's Mental Health, 22*(3), 349–355. https://doi.org/10.1007/s00737-018-0893-3

Jairaj, C., O'Leary, N., Doolin, K., et al. (2020). The hypothalamic-pituitary-adrenal axis in the perinatal period: Its relationship with major depressive disorder and early life adversity. *World Journal of Biological Psychiatry, 21*(7), 552–563. https://doi.org/10.1080/15622975.2020.1740318

Jairaj, C., and Rucker, J. J. (2022). Postpartum depression: A role for psychedelics? *Journal of Psychopharmacology (Oxford, England), 36*(8), 920–931. https://doi.org/10.1177/02698811221093793

Janikian, M. (2019). *Your Psilocybin Mushroom Companion: An Informative, Easy-to-Use Guide to Understanding Magic Mushrooms*. Simon and Schuster.

Janikian, M. (2020, April 6). Types of magic mushrooms: 10 shroom strains you should know about. (n.d.). *Double Blind Mag*. https://doubleblindmag.com/mushrooms/types/psilocybe-cubensis-magic-mushrooms/

Jelen, L., and Young, A. (2022). New antidepressants: New day or false dawn? *European Neuropsychopharmacology, 63*, 1–3. https://doi.org/10.1016/j.euroneuro.2022.07.004

Jo, W.-S., Hossain, Md. A., and Park, S.-C. (2014). Toxicological profiles of poisonous, edible, and medicinal mushrooms. *Mycobiology*, 42(3), 215–220. https://doi.org/10.5941/MYCO.2014.42.3.215

Johns Hopkins University. (2023). Effects of psilocybin in post-treatment Lyme Disease (Clinical Trial Registration NCT05305105). ClinicalTrials.gov. https://clinicaltrials.gov/study/NCT05305105

Johns Hopkins University Center for Psychedelic and Consciousness Research. (n.d.). Academic publications. Retrieved September 3, 2021, from https://hopkinspsychedelic.org/publications

Johnson, M. W., Garcia-Romeu, A., Cosimano, M. P., and Griffiths, R. R. (2014). Pilot study of the 5-HT2AR agonist psilocybin in the treatment of tobacco addiction. *Journal of Psychopharmacology (Oxford, England)*, 28(11), 983–992. https://doi.org/10.1177/0269881114548296

Johnson, M. W., Garcia-Romeu, A., and Griffiths, R. R. (2017). Long-term follow-up of psilocybin-facilitated smoking cessation. *American Journal of Drug and Alcohol Abuse*, 43(1), 55–60. https://doi.org/10.3109/00952990.2016.1170135

Johnson, M. W., and Griffiths, R. R. (2017). Potential therapeutic effects of psilocybin. *Neurotherapeutics*, 14(3), 734–740. https://doi.org/10.1007/s13311-017-0542-y

Johnson, M. W., Sewell, R. A., and Griffiths, R. R. (2012). Psilocybin dose-dependently causes delayed, transient headaches in healthy volunteers. *Drug and Alcohol Dependence*, 123(1–3), 132–140. https://doi.org/10.1016/j.drugalcdep.2011.10.029

Johnstad, P. G. (2018). Powerful substances in tiny amounts: An interview study of psychedelic microdosing. *Nordisk Alkohol- & Narkotikatidskrift: NAT*, 35(1), 39–51. https://doi.org/10.1177/1455072517753339

Jones, D. T., and Graff-Radford, J. (2021). Executive dysfunction and the prefrontal cortex. *Continuum (Minneapolis, Minn.)*, 27(6), 1586–1601. https://doi.org/10.1212/CON.0000000000001009

Jones, E. (2023). Dutch newspapers on war victims and their LSD-treatment by Jan Bastiaans, from KZ-syndrome to PTSD. *Medicine, Conflict and Survival*, 39(3), 313–315. https://doi.org/10.1080/13623699.2023.2233830

Jones, G., Lipson, J., and Nock, M. K. (2022). Associations between classic psychedelics and nicotine dependence in a nationally representative sample. *Scientific Reports*, 12(1), 10578. https://doi.org/10.1038/s41598-022-14809-3

Kang, K., Orlandi, S., Leung, J., et al. (2023, May 10). Electroencephalographic interbrain synchronization in children with disabilities, their parents, and neurologic music therapists. *European Journal of Neuroscience*, 58(1), 2367–2383. https://onlinelibrary.wiley.com/doi/abs/10.1111/ejn.16036

Kansas State Legislature. (2022). House Bill 2465. http://kslegislature.org/li_2022/b2021_22/measures/documents/hb2465_00_0000.pdf

Katsnelson, A. (2022, May 31). Tripping over the potential of psychedelics for autism. Spectrum. https://www.spectrumnews.org/news/tripping-over-the-potential-of-psychedelics-for-autism/

Kawai, N., Honda, M., Nishina, E., et al. (2017). Electroencephalogram characteristics during possession trances in healthy individuals. *Neuroreport*, 28(15), 949.

Kaye, W. (2022). Evaluation of psilocybin in anorexia nervosa: Safety and efficacy (Clinical Trial Registration NCT04661514). ClinicalTrials. gov. https://clinicaltrials.gov/study/NCT04661514

Kelly, E., Meng, F., Fujita, H., et al. (2020). Regulation of autism-relevant behaviors by cerebellar–prefrontal cortical circuits. *Nature Neuroscience*, 23(9), 1102–1110. https://doi.org/10.1038/s41593-020-0665-z

Kelmendi, B. (2023). Psilocybin treatment in obsessive-compulsive disorder: A preliminary efficacy study and exploratory investigation of neural correlates. (Clinical Trial Registration NCT03356483). ClinicalTrials. gov. https://clinicaltrials.gov/study/NCT03356483

Kelmendi, B., Kichuk, S. A., DePalmer, G., et al. (2022). Single-dose psilocybin for treatment-resistant obsessive-compulsive disorder: A case report. *Heliyon*, 8(12), e12135. https://doi.org/10.1016/j.heliyon.2022.e12135

Kemp, A. H., Quintana, D. S., Gray, M. A., et al. (2010). Impact of depression and antidepressant treatment on heart rate variability: A review and meta-analysis. *Synaptic Development in Mood Disorders*, 67(11), 1067–1074. https://doi.org/10.1016/j.biopsych.2009.12.012

Kendrick, B. (2000). *The Fifth Kingdom*. Focus Pub.

Kenney, A. (2023, June 21a). Colorado decriminalized psilocybin. Here's what happens next. *Colorado Sun*. https://coloradosun.com/2023/06/18/colorado-decriminalized-psilocybin-whats-next/

Kenney, A. (2023, June 21b). What to know about Colorado's psychedelic law. *Colorado Public Radio News*. https://www.cpr.org/2023/06/21/colorado-psychedelic-law-for-psilocybin-mushrooms/

Kenney, A. (2023, July 4). A gray market emerges in Colorado after voters approved psychedelic substances. *Morning Edition*. https://www.npr.org/2023/07/04/1185922732/a-gray-market-emerges-in-colorado-after-voters-approved-psychedelic-substances

Kerbel, J. (2021, September 28). Understanding and measuring magic mushroom potency. Frshminds. https://frshminds.com/understanding-and-measuring-magic-mushroom-potency/

Kerbel, J. (2021, November 8). Blame it all on the *Psilocybe mexicana*. Frshminds. https://frshminds.com/psilocybe-mexicana/

Kerbel, J. (2021, November 19). Penis Envy mushrooms: What's in a name. Frshminds. https://frshminds.com/penis-envy-mushrooms/

Kerbel, J. (2022, August 21). Magic mushroom species list. Frshminds. https://frshminds.com/magic-mushroom-species-list/

Kerbel, J. (2022, September 13). Magic mushrooms of South and Central America. Frshminds. https://frshminds.com/magic-mushrooms-of-south-and-central-america/

Kiernan, J. A. (2012). Anatomy of the temporal lobe. *Epilepsy Research and Treatment*, 2012, 176157. https://doi.org/10.1155/2012/176157

Kinderlehrer, D. A. (2023). The effectiveness

of microdosed psilocybin in the treatment of neuropsychiatric Lyme disease: A case study. *International Medical Case Reports Journal*, 16, 109–115. https://doi.org/10.2147/IMCRJ.S395342

Kiraga, M. K., Kuypers, K. P. C., Uthaug, M. V., et al. (2022). Decreases in state and trait anxiety post-psilocybin: A naturalistic, observational study among retreat attendees. *Frontiers in Psychiatry*, 13. https://www.frontiersin.org/articles/10.3389/fpsyt.2022.883869

Kirk, P., Cannon, P. F., Minter, D. W., and Stalpers, J. A. (2008). *Dictionary of the Fungi* (10th ed.). CABI.

Kits van Waveren, E. (1985). *The Dutch, French, and British Species of* Psathyrella. Rijksherbarium.

Köhler, S., Cierpinsky, K., Kronenberg, G., and Adli, M. (2016). The serotonergic system in the neurobiology of depression: Relevance for novel antidepressants. *Journal of Psychopharmacology*, 30(1), 13–22. https://doi.org/10.1177/0269881115609072

Köhler, U. (1995). Rectangular mushroom stones from Oaxaca, Mexico. *Mexicon*, 17(4), 70–73.

Koike, Y., Wada, K., Kusano, G., et al. (1981). Isolation of psilocybin from *Psilocybe argentipes* and its determination in specimens of some mushrooms. *Journal of Natural Products*, 44(3), 362–365. https://doi.org/10.1021/np50015a023

Kometer, M., Pokorny, T., Seifritz, E., and Volleinweider, F. X. (2015). Psilocybin-induced spiritual experiences and insightfulness are associated with synchronization of neuronal oscillations. *Psychopharmacology*, 232(19), 3663–3676. https://doi.org/10.1007/s00213-015-4026-7

Korr, H., and Schmitz, C. (1999). Facts and fictions regarding post-natal neurogenesis in the developing human cerebral cortex. *Journal of Theoretical Biology*, 200(3), 291–297. https://doi.org/10.1006/jtbi.1999.0992

Kraehenmann, R. (2017). Dreams and psychedelics: Neurophenomenological comparison and therapeutic implications. *Current Neuropharmacology*, 15(7), 1032–1042. https://www.ingentaconnect.com/content/ben/cn/2017/00000015/00000007/art00009

Kraehenmann, R., Pokorny, D., Vollenweider, L., et al. (2017). Dreamlike effects of LSD on waking imagery in humans depend on serotonin 2A receptor activation. *Psychopharmacology*, 234(13), 2031–2046. https://doi.org/10.1007/s00213-017-4610-0

Kraehenmann, R., Preller, K. H., Scheidegger, M., et al. (2015). Psilocybin-induced decrease in amygdala reactivity correlates with enhanced positive mood in healthy volunteers. *Biological Psychiatry*, 78(8), 572–581. https://doi.org/10.1016/j.biopsych.2014.04.010

Kraehenmann, R., Schmidt, A., Friston, K., et al. (2016). The mixed serotonin receptor agonist psilocybin reduces threat-induced modulation of amygdala connectivity. *NeuroImage: Clinical*, 11, 53–60. https://doi.org/10.1016/j.nicl.2015.08.009

Krediet, E., Bostoen, T., Breeksema, J., et al. (2020). Reviewing the potential of psychedelics for the treatment of PTSD. *International Journal of Neuropsychopharmacology*, 23(6), 385–400. https://doi.org/10.1093/ijnp/pyaa018

Kühner, R. K. (1972). Agaricales de la zone alpine: Genres *Galera earle* et *Phaeogalera gen. nov. Bulletin Trimestriel de La Société Mycologique de France*, 88, 41–153.

Kuo, M. (2007, April). The genus *Inocybe*. MushroomExpert.com. https://www.mushroomexpert.com/inocybe.html

Kuypers, K. P. C. (2020). The therapeutic potential of microdosing psychedelics in depression. *Therapeutic Advances in Psychopharmacology*, 10, 1–15.

Kuypers, K. P. C., Ng, L., Erritzoe, D., et al. (2019). Microdosing psychedelics: More questions than answers? An overview and suggestions for future research. *Journal of Psychopharmacology*, 33(9), 1093–1057.

Laird, K. T., Lavretsky, H., Paholpak, P., et al. (2019). Clinical correlates of resilience factors in geriatric depression. *International Psychogeriatrics*, 31(2), 193–202. https://doi.org/10.1017/S1041610217002873

Laird, K. T., Lavretsky, H., Wu, P., et al. (2019). Neurocognitive correlates of resilience in late-life depression. *American Journal of Geriatric Psychiatry*, 27(1), 12–17. https://doi.org/10.1016/j.jagp.2018.08.009

LaMaison, J.-L. (1998). *The Great Encyclopedia of Mushrooms*. Konemann.

Lanius, R. A., Bluhm, R., Lanius, U., and Pain, C. (2006). A review of neuroimaging studies in PTSD: Heterogeneity of response to symptom provocation. *Journal of Psychiatric Research*, 40(8), 709–729. https://doi.org/10.1016/j.jpsychires.2005.07.007

Largent, D., and Baroni, T. J. (1988). *How to Identify Mushrooms to Genus VI: Modern Genera*. Mad River Press.

Lea, T., Amada, N., Jungaberle, H., et al. (2020). Perceived outcomes of psychedelic microdosing as self-managed therapies for mental and substance use disorders. *Psychopharmacology*, 237(5), 1521–1532. https://doi.org/10.1007/s00213-020-05477-0

Lebedev, A. V., Kaelen, M., Lövdén, M., et al. (2016). LSD-induced entropic brain activity predicts subsequent personality change. *Human Brain Mapping*, 37(9), 3203–3213.

Lechter, A. (2008). *Shroom: A Cultural History of the Magic Mushroom*. Harper Collins.

Ledwos, N., Rodas, J. D., Husain, M. I., et al. (2023). Therapeutic uses of psychedelics for eating disorders and body dysmorphic disorder. *Journal of Psychopharmacology*, 37(1), 3–13. https://doi.org/10.1177/02698811221140009

Leech, R., and Sharp, D. J. (2014). The role of the posterior cingulate cortex in cognition and disease. *Brain: A Journal of Neurology*, 137(Pt 1), 12–32. https://doi.org/10.1093/brain/awt162

Leschik, J., Lutz, B., and Gentile, A. (2021). Stress-related dysfunction of adult hippocampal neurogenesis—an attempt for understanding resilience? *International Journal of Molecular Sciences*, 22(14). https://doi.org/10.3390/ijms22147339

Leung, A., and Paul, A. G. (1967). Baeocystin, a mono-methyl analog of psilocybin from *Psilocybe baeocystis* saprophytic culture. *J Pharm Sci*, 56(1), 146. https://doi.org/10.1002/jps.2600560132

Leung, A., and Paul, A. G. (1968). Baeocystin and norbaeocystin: New analogs of psilocybin from *Psilocybe baeocystis*. *J*

Pharm Sci, 57(10), 1667–1671. https://doi.org/10.1002/jps.2600571007

Levinas, E. (1969). *Totality and Infinity: An Essay on Exteriority* (A. Lingis, Trans.). Duquesne University Press.

Lewis-Healey, E. (2021, May 25). What is changa? The psychedelic you've likely never heard of (yet). *Psychedelic Spotlight*. https://psychedelicspotlight.com/what-is-changa/

Lima da Cruz, R. V., Moulin, T. C., Petiz, L. L., and Leão, R. N. (2018). A single dose of 5-MeO-DMT stimulates cell proliferation, neuronal survivability, morphological, and functional changes in adult mice ventral dentate gyrus. *Frontiers in Molecular Neuroscience*, 11. https://doi.org/10.3389/fnmol.2018.00312

Lincoff, G. (2008). *National Audubon Society Field Guide to North American Mushrooms*. Alfred A. Knopf.

Ling, S., Ceban, F., Lui, L. M. W., et al. (2022). Molecular mechanisms of psilocybin and implications for the treatment of depression. *CNS Drugs*, 36(1), 17–30. https://doi.org/10.1007/s40263-021-00877-y

Loneragan, M. (n.d.). A therapy session with the "Golden Teacher." You:Time. Retrieved June 15, 2023, from https://youtime.com/think/a-therapy-session-with-the-golden-teacher

Lowe, H., Toyang, N., Steele, B., et al. (2022). Psychedelics: Alternative and potential therapeutic options for treating mood and anxiety disorders. *Molecules (Basel, Switzerland)*, 27(8), 2520. https://doi.org/10.3390/molecules27082520

Lowy, B. (1971). New records of mushroom stones from Guatemala. *Mycologia*, 63(5), 983–993. https://doi.org/10.1080/00275514.1971.12019194

Lubiano, K. (2022, June 1). Tidal Wave: Psilocybin Cup winner 2021 for highest potency. Tripsitter. https://tripsitter.com/magic-mushrooms/strains/tidal-wave/

Lubiano, K. (2022, October 28). Enigma magic mushrooms: The "blob mutation" mushrooms. Tripsitter. https://tripsitter.com/magic-mushrooms/strains/enigma/

Lucherini Angeletti, L., Innocenti, M., Felciai, F., et al. (2022). Anorexia nervosa as a disorder of the subcortical-cortical interoceptive-self. *Eating and Weight Disorders: EWD*, 27(8), 3063–3081. https://doi.org/10.1007/s40519-022-01510-7

Lyes, M., Yang, K. H., Castellanos, J., and Furnish, T. (2023). Microdosing psilocybin for chronic pain: A case series. *Pain*, 164(4), 698–702. https://doi.org/10.1097/j.pain.0000000000002778

MacLean, K. A., Johnson, M. W., and Griffiths, R. R. (2011). Mystical experiences occasioned by the hallucinogen psilocybin lead to increases in the personality domain of openness. *Journal of Psychopharmacology*, 25(11), 1453–1461.

Mahmood, Z. A. (2013). *Natural Products*. Colorcon Limited. Table 18.1: Psilocybin and psilocin content of some major species of . . . Available on ResearchGate, https://www.researchgate.net/figure/1-Psilocybin-and-psilocin-content-of-some-major-species-of-Psilocybe_tbl1_278709278

Mainieri, A. G., Peres, J. F. P., Moreira-Almeida, A., et al. (2017). Neural correlates of psychotic-like experiences during spiritual-trance state. *Psychiatry Research: Neuroimaging*, 266, 101–107.

Mandrake, K. (2021, May 5). *Psilocybe mexicana*: What you should know about the magic mushroom that changed history. *Double Blind Mag.* https://doubleblindmag.com/mushrooms/types/psilocybe-mexicana/

Mandrake, K. (2022, February 24). Meet the Ohio Valley shroom taking over the world. *DoubleBlind Mag.* https://doubleblindmag.com/psilocybe-ovoideocystidiata/

Mandrake, K. (2023, April 13). *Psilocybe serbica* and the case of mistaken identity. *DoubleBlind Mag.* https://doubleblindmag.com/psilocybe-serbica-psilocybe-bohemica/

Mandrake, K. (2023, April 20). *Psilocybe baeocystis* was once mistaken as deadly—it's just psychedelic. *DoubleBlind Mag.* https://doubleblindmag.com/psilocybe-baeocystis/

Mandy, W. (2018). The Research Domain Criteria: A new dawn for neurodiversity research? *Autism, 22*(6), 642–644. https://doi.org/10.1177/1362361318782586

Mans, K., Kettner, H., Erritzoe, D., et al. (2021). Sustained, multifaceted improvements in mental well-being following psychedelic experiences in a prospective opportunity sample. *Frontiers in Psychiatry, 12,* 647909. https://doi.org/10.3389/fpsyt.2021.647909

Marcano, V., Méndez, A. M., Castellano, F., et al. (1994). Occurrence of psilocybin and psilocin in *Psilocybe pseudobullacea* (Petch) Pegler from the Venezuelan Andes. *Journal of Ethnopharmacology, 43*(2), 157–159. https://doi.org/10.1016/0378-8741(94)90013-2

Marchese, D. (2023, April 7). A psychedelics pioneer takes the ultimate trip. *New York Times.* https://www.nytimes.com/interactive/2023/04/03/magazine/roland-griffiths-interview.html

Markey, E. (2023, April 1). *Psilocybe cubensis.* PsyTech. https://psytechglobal.com/psilocybe-cubensis/

Markey, E. (2023, May 1). The bright wisdom of the Golden Teacher mushroom. PsyTech. https://psytechglobal.com/golden-teachers/

Marley, J. (2022, August 29). Alacabenzi magic mushroom strain: Mild, euphoric, and insightful. *Tripsitter.* https://tripsitter.com/magic-mushrooms/strains/alacabenzi/

Marshall, C. (2021, January 27). Algerian cave paintings suggest humans did magic mushrooms 9,000 years ago. Open Culture. https://www.openculture.com/2021/01/algerian-cave-paintings-suggest-humans-did-magic-mushrooms-9000-years-ago.html

Marstaller, L., Fynes-Clinton, S., Burianová, H., and Reutens, D. C. (2020). Salience and default-mode network connectivity during threat and safety processing in older adults. *Human Brain Mapping, 42*(1), 14–23. https://doi.org/10.1002/hbm.25199

Martial, C., Cassol, H., Charland-Verville, V., et al. (2019). Neurochemical models of near-death experiences: A large-scale study based on the semantic similarity of written reports. *Consciousness and Cognition, 69,* 52–69. https://doi.org/10.1016/j.concog.2019.01.011

Martin, D. (2004, February 22). Humphry Osmond, 86, who sought medicinal value in psychedelic drugs, dies. *New York Times*. https://www.nytimes.com/2004/02/22/us/humphry-osmond-86-who-sought-medicinal-value-in-psychedelic-drugs-dies.html

Mason, N. L., Kuypers, K. P. C., Müller, F., et al. (2020). Me, myself, bye: Regional alterations in glutamate and the experience of ego dissolution with psilocybin. *Neuropsychopharmacology*, *45*(12), Article 12. https://doi.org/10.1038/s41386-020-0718-8

Mastinu, A., Anyanwu, M., Carone, M., et al. (2023). The bright side of psychedelics: Latest advances and challenges in neuropharmacology. *International Journal of Molecular Sciences*, *24*(2), 1329. https://doi.org/10.3390/ijms24021329

Matheny, P. B., Curtis, J. M., Hofstetter, V., et al. (2006). Major clades of *Agaricales*: A multilocus phylogenetic overview. *Mycologia*, *98*(6), 982–995. https://doi.org/10.1080/15572536.2006.11832627

Matsushima, Y., Shirota, O., Kikura-Hanajiri, R., et al. (2009). Effects of *Psilocybe argentipes* on marble-burying behavior in mice. *Bioscience, Biotechnology, & Biochemistry*, *73*(8), 1866–1868. https://doi.org/10.1271/bbb.90095

May, P. (1999, October). Psilocybin and mescaline. University of Bristol. http://www.chm.bris.ac.uk/motm/psilocybin/psilocybinv.htm

McAdams, C. J., and Smith, W. (2015). Neural correlates of eating disorders: Translational potential. *Neuroscience and Neuroeconomics*, *4*, 35–49. https://doi.org/10.2147/NAN.S76699

McAlonan, D. G. (2022). Modulation of serotonin pathways using psilocybin in adults with and without autism spectrum disorder (ASD) (Clinical Trial Registration NCT05651126). ClinicalTrials.gov. https://clinicaltrials.gov/study/NCT05651126

McElroy, C. (2023, January 16). How strong is the average magic mushroom? Tripsitter. https://tripsitter.com/magic-mushrooms/average-potency/

McElroy, C. (2023, January 24). *Psilocybe azurescens* 101: The "Flying Saucer" shrooms. Tripsitter. https://tripsitter.com/magic-mushrooms/species/psilocybe-azurescens/

McElroy, C. (2023, May 23). Blue Meanies mushrooms: A definitive guide to *Panaeolus cyanescens*. Tripsitter. https://tripsitter.com/magic-mushrooms/species/panaeolus-cyanescens/

McElroy, C. (2023, June 18). PF Classic: An OG strain of *Psilocybe cubensis*. Tripsitter. https://tripsitter.com/magic-mushrooms/strains/pf-classic/

McElroy, C. (2023, June 20). *Psilocybe baeocystis*: Oregon's gateway to altered states of consciousness. Tripsitter. https://tripsitter.com/magic-mushrooms/species/psilocybe-baeocystis/

McIntyre, R. S. (2023). Serotonin 5-HT2B receptor agonism and valvular heart disease: Implications for the development of psilocybin and related agents. *Expert Opinion on Drug Safety*, *22*(10), 881–883. https://doi.org/10.1080/14740338.2023.2248883

McKenna, T. (1992). *Food of the Gods: The Search for the Original Tree of Knowledge, A Radical History of Plants, Drugs, and Human Evolution*. Bantam Books.

McKernan, K., Kane, L., Helbert, Y., et al. (2021). A whole genome atlas of 81

Psilocybe genomes as a resource for psilocybin production. [version 2; peer review: 1 not approved]. *F1000Research*, *10*(961). https://doi.org/10.12688/f1000research.55301.2

McKnight, K., Rohrer, J., McKnight Ward, K., and McKnight, K. H. (2021). *Peterson Field Guide to Mushrooms of North America* (2nd ed.). Mariner Books.

McLeod, E. (2022, April 12). Maryland approves bill expanding psychedelics research, access for veterans with PTSD. Outlaw Report. https://outlawreport.com/maryland-approves-bill-expanding-psychedelics-research-access-for-veterans-with-ptsd/

McTaggart, A. R., James, T. Y., Slot, J. C., et al. (2023). Genome sequencing progenies of magic mushrooms (*Psilocybe subaeruginosa*) identifies tetrapolar mating and gene duplications in the psilocybin pathway. *Fungal Genetics and Biology*, *165*, 103769. https://doi.org/10.1016/j.fgb.2022.103769

Medical News Today. (n.d.). What are Penis Envy mushrooms? https://www.medicalnewstoday.com/articles/penis-envy-mushrooms

Mentlein, R., and Kendall, M. D. (2000). The brain and thymus have much in common: A functional analysis of their microenvironments. *Immunology Today*, *21*(3), 133–140. https://doi.org/10.1016/s0167-5699(99)01557-1

Mérida Ponce, J. P., Hernández Calderón, M. A., Comandini, O., et al. (2019). Ethno-mycological knowledge among Kaqchikel, indigenous Maya people of Guatemalan highlands. *Journal of Ethnobiology and Ethnomedicine*, *15*(1), 36. https://doi.org/10.1186/s13002-019-0310-7

Merlin, M. D., and Allen, J. W. (1993). Species identification and chemical analysis of psychoactive fungi in the Hawaiian Islands. *Journal of Ethnopharmacology*, *40*(1), 21–40. https://doi.org/10.1016/0378-8741(93)90086-K

Metzner, R., and Darling, D. (2005). *Sacred Mushroom of Visions: Teonanácatl : A Sourcebook on the Psilocybin Mushroom*. Park Street Press.

Micro Zoomers. (n.d.-a). *Alacabenzi cubensis*. Retrieved June 15, 2023, from https://microzoomers.co/strains/alcabenzi/

Micro Zoomers. (n.d.-b). *Psilocybe*. Retrieved June 15, 2023, from https://microzoomers.co/strains/lists/genus/psilocybe/

Mikhail, A. (2023, June 27). Silicon Valley elites are reportedly taking ketamine and attending psychedelic parties to bolster their focus and creativity. Here's what the drugs do to your brain. *Fortune*. https://fortune.com/well/2023/06/27/silicon-valley-elites-ketamine-psychedelics-effects-on-brain/

Miller, G. (n.d.). Timothy Leary's transformation from scientist to psychedelic celebrity. *Wired*. Retrieved September 19, 2023, from https://www.wired.com/2013/10/timothy-leary-archives/

Miller, O. K., and Miller, H. H. (1981). *Mushrooms in Color: How to Know Them, Where to Find Them, What to Avoid*. E. P. Dutton.

Minzenberg, M. J., Laird, A. R., Thelen, S., et al. (2009). Meta-analysis of 41 functional neuroimaging studies of executive function in schizophrenia. *Archives of General Psychiatry*, *66*(8), 811–822.

Mitchell, J. M., Ot'alora G., M., van der Kolk, B., et al. (2023). MDMA-assisted therapy for moderate to severe PTSD: A randomized, placebo-controlled phase 3 trial. *Nature Medicine*, 1–8. https://doi.org/10.1038/s41591-023-02565-4

MND Staff. (2021, July 20). Sonora's traditional toad medicine "removes the madness from your mind." *Mexico News Daily*. https://mexiconewsdaily.com/news/sonoras-traditional-toad-medicine-removes-the-madness-from-your-mind/

Mohandas, E. (2008). Neurobiology of spirituality. *Mens Sana Monographs*, 6(1), 63–80. https://doi.org/10.4103/0973-1229.33001

Moncalvo, J. M., Vilgalys, R., Redhead, S. A., et al. (2002). One hundred and seventeen clades of euagarics. *Molecular Phylogenetics and Evolution*, 23(3), 357–400. https://doi.org/10.1016/S1055-7903(02)00027-1

Monroy, M., and Keltner, D. (2023). Awe as a pathway to mental and physical health. *Perspectives on Psychological Science: A Journal of the Association for Psychological Science*, 18(2), 309–320. https://doi.org/10.1177/17456916221094856

Montoya, A., Hernández-Totomoch, O., Estrada-Torres, A., et al. (2003). Traditional knowledge about mushrooms in a Nahua community in the state of Tlaxcala, México. *Mycologia*, 95(5), 793–806. https://doi.org/10.1080/15572536.2004.11833038

Moreno, F. A. (2023). Psilocybin for treatment of obsessive compulsive disorder (Clinical Trial Registration NCT03300947). ClinicalTrials.gov. https://clinicaltrials.gov/study/NCT03300947

Moreno, F. A., Wiegand, C. B., Taitano, E. K., and Delgado, P. L. (2006). Safety, tolerability, and efficacy of psilocybin in 9 patients with obsessive-compulsive disorder. *The Journal of Clinical Psychiatry*, 67(11), 1735–1740. https://doi.org/10.4088/jcp.v67n1110

Morton, E., Sakai, K., Ashtari, A., et al. (2023). Risks and benefits of psilocybin use in people with bipolar disorder: An international web-based survey on experiences of "magic mushroom" consumption. *Journal of Psychopharmacology*, 37(1), 49–60.

Moser, M., and Horak, E. (1968). Psilocybe serbica spec.nov., eine neue Psilocybin und Psilocin bildende Art aus Serbien. *Zeitschrift Für Pilzkunde*, 34(3), 137–144.

Moses-Kolko, E. L., Perlman, S. B., Wisner, K. L., et al. (2010). Abnormally reduced dorsomedial prefrontal cortical activity and effective connectivity with amygdala in response to negative emotional faces in postpartum depression. *The American Journal of Psychiatry*, 167(11), 1373–1380. https://doi.org/10.1176/appi.ajp.2010.09081235

Moskowitz, L., and Weiselberg, E. (2017). Anorexia nervosa/atypical anorexia nervosa. *Current Problems in Pediatric and Adolescent Health Care*, 47(4), 70–84. https://doi.org/10.1016/j.cppeds.2017.02.003

Mukerji, K. G., and Manoharachary, C. (2010). *Taxonomy and Ecology of Indian Fungi*. I. K. International Pvt. P. 204.

Muraresku, B. C. (2020). *The Immortality Key: The Secret History of the Religion with No Name*. St. Martin's Publishing Group.

Murrill, W. A. (1923). Dark-spored agarics: V. *Psilocybe. Mycologia*, 15(1), 1–22. https://doi.org/10.2307/3753647

Musha, M., Kusano, G., Tanaka, F. et al. (1988). Poisoning by the hallucinogenic mushroom hikageshibiretake *Psilocybe argentipes* with special regard to the subjective experiences during psilocybin intoxication. *Psychiatria et Neurologia Japonica*, 90(4), 313–333.

MushMagic. (n.d.). How to reuse your spent mycelium cakes. Retrieved August 9, 2023, from https://www.mushmagic.com/blog-how-to-reuse-your-spent-mycelium-cakes–n125

Mushly. (n.d.-a). Orissa India magic mushrooms—*Psilocybe cubensis*. Retrieved October 12, 2023, from https://mushly.com/psychedelic-mushrooms/orissa-india-mushrooms

Mushly. (n.d.-b). PF Classic magic mushrooms—*Psilocybe cubensis*. Retrieved October 12, 2023, from https://mushly.com/psychedelic-mushrooms/pf-classic

Mushroom Appreciation. (2022, February 27). Poisonous mushrooms: Facts, myths, and identification information. https://www.mushroom-appreciation.com/poisonous-mushrooms.html

Mushroom Health Guide. (2020, February 11). Foraging & 3 keys of a mushroom hunter. https://mushroomhealthguide.com/3-keys-of-a-mushroom-hunter/

Mushroom Observer. (n.d.). Observation 509119: *Psilocybe liniformans Guzmán & Bas*. Retrieved June 24, 2023, from https://mushroomobserver.org/observations/509119

Muttoni, S., Ardissino, M., and John, C. (2019). Classical psychedelics for the treatment of depression and anxiety: A systematic review. *Journal of Affective Disorders*, 258, 11–24. https://doi.org/10.1016/j.jad.2019.07.076

MycoBank. (n.d.-a). *Diatrypella stigma*. Retrieved June 24, 2023, from https://www.mycobank.org/page/Name%20details%20page/321934

MycoBank. (n.d.-b). *Psilocybe*. (n.d.). International Mycological Association. https://www.mycobank.org/page/Name%20details%20page/49165

Mycology Wiki. (n.d.). *Psilocybe cubensis*. Retrieved June 16, 2023, from https://mycology.fandom.com/wiki/Psilocybe_cubensis

Mycophiliac. (2023, June 19). *Psilocybe silvatica*. Mycophiliac. https://www.mycophiliac.com/p/psilocybe-silvatica

Natarajan, K., and Raman, N. (1985). A new species of *Psilocybe* from India. *Mycologia*, 77(1), 158–161. https://doi.org/10.1080/00275514.1985.12025076

National Audubon Society. (2023). *National Audubon Society Mushrooms of North America*. Knopf Publishers.

National Institute of Mental Health. (n.d.-a). Any anxiety disorder. Retrieved July 23, 2023, from https://www.nimh.nih.gov/health/statistics/any-anxiety-disorder

National Institute of Mental Health. (n.d.-b). Major depression. Retrieved August 7, 2023, from https://www.nimh.nih.gov/health/statistics/major-depression

NatureServe Explorer. (n.d.). *Conocybe cyanopus*. Retrieved June 25, 2023, from https://explorer.natureserve.org/Taxon/ELEMENT_GLOBAL.2.1063486/Conocybe_cyanopus

Nayak, S. M., and Griffiths, R. R. (2022). A single belief-changing psychedelic experience is associated with increased attribution of consciousness to living and non-living entities. *Frontiers in Psychology*, *13*, 852248. https://doi.org/10.3389/fpsyg.2022.852248

Nayak, S. M., Gukasyan, N., Barrett, F. S., et al. (2021). Classic psychedelic coadministration with lithium, but not lamotrigine, is associated with seizures: An analysis of online psychedelic experience reports. *Pharmacopsychiatry*. https://doi.org/10.1055/a-1524-2794

NBN Atlas Scotland. (n.d.). *Psilocybe semilanceata (Fr.) P. Kumm.* magic mushroom. https://scotland-species.nbnatlas.org/species/NBNSYS0000021551

Nebigil, C. G., Jaffré, F., Messaddeq, N., et al. (2003). Overexpression of the serotonin 5-HT2B receptor in heart leads to abnormal mitochondrial function and cardiac hypertrophy. *Circulation*, *107*(25), 3223–3229. https://doi.org/10.1161/01.CIR.0000074224.57016.01

Nestler, E., Barrot, M., DiLeone, R., et al. (2002). Neurobiology of depression. *Neuron*. *34*(1), 13–25.

Nguyen, S. A., and LAvretsky, H. (2020). Emerging complementary and integrative therapies for geriatric mental health. *Current Treatment Options in Psychiatry*, *7*(4), 447–470. https://doi.org/10.1007/s40501-020-00229-5

Nguyen, T. (2023, October 7). California Gov. Gavin Newsom vetoes bill that would have decriminalized psychedelic mushrooms. AP News. https://apnews.com/article/psychedelics-magic-mushrooms-psilocybin-gavin-newsom-california-df0acc070df06de668ef69aafc1f13e1

Nichols, D. E. (2004). Hallucinogens. *Pharmacology & Therapeutics*, *101*(2), 131–181. https://doi.org/10.1016/j.pharmthera.2003.11.002

Nikolič, M., Viktorin, V., Zach, P., et al. (2023). Psilocybin intoxication did not affect daytime or sleep-related declarative memory consolidation in a small sample exploratory analysis. *European Neuropsychopharmacology*, *74*, 78–88. https://doi.org/10.1016/j.euroneuro.2023.04.019

Nkadimeng, S. M., Steinmann, C. M. L., and Eloff, J. N. (2020). Effects and safety of *Psilocybe cubensis* and *Panaeolus cyanescens* magic mushroom extracts on endothelin-1-induced hypertrophy and cell injury in cardiomyocytes. *Scientific Reports*, *10*(1). https://doi.org/10.1038/s41598-020-79328-5

Nkadimeng, S. M., Steinmann, C. M. L., and Eloff, J. N. (2021). Anti-inflammatory effects of four psilocybin-containing magic mushroom water extracts in vitro on 15-lipoxygenase activity and on lipopolysaccharide-induced cyclooxygenase-2 and inflammatory cytokines in human u937 macrophage cells. *Journal of Inflammation Research*, *14*, 3729–3738. https://doi.org/10.2147/JIR.S317182

Noorani, T., Garcia-Romeu, A., Swift, T. C., et al. (2018). Psychedelic therapy for smoking cessation: Qualitative analysis of participant accounts. *Journal of Psychopharmacology (Oxford, England)*, *32*(7), 756–769. https://doi.org/10.1177/0269881118780612

North American Mycological Association. (n.d.). How to make a spore print.

Retrieved August 9, 2023, from https://namyco.org/how_to_spore_prints.php

Northoff, G., and Heinzel, A. (2006). First-person neuroscience: A new methodological approach for linking mental and neuronal states. *Philosophy, Ethics, and Humanities in Medicine, 1*(1), 1–10.

Norvell, L. L. (2010). Report of the nomenclature committee for fungi: 15. *TAXON, 59*(1), 291–293. https://doi.org/10.1002/tax.591029

Nunez, P. L. (2012). *Brain, Mind, and the Structure of Reality*. Oxford University Press.

Nunez, P. L. (2016). *The New Science of Consciousness: Exploring the Complexity of Brain, Mind, and Self*. Prometheus Books.

Nygart, V. A., Pommerencke, L. M., Haijen, E. C. H. M., and Erritzoe, D. (2022). Antidepressant effects of a psychedelic experience in a large prospective naturalistic sample. *Journal of Psychopharmacology, 36*(8), 932–942.

Oaklander, M. (2021, April 5). Inside ibogaine, one of the most promising and perilous psychedelics for addiction. *Time*. https://time.com/5951772/ibogaine-drug-treatment-addiction/

Oláh, G.-M. (1973). The fine structure of *Psilocybe quebecensis. Mycopathologia et Mycologia Applicata, 49*(4), 321–338. https://doi.org/10.1007/BF02050725

Olza, I., Uvnas-Moberg, K., Ekström-Bergström, A., et al. (2020). Birth as a neuro-psycho-social event: An integrative model of maternal experiences and their relation to neurohormonal events during childbirth. *PLOS ONE, 15*(7), e0230992. https://doi.org/10.1371/journal.pone.0230992

Omissi, A. (2016). The cap of liberty: Roman slavery, cultural memory, and magic mushrooms. *Folklore, 127*(3), 270–285. https://doi.org/10.1080/0015587X.2016.1155371

Ona, G., Kohek, M., and Bouso, J. C. (2022). The illusion of knowledge in the emerging field of psychedelic research. *New Ideas in Psychology, 67*, 100967. https://doi.org/10.1016/j.newideapsych.2022.100967

Osarenkhoe, O. O., John, O. A., and Theophilus, D. A. (2014). Ethnomycological conspectus of West African mushrooms: An awareness document. *Advances in Microbiology, 4*(1). https://www.scirp.org/html/8-2270260_42265.htm

Oss, O. T., and Oeric, O. N. (1976). *Psilocybin, Magic Mushroom Grower's Guide: A Handbook for Psilocybin Enthusiasts*. And/Or Press.

Ott, J., and Bigwood, J. (1978). *Teonanácatl: Hallucinogenic Mushrooms of North America: Extracts from the Second International Conference on Hallucinogenic Mushrooms, Held October 27–30, 1977, near Port Townsend, Washington*. Madrona Publishers.

Oughli, H., Simmons, S., Ngyuen, S., and Lavretsky, H. (2021). Resilience and mind-body interventions in late-life depression. *MD Edge Psychiatry, 21*(12), 29–35. https://www.mdedge.com/psychiatry/article/259827/geriatrics/resilience-and-mind-body-interventions-late-life-depression

Oyetayo, O. V. (2011). Medicinal uses of mushrooms in Nigeria: Towards full and sustainable exploitation. *African Journal*

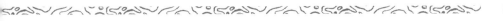

of Traditional, Complementary, and Alternative Medicines, 8(3), 267–274.

Pace, B. A., and Devenot, N. (2021). Right-wing psychedelia: Case studies in cultural plasticity and political pluripotency. *Frontiers in Psychology, 12*. https://www.frontiersin.org/articles/10.3389/fpsyg.2021.733185

Pallay, A. (2022, March 7). Meet the fast-growing mushroom cultivators love. *DoubleBlind Mag*. https://doubleblindmag.com/the-ultimate-guide-to-z-strain-mushrooms/

Papo, D. (2016). Commentary: The entropic brain: A theory of conscious states informed by neuroimaging research with psychedelic drugs. *Frontiers in Human Neuroscience, 10*, 423.

Passie, T., Guss, J., and Krähenmann, R. (2022). Lower-dose psycholytic therapy—a neglected approach. *Frontiers in Psychiatry, 13*. https://www.frontiersin.org/articles/10.3389/fpsyt.2022.1020505

Passie, T., Karst, M., Borsutzky, M., et al. (2003). Effects of different subanaesthetic doses of (S)-ketamine on psychopathology and binocular depth inversion in man. *Journal of Psychopharmacology, 17*(1), 51–56.

Passie, T., Seifert, J., Schneider, U., and Emrich, H. M. (2002). The pharmacology of psilocybin. *Addiction Biology, 7*(4), 357–364. https://doi.org/10.1080/1355621021000005937

Patel, A. (2023, May 20). Can psychedelics prevent cocaine use? PsyTech. https://psytechglobal.com/can-psychedelics-prevent-cocaine-use/

Patocka, J., Wu, R., Nepovimova, E., et al. (2021). Chemistry and toxicology of major bioactive substances in *Inocybe*

mushrooms. *International Journal of Molecular Sciences, 22*(4), 2218. https://doi.org/10.3390/ijms22042218

Peck, S. K., Shao, S., Gruen, T., et al. (2023). Psilocybin therapy for females with anorexia nervosa: A phase 1, open-label feasibility study. *Nature Medicine, 29*(8), 1947–1953. https://doi.org/10.1038/s41591-023-02455-9

Perez, E. (2022, June 12). The best mushroom strain for psilocybin-assisted therapy. Psychedelic Passage. https://www.psychedelicpassage.com/the-best-mushroom-strain-for-psilocybin-assisted-therapy/

Persinger, M. A. (1993). Vectorial cerebral hemisphericity as differential sources for the sensed presence, mystical experiences and religious conversions. *Perceptual and Motor Skills, 76*(3), 915–930.

Pfister, D. H. (1988). R. Gordon Wasson—1898–1986. *Mycologia, 80*(1), 11–13. https://doi.org/10.1080/00275514.1988.12025491

Phillips, R. (2005). *Mushrooms and Other Fungi of North America*. Firefly Books.

Pilger, G. (2023, August 28). The weirdest magic mushroom strain might be the Enigma. *HealingMaps*. https://healingmaps.com/the-weirdest-magic-mushroom-strain-might-be-the-enigma/

Pisano, V. D., Putnam, N. P., Kramer, H. M., et al. (2017). The association of psychedelic use and opioid use disorders among illicit users in the United States. *Journal of Psychopharmacology, 31*(5). https://journals.sagepub.com/doi/abs/10.1177/0269881117691453

Polito, V. (2019). Motives and side-effects of microdosing with psychedelics among users. *International Journal of Neuropsychopharmacology, 22*(7). https://doi.org/10.1093/ijnp/pyz029

Polito, V., and Liknaitzky, P. (2022). The emerging science of microdosing: A systematic review of research on low dose psychedelics (1955–2021) and recommendations for the field. *Neuroscience & Biobehavioral Reviews, 139*, 104706. https://doi.org/10.1016/j.neubiorev.2022.104706

Posada-Quintero, H. F., Reljin, N., Bolkhovsky, J. B., et al. (2019). Brain activity correlates with cognitive performance deterioration during sleep deprivation. *Frontiers in Neuroscience, 13*. https://www.frontiersin.org/article/10.3389/fnins.2019.01001

Powell, S. G. (2011). *The Psilocybin Solution: The Role of Sacred Mushrooms in the Quest for Meaning*. Park Street Press.

Preuss, T. M., and Wise, S. P. (2022). Evolution of prefrontal cortex. *Neuropsychopharmacology, 47*(1), 3–19. https://doi.org/10.1038/s41386-021-01076-5

Prochazkova, L., Lippelt, D. P., Colzato, L. S., et al. (2018). Exploring the effect of microdosing psychedelics on creativity in an open-label natural setting. *Psychopharmacology, 235*(12), 3401–3413. https://doi.org/10.1007/s00213-018-5049-7

Psillow. (2019a, December 30). *Psilocybe caerulescens*. https://psillow.com/species/psilocybe-caerulescens/

Psillow. (2019b, December 30). *Psilocybe quebecensis*. https://psillow.com/species/psilocybe-quebecensis/

Psilocybe. (2012). *Farlex Partner Medical Dictionary*. http://medical-dictionary.thefreedictionary.com/Psilocybe

Psilosophy. (n.d.). Entheogenic mushrooms—philosophy of cultivation. Retrieved June 18, 2023, from http://www.en.psilosophy.info/

Psilosophy. (n.d.). *Psilocybe cubensis* "B+." Retrieved June 12, 2023, from http://www.en.psilosophy.info/species/psilocybe_cubensis_b+.htm

Psilosophy. (n.d.). *Psilocybe cubensis* "PF Classic." Retrieved October 12, 2023, from http://www.en.psilosophy.info/species/psilocybe_cubensis_pf_classic.htm

Psychedelic Science Review. (2018, November 19). Baeocystin. https://psychedelicreview.com/compound/baeocystin/

Psychedelic Science Review. (2018, December 20a). Early inhabitants of Algeria create cave art that shows mushrooms. https://psychedelicreview.com/event/cave-art-in-algeria-the-mushroom-shaman/

Psychedelic Science Review. (2018, December 20b). English doctor makes first medical documentation of the effects of psychedelic mushrooms. https://psychedelicreview.com/event/first-medical-documentation-of-the-effects-of-psychedelic-mushrooms/

Psychedelic Science Review. (2019, January 18). R. Gordon Wasson. https://psychedelicreview.com/person/r-gordon-wasson/

Psychology Today. (n.d.) Acceptance and Commitment Therapy. Retrieved September 23, 2023, from https://www.psychologytoday.com/us/therapy-types/acceptance-and-commitment-therapy

PsychonautWiki. (n.d.). Experience: 2.5g Psilocybe Cubensis B+ strain—epiphany of nondualistic reality. Retrieved June 15, 2023, from https://psychonautwiki. org/wiki/Experience:2.5g_Psilocybe_ Cubensis_B%2B_strain_-_epiphany_of_ nondualistic_reality

PsychonautWiki. (n.d.). *Psilocybe cyanescens*. Retrieved June 18, 2023, from https:// psychonautwiki.org/wiki/Psilocybe_ cyanescens

Puls, M. (n.d.). How magical are Australia's native magic mushrooms? University of Queensland. Retrieved June 20, 2023, from https://stories.uq.edu.au/ how-magical-are-australia-s-native-magic-mushrooms/index.html

Radiolab. (2022, June 30). My thymus, myself. WNYC Studios. Retrieved October 22, 2023, from https://www.radiolab.org/ podcast/my-thymus-myself

Raichle, M. E., MacLeod, A. M., Snyder, A. Z., et al. (2001, January 16). A default mode of brain function. *Proceedings of the National Academy of Sciences USA*, 98(2), 676–682. https://doi.org/10.1073/ pnas.98.2.676

Raufman, J.-P., Samimi, R., Shah, N., et al. (2008). Genetic ablation of M3 muscarinic receptors attenuates murine colon epithelial cell proliferation and neoplasia. *Cancer Research*, 68(10), 3573–3578. https://doi.org/10.1158/0008-5472.CAN-07-6810

Raut, S. B., Marathe, P. A., van Eijk, L., et al. (2022). Diverse therapeutic developments for post-traumatic stress disorder (PTSD) indicate common mechanisms of memory modulation. *Pharmacology & Therapeutics*, 239, 108195. https://doi. org/10.1016/j.pharmthera.2022.108195

Redhead, S., Moncalvo, J. M., Vilgalys, R., et al. (2007). Propose to conserve the name *Psilocybe* (Basidiomycota) with a conserved type. *Taxon*, 56(1), 255–257.

Repke, D. B., Leslie, D. T., and Guzmán, G. (1977). *Psilocybe, Conocybe*, and *Panaeolus*. *Lloydia*, 40, 566–578.

Riga, M. S., Soria, G., Tudela, R., et al. (2014). The natural hallucinogen 5-MeO-DMT, component of ayahuasca, disrupts cortical function in rats: Reversal by antipsychotic drugs. *International Journal of Neuropsychopharmacology*, 17(8), 1269–1282. https://doi.org/10.1017/ S1461145714000261

Riggio, H. R., and Riggio, R. E. (2002). Emotional expressiveness, extraversion, and neuroticism: A meta-analysis. *Journal of Nonverbal Behavior*, 26(4), 195–218. https://doi.org/10.1023/A:1022117500440

Roberts, T., and Jesse, R. (1997). Recollections of the Good Friday experiment: An interview with Huston Smith. *Journal of Transpersonal Psychology*, 29(2), 99–110.

Rockefeller, A. (2011a). A fruit body of the psychedelic mushroom *Psilocybe yungensis Singer & A.H.Sm* (1958). https://commons.wikimedia.org/wiki/ File:Psilocybe_yungensis_163986.jpg

Rockefeller, A. (2011b). Microscopy showing the pileipellis, pileus trama, and lamellar trama at 100x magnification, from the mushroom *Psilocybe yungensis Singer & A.H.Sm*. https://commons.wikimedia.org/ wiki/File:Psilocybe_yungensis_171250.jpg

Rockefeller, A. (2011c). Spores and cheilocystidia from the psychedelic mushroom *Psilocybe yungensis Singer & A.H.Sm*. https://commons.wikimedia.org/ wiki/File:Psilocybe_yungensis_171324.jpg

Rockefeller, A. (2013). *Psilocybe yungensis from Western Jalisco, Mexico.* https://commons.wikimedia.org/wiki/File:Psilocybe.yungensis.Jalisco.jpg

Rodríguez-Cano, B. J., Kohek, M., Ona, G., et al. (2023). Underground ibogaine use for the treatment of substance use disorders: A qualitative analysis of subjective experiences. *Drug and Alcohol Review, 42*(2), 401–414. https://doi.org/10.1111/dar.13587

Rogers, R. (2011). *The Fungal Pharmacy: The Complete Guide to Medicinal Mushrooms and Lichens of North America.* North Atlantic Books.

Rootman, J. M., Kiraga, M., Kryskow, P., et al. (2022). Psilocybin microdosers demonstrate greater observed improvements in mood and mental health at one month relative to non-microdosing controls. *Scientific Reports, 12*(1), Article 1. https://doi.org/10.1038/s41598-022-14512-3

Rootman, J. M., Kryskow, P., Harvey, K., et al. (2021). Adults who microdose psychedelics report health related motivations and lower levels of anxiety and depression compared to non-microdosers. *Scientific Reports, 11*(1), Article 1. https://doi.org/10.1038/s41598-021-01811-4

Ross, S. (2019). Microdosing psychedelics: Too much hype, almost no rigorous research. *Journal of Psychopharmacology, 33*(9), 1050–1051.

Rothman, R. B., Baumann, M. H., Savage, J. E., et al. (2000). Evidence for possible involvement of 5-HT2B receptors in the cardiac valvulopathy associated with fenfluramine and other serotonergic medications. *Circulation, 102*(23), 2836–2841. https://doi.org/10.1161/01.CIR.102.23.2836

Ruch, D. G., and Motta, J. J. (1987). Ultrastructure and cytochemistry of dormant basidiospores of *Psilocybe cubensis. Mycologia, 79*(3), 387–398. https://doi.org/10.1080/00275514.1987.12025395

Rucker, J. J., Jelen, L. A., Flynn, S., et al. (2016). Psychedelics in the treatment of unipolar mood disorders: A systematic review. *Journal of Psychopharmacology (Oxford, England), 30*(12), 1220–1229. https://doi.org/10.1177/0269881116679368

Rucker, J. J., Marwood, L., Ajantaival, R.-L. J., et al. (2022). The effects of psilocybin on cognitive and emotional functions in healthy participants: Results from a phase 1, randomised, placebo-controlled trial involving simultaneous psilocybin administration and preparation. *Journal of Psychopharmacology (Oxford, England), 36*(1), 114–125. https://doi.org/10.1177/02698811211064720

Rudden, M., Busch, F. N., Milrod, B., et al. (2003). Panic disorder and depression: A psychodynamic exploration of comorbidity. *International Journal of Psycho-Analysis, 84*(4), 997–1015.

Ryan, R. S., Copello, A., and Fox, A. P. (2023). Experiences of microdosing psychedelics in an attempt to support wellbeing and mental health. *BMC Psychiatry, 23*(1), 160. https://doi.org/10.1186/s12888-023-04628-9

Sadibolova, R., Murray-Lawson, C., Neiloufar Family, et al. (2023, April 16). LSD microdosing attenuates the impact of temporal priors in

time perception. BioRxiv. https://doi.
org/10.1101/2023.04.14.536983

Salvat-Pujol, N., Labad, J., Urretavizcaya, M.,
et al. (2017). Hypothalamic-pituitary-
adrenal axis activity and cognition in
major depression: The role of remission
status. *Psychoneuroendocrinology*,
76, 38–48. https://doi.org/10.1016/j.
psyneuen.2016.11.007

Samorini, G., and Camilla, G. (1995).
Rappresentiazioni fungine nell'arte greca.
Annalu Del Museo Civico Roverto, 10,
307–326.

Sansalone, G., Profico, A., Wroe, S., et al.
(2023). Homo sapiens and Neanderthals
share high cerebral cortex integration into
adulthood. *Nature Ecology & Evolution*,
7(1), Article 1. https://doi.org/10.1038/
s41559-022-01933-6

Sanz, C., Pallavicini, C., Carrillo, F.,
et al. (2021). The entropic tongue:
Disorganization of natural language
under LSD. *Consciousness and Cognition*,
87, 103070.

Sarparast, A., Thomas, K., Malcolm, B.,
and Stauffer, C. S. (2022). Drug-
drug interactions between psychiatric
medications and MDMA or psilocybin: A
systematic review. *Psychopharmacology*,
239(6), 1945–1976. https://doi.
org/10.1007/s00213-022-06083-y

Schindler, E. A. D. (2022). Psychedelics
as preventive treatment in
headache and chronic pain
disorders. *Neuropharmacology*, 215,
109166. https://doi.org/10.1016/j.
neuropharm.2022.109166

Schindler, E. A. D., Sewell, R. A., Gottschalk,
C. H., et al. (2021). Exploratory controlled
study of the migraine-suppressing effects
of psilocybin. *Neurotherapeutics: The
Journal of the American Society for
Experimental NeuroTherapeutics*, 18(1),
534–543. https://doi.org/10.1007/s13311-
020-00962-y

Schmoldt, A., Benthe, H. F., and Haberland,
G. (1975). Digitoxin metabolism by
rat liver microsomes. *Biochemical
Pharmacology*, 24(17), 1639–1641.

Schoch, C. L., Ciufo, S., Domrachev,
M., et al. (2020). NCBI taxonomy: A
comprehensive update on curation,
resources and tools. *Database*, 2020,
baaa062. https://doi.org/10.1093/database/
baaa062

ScienceDirect. (n.d.-a). Peyote. Retrieved
July 7, 2023, from https://www.
sciencedirect.com/topics/
neuroscience/peyote

Science Direct. (n.d.-b). *Psilocybe cubensis*—
an overview. Retrieved June 24, 2023,
from https://www.sciencedirect.com/
topics/neuroscience/psilocybe-cubensis

Science Direct. (n.d.-c.). *Psilocybe
semilanceata*—an overview. Retrieved
October 11, 2023, from https://www.
sciencedirect.com/topics/neuroscience/
psilocybe-semilanceata

Science Direct. (n.d.-d). *Psilocybe*—an
overview. https://www.sciencedirect.
com/topics/biochemistry-genetics-and-
molecular-biology/psilocybe

Sebek, Š. (1983). Böhmischer Kahlkopf—
Psilocybe bohemica. *Ceská Mykologie*,
37(3), 177–181.

Seo, Z. (n.d.). Most potent mushroom
strains: Your essential ranking need.
Retrieved October 11, 2023, from https://
www.zoomiescanada.ca/the-strongest-
mushroom-strains-ranked-by-potency/

Shāfaa. (n.d.). PF Classic magic mushrooms: Mind-altering experience. Retrieved June 15, 2023, from https://shafaa.ca/product/pf-classic-magic-mushrooms-3-5-to-28-g/

Sheldrake, M. (2020). *Entangled Life: How Fungi Make Our World, Change Our Minds, and Shape Our Futures.* Random House.

Shipley, M. (2014). "A necessary but not sufficient condition": Psychedelic mysticism, perrenial liminality, and the limits of supernatural theism. *Preternature, 3*(2).

Shorey, S., Chee, C. Y. I., Ng, E. D., et al. (2018). Prevalence and incidence of postpartum depression among healthy mothers: A systematic review and meta-analysis. *Journal of Psychiatric Research, 104,* 235–248. https://doi.org/10.1016/j.jpsychires.2018.08.001

Shroomery. (n.d.-a). B+. Retrieved June 12, 2023, from https://www.shroomery.org/9106/B

Shroomery. (n.d.-b). *Psilocybe fimetaria.* Retrieved October 13, 2023, from https://www.shroomery.org/12504/Psilocybe-fimetaria

Shroomery. (n.d.-c). *Psilocybe ovoideocystidiata.* Retrieved June 25, 2023, from https://www.shroomery.org/12508/Psilocybe-ovoideocystidiata

Shroomery. (n.d.-d). *Psilocybe yungensis.* Retrieved June 25, 2023, from https://www.shroomery.org/12518/Psilocybe-yungensis

Shroomery. (n.d.-e). South America. Retrieved June 25, 2023, from https://www.shroomery.org/12258/South-America

Shulman, G. L., Fiez, J. A., Corbetta, M., et al. (1997). Common blood flow changes across visual tasks: II. Decreases in cerebral cortex. *Journal of Cognitive Neuroscience, 9*(5), 648–663. https://doi.org/10.1162/jocn.1997.9.5.648

Shultes, R. E. (1976). *Hallucinogenic Plants.* Golden Press. Available online at https://erowid.org/library/books_online/golden_guide/g01-10.shtml

Siebert, A. (2021, February 25). NYU establishes Center for Psychedelic Medicine with $10 million from MindMed, philanthropists. *Forbes.* Retrieved October 10, 2023, from https://www.forbes.com/sites/amandasiebert/2021/02/25/nyu-langone-establishes-center-for-psychedelic-medicine-with-10-million-from-mindmed-philanthropists/

Simeon, D., Kozin, D. S., Segal, K., et al. (2008). De-constructing depersonalization: Further evidence for symptom clusters. *Psychiatry Research, 157*(1), 303–306. https://doi.org/10.1016/j.psychres.2007.07.007

Simms, D. (2022, April 27). What is the B+ shroom strain? Everything you need to know. *Tripsitter.* https://tripsitter.com/magic-mushrooms/strains/b-plus/

Simms, D. (2022, July 9). Orissa India shroom strain: One of the largest and most potent *cubensis* strains. *Tripsitter.* https://tripsitter.com/magic-mushrooms/strains/orissa-india/

Simon, J. J., Stopyra, M. A., and Friederich, H.-C. (2019). Neural processing of disorder-related stimuli in patients with anorexia nervosa: A narrative review of brain imaging studies. *Journal of Clinical Medicine, 8*(7), 1047. https://doi.org/10.3390/jcm8071047

Singer, R. (1951). Diagnoses fungorum novorum agaricalium. *Lilloa, 22,* 472, 506.

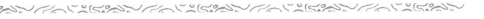
Singer, R. (1953). Four years of mycological work in southern South America. *Mycologia*, 45(6), 865–891. https://doi.org/10.1080/00275514.1953.12024322

Singer, R. (1958). Mycological investigations on Teonanácatl, the Mexican hallucinogenic mushroom. Part I. The history of Teonanácatl, field work, and culture work. *Mycologia*, 50(2), 239–261. https://doi.org/10.1080/00275514.1958.12024725

Singer, R., and Smith, A. H. (1946). Proposals concerning the nomenclature of the gill fungi including a list of proposed lectotypes and genera conservanda. *Mycologia*, 38(3), 240–299. https://doi.org/10.1080/00275514.1946.12024058

Singer, R., and Smith, A. H. (1958a). Mycological investigations on Teonanacatl, the Mexican hallucinogenic mushroom. Part II. A taxonomic monograph of *Psilocybe*, section Caerulescentes. *Mycologia*, 50(2), 262–303. https://doi.org/10.2307/3756197

Singer, R., and Smith, A. H. (1958b). New species of *Psilocybe*. *Mycologia*, 50(1), 141–142. https://doi.org/10.2307/3756045

Smith, A. H. (1937). New and unusual agarics from the western United States. *Mycologia*, 29(1), 45–59. https://doi.org/10.2307/3754199

Smith, A. H. (1941). Studies of North American agarics–I. *Contributions of the University of Michigan Herbarium*, 5, 5–73.

Smith, A. H. (1948). Studies in the dark-spored Agarics. *Mycologia*, 40(6), 669–707. https://doi.org/10.1080/00275514.1948.12017737

Smith, A. H. (1951). The North American species of *Naemalotoma*. *Mycologia*, 43(5), 467–521. https://doi.org/10.1080/00275514.1951.12024150

Smith, A. H. (1975). *A Field Guide to Western Mushrooms*. University of Michigan Press.

Smith, A. H. (1977). Comments on hallucinogenic agarics and the hallucinations of those who study them. *Mycologia*, 69(6), 1196–1200. https://doi.org/10.1080/00275514.1977.12020180

Smith, S. M., and Vale, W. W. (2006). The role of the hypothalamic-pituitary-adrenal axis in neuroendocrine responses to stress. *Dialogues in Clinical Neuroscience*, 8(4), 383–395. https://doi.org/10.31887/DCNS.2006.8.4/ssmith

Snelders, S. (1998). The LSD therapy career of Jan Bastiaans, M.D. *Newsletter of the Multidisciplinary Association for Psychedelic Studies*, 8(1), 18–20. https://maps.org/news-letters/v08n1/08118sne.html

Solomon, A., and Wane, N. N. (2005). Indigenous Healers and Healing in a Modern World. In R. Moodley and W. West (Eds.), *Integrating Traditional Healing Practices into Counseling and Psychotherapy*. Sage.

Sorrells, S. F., Paredes, M. F., Cebrian-Silla, A., et al. (2018). Human hippocampal neurogenesis drops sharply in children to undetectable levels in adults. *Nature*, 555(7696), Article 7696. https://doi.org/10.1038/nature25975

Sosa, A. (2023, October 7). Newsom vetoes bill to decriminalize "magic mushrooms" in California. *Los Angeles Times*. https://www.latimes.com/california/story/2023-10-07/gavin-newsom-psychedelics-magic-mushrooms-sb-58-veto-drugs-california

Species Fungorum. (n.d.). *Psilocybe caerulescens*. http://www.speciesfungorum.org/Names/SynSpecies.asp?RecordID=259270

Spriggs, M. J., Giribaldi, B., Lyons, T., et al. (2023). Body mass index (BMI) does not predict responses to psilocybin. *Journal of Psychopharmacology*, 37(1), 107–116. https://doi.org/10.1177/02698811221131994

Squire, L. R., Genzel, L., Wixted, J. T., and Morris, R. G. (2015). Memory consolidation. *Cold Spring Harbor Perspectives in Biology*, 7(8), a021766. https://doi.org/10.1101/cshperspect.a021766

Stahl, S. M. (2018, June 29). Beyond the dopamine hypothesis of schizophrenia to three neural networks of psychosis: Dopamine, serotonin, and glutamate. *CNS Spectrums*, 23(3), 187–191. https://doi.org/10.1017/S1092852918001013

Stamets, P. (1996). *Psilocybin Mushrooms of the World: An Identification Guide*. Clarkson Potter/Ten Speed.

Stamets, P. (2000). *Growing Gourmet and Medicinal Mushrooms* (3rd rev. ed.). Ten Speed Press.

Stamets, P. (2011). *Mycelium Running: How Mushrooms Can Help Save the World*. Clarkson Potter/Ten Speed.

Stamets, P. (2020). *Fantastic Fungi: How Mushrooms Can Heal, Shift Consciousness, and Save the Planet*. Simon and Schuster.

Stamets, P., and Gartz, J. (1995). A new caerulescent *Psilocybe* from the Pacific Coast of Northwestern America. *Integration*, 6, 21–28.

Stamets, P., and Yao, C. D. W. (2002). *Mycomedicinals: An Informational Booklet on Medicinal Mushrooms*. MycoMedia.

Starr, J. M., Farrall, A. J., Armitage, P., et al. (2009). Blood–brain barrier permeability in Alzheimer's disease: A case–control MRI study. *Psychiatry Research: Neuroimaging*, 171(3), 232–241.

Stauffer, C. S., Anderson, B. T., Ortigo, K. M., and Woolley, J. (2021). Psilocybin-assisted group therapy and attachment: Observed reduction in attachment anxiety and influences of attachment insecurity on the psilocybin experience. *ACS Pharmacology & Translational Science*, 4(2), 526–532. https://doi.org/10.1021/acsptsci.0c00169

Stein, S. I. (1959). Clinical observations on the effects of *Panaeolus venenosus* versus *Psilocybe caerulescens* mushrooms. *Mycologia*, 51(1), 49–50. https://doi.org/10.1080/00275514.1959.12024795

Steinhardt, J. (2021, February 12). Hackers, mason jars, and the psychedelic science of DIY shrooms. *Wired*. https://www.wired.com/story/hackers-mason-jars-psychedelic-science-diy-shrooms/

Stocks, D. L., and Hess, W. M. (1970). Ultrastructure of dormant and germinated basidiospores of a species of *Psilocybe*. *Mycologia*, 62(1), 176–191. https://doi.org/10.1080/00275514.1970.12018952

Strassman R. J. (1996). Human psychopharmacology of N,N-dimethyltryptamine. *Behavioural Brain Research*, 73(1–2), 121–124. https://doi.org/10.1016/0166-4328(96)00081-2.

Strauss, D., Ghosh, S., Murray, Z., and Gryzenhout, M. (2022). An overview on the taxonomy, phylogenetics and ecology of the psychedelic genera *Psilocybe*,

Panaeolus, Pluteus, and *Gymnopilus. Frontiers in Forests and Global Change, 5.* https://www.frontiersin.org/articles/10.3389/ffgc.2022.813998

Strauss, D., Ghosh, S., Murray, Z., and Gryzenhout, M. (2023). Global species diversity and distribution of the psychedelic fungal genus *Panaeolus. Heliyon, 9*(6), e16338. https://doi.org/10.1016/j.heliyon.2023.e16338

Sughrue, M. (2022, July 5). What are brain networks? Omniscient Neurotechnology. https://www.o8t.com/blog/brain-networks

Surapaneni, P., Vinales, K. L., Najib, M. Q., and Chaliki, H. P. (2011). Valvular heart disease with the use of fenfluramine-phentermine. *Texas Heart Institute Journal, 38*(5), 581-583.

Szigeti, B., Kartner, L., Blemings, A., et al. (2021). Self-blinding citizen science to explore psychedelic microdosing. *eLife, 10.*

Tagliazucchi, E., Dehaene, S., Deco, G., et al. (2019). Human consciousness is supported by dynamic complex patterns of brain signal coordination. *Science Advances, 5*(2). https://pubmed.ncbi.nlm.nih.gov/30775433/

Tavares, I. (2022, April 29). *The Penis Envy mushroom.* Frshminds. https://frshminds.com/penis-envy-mushroom/

Thiers, H. D. (1987). Alexander H. Smith, 1904–1986. *Mycologia, 79*(6), 811–818. https://doi.org/10.1080/00275514.1987.12025468

Thomas, K. (2022, April 13). Safety first: potential heart health risks of microdosing. Harvard Health and Law Bill of Health. https://blog.petrieflom.law.harvard.edu/2022/04/13/safety-first-potential-heart-health-risks-of-microdosing/

Thomas, K. S., Birch, R. E., Jones, C. R. G., and Vanderwert, R. E. (2022). Neural correlates of executive functioning in anorexia nervosa and obsessive-compulsive disorder. *Frontiers in Human Neuroscience, 16,* 841633. https://doi.org/10.3389/fnhum.2022.841633

Thursby, E., and Juge, N. (2017). Introduction to the human gut microbiota. *Biochemical Journal, 474*(11), 1823–1836. https://doi.org/10.1042/BCJ20160510

Toda, T., Parylak, S., Linker, S. B., and Gage, F. H. (2019). The role of adult hippocampal neurogenesis in brain health and disease. *Molecular Psychiatry, 24*(1), 67–87. https://doi.org/10.1038/s41380-018-0036-2

Tondo, G., Boccalini, C., Vanoli, E. G., et al. (2022). Brain metabolism and amyloid load in individuals with subjective cognitive decline or pre-mild cognitive impairment. *Neurology, 99*(3), e258–269. https://doi.org/10.1212/WNL.0000000000200351

Torrado Pacheco, A., Olson, R. J., Garza, G., and Moghaddam, B. (2023). Acute psilocybin enhances cognitive flexibility in rats. *Neuropsychopharmacology, 48*(7), 1011–1020. https://doi.org/10.1038/s41386-023-01545-z

Tóth, A., Hausknecht, A., Krisai-Greilhuber, I., et al. (2013). Iteratively refined guide trees help improving alignment and phylogenetic inference in the mushroom family Bolbitiaceae. *PLOS ONE, 8*(2), e56143. https://doi.org/10.1371/journal.pone.0056143

Tralamazza, S. M., Rocha, L. O., Oggenfuss, U., et al. (2019). Complex evolutionary origins of specialized metabolite gene cluster diversity among the plant pathogenic fungi of the *Fusarium graminearum* species complex. *Genome Biology and Evolution, 11*(11). https://doi.org/10.1093/gbe/evz225

Treaster, J. B. (1994, May 7). Use of drugs is legalized by Colombia. *New York Times.* https://www.nytimes.com/1994/05/07/world/use-of-drugs-is-legalized-by-colombia.html

Trip, M. (2021). *Magic Mushrooms Guide: The Most Complete Bible to Cultivation and Safe Use of Psilocybin Mushrooms with All the Benefits and Side Effects.* Robert Murray.

Trippy Spot. (2021, June 2). *Psilocybe quebecensis.* https://trippyspot.com/shop/mushrooms/dried-magic-mushrooms/psilocybe-quebecensis/

Trudell, S., and Ammirati, J. (2009). *Mushrooms of the Pacific Northwest: Timber Press Field Guide (Timber Press Field Guides).* Timber Press, p. 208.

Tullis, P. (2021). How ecstasy and psilocybin are shaking up psychiatry. *Nature, 589*(7843), 506–509. https://doi.org/10.1038/d41586-021-00187-9

Twomey, S. (2010). Phineas Gage: Neuroscience's most famous patient. *Smithsonian Magazine.* https://www.smithsonianmag.com/history/phineas-gage-neurosciences-most-famous-patient-11390067/

Ultimate Mushroom. (n.d.-a). *Gymnopilus junonius.* Retrieved June 26, 2023, from https://ultimate-mushroom.com/inedible/3-gymnopilus-junonius.html

Ultimate Mushroom. (n.d.-b). *Pholiotina rugosa.* Retrieved June 26, 2023, from https://ultimate-mushroom.com/poisonous/793-pholiotina-rugosa.html

University of Chicago. (2023). An open label study of single-dose psilocybin for major depressive disorder with co-occurring borderline personality disorder (Clinical Trial Registration NCT05399498). ClinicalTrials.gov. https://clinicaltrials.gov/study/NCT05399498

Urban Spore. (n.d.). PF Tek. Retrieved August 9, 2023, from https://urbanspore.com.au/how-to-grow-mushrooms/pf-tek/

van Amsterdam, J., Opperhuizen, A., and van den Brink, W. (2011). Harm potential of magic mushroom use: A review. *Regulatory Toxicology and Pharmacology, 59*(3), 423–429. https://doi.org/10.1016/j.yrtph.2011.01.006

Van Court, R. C., Wiseman, M. S., Meyer, K. W., et al. (2022). Diversity, biology, and history of psilocybin-containing fungi: Suggestions for research and technological development. *Fungal Biology, 126*(4), 308–319. https://doi.org/10.1016/j.funbio.2022.01.003

van de Peppel, L. J. J., Aime, M. C., Læssøe, T., et al. (2022). Four new genera and six new species of lyophylloid agarics (*Agaricales, Basidiomycota*) from three different continents. *Mycological Progress, 21*(10), 85. https://doi.org/10.1007/s11557-022-01836-7

van der Kolk, B. A. (2014). *The Body Keeps the Score: Brain, Mind, and Body in the Healing of Trauma.* Viking.

van Elk, M., and Snoek, L. (2020). The relationship between individual differences in gray matter volume and religiosity and mystical experiences: A preregistered voxel-based morphometry study. *European Journal of Neuroscience, 51*(3), 850–865. https://doi.org/10.1111/ejn.14563

Van Overwalle, F. (2009). Social cognition and the brain: A meta-analysis. *Human Brain Mapping*, 30(3), 829–858. https://doi.org/10.1002/hbm.20547

Via, E., Goldberg, X., Sánchez, I., et al. (2018). Self and other body perception in anorexia nervosa: The role of posterior DMN nodes. *World Journal of Biological Psychiatry*, 19(3), 210–224. https://doi.org/10.1080/15622975.2016.1249951

Vo, K. T. (2017). *Amanita phalloides* mushroom poisonings—Northern California, December 2016. *MMWRL Morbidity and Mortality Weekly Report*, 66. https://doi.org/10.15585/mmwr.mm6621a1

Vollenweider, F. X., Vollenweider-Scherpenhuyzen, M. F., Bäbler, A., et al. (1998). Psilocybin induces schizophrenia-like psychosis in humans via a serotonin-2 agonist action. *Neuroreport*, 9(17), 3897–3902. https://doi.org/10.1097/00001756-199812010-00024

Wall, M., Demetriou, L., Giribaldi, B., et al. (2023). Reduced brain responsiveness to emotional stimuli with escitalopram but not psilocybin therapy for depression. *MedRxiv, Preprint*. https://doi.org/10.1101/2023.05.29.23290667

Wang, X., Xie, H., Chen, T., et al. (2021). Cortical volume abnormalities in posttraumatic stress disorder: An ENIGMA-psychiatric genomics consortium PTSD workgroup mega-analysis. *Molecular Psychiatry*, 26(8), Article 8. https://doi.org/10.1038/s41380-020-00967-1

Washington, S. D., Gordon, E. M., Brar, J., et al. (2014). Dysmaturation of default network in autism. *Human Brain Mapping*, 35(4), 1284–1296. https://doi.org/10.1002/hbm.22252

Wasson, R. G. (1957, May 13). Seeking the Magic Mushroom. *Life*, 42(19), 100–120.

Wasson, R. G. (1970, September 26). Drugs: The sacred mushroom. *New York Times*, 21.

Wasson, R. G. (1980). *The Wondrous Mushroom: Mycolatry in Mesoamerica*. McGraw-Hill.

Watson, C. (2022). The psychedelic remedy for chronic pain. *Nature*, 609(7929), S100–S102. https://doi.org/10.1038/d41586-022-02878-3

Whelan, T., Daly, E., Puts, N., et al. (2023). Bridging the translational neuroscience gap: Development of the 'shiftability' paradigm and an exemplar protocol to capture psilocybin-elicited 'shift' in neurobiological mechanisms in autism. *MedRxiv*. https://doi.org/10.1101/2023.05.25.23290521

Whinkin, E., Opalka, M., Watters, C., et al. (2023). Psilocybin in palliative care: An update. *Current Geriatrics Reports*, 12(2), 50–59. https://doi.org/10.1007/s13670-023-00383-7

Whitehead, N. (2014, February 8). Ninety-eight percent of fungi remain unidentified. Science.org. https://www.science.org/content/article/ninety-eight-percent-fungi-remain-unidentified

Widiger, T. A., and Oltmanns, J. R. (2017). Neuroticism is a fundamental domain of personality with enormous public health implications. *World Psychiatry*, 16(2), 144–145. https://doi.org/10.1002/wps.20411

Wieczorek, P. P., Witkowska, D., Jasicka-Misiak, I., et al. (2015). Bioactive alkaloids of hallucinogenic mushrooms.

In *Studies in Natural Products Chemistry* (Vol. 46, pp. 133–168). Elsevier. https://doi.org/10.1016/B978-0-444-63462-7.00005-1

Wikidoc. (n.d.). *Psilocybe tampanensis*. (n.d.). Retrieved June 18, 2023, from https://www.wikidoc.org/index.php/Psilocybe_tampanensis

Wikidoc. (n.d.). *Psilocybe weilii*. (n.d.). Retrieved June 25, 2023, from https://www.wikidoc.org/index.php/Psilocybe_weilii

Wikidoc. (n.d.). *Psilocybe zapotecorum*. Retrieved June 18, 2023, from https://www.wikidoc.org/index.php/Psilocybe_zapotecorum

Wikipedia. (n.d.-a). Echo and Narcissus. https://en.wikipedia.org/w/index.php?title=Echo_and_Narcissus

Wikipedia. (n.d.-b). *Gymnopilus*. https://en.wikipedia.org/w/index.php?title=Gymnopilus

Wikipedia. (n.d.-c). *Psilocybe quebecensis*. https://en.wikipedia.org/w/index.php?title=Psilocybe_quebecensis

Wilson, J. R. (n.d.). EO/IR sensors boost situational awareness. *Military & Aerospace Electronics*. Retrieved May 15, 2019, from https://www.militaryaerospace.com/communications/article/16709096/eoir-sensors-boost-situational-awareness

Wilson, R. S., Capuano, A. W., Boyle, P. A., et al. (2014). Clinical-pathologic study of depressive symptoms and cognitive decline in old age. *Neurology*, 83(8), 702. https://doi.org/10.1212/WNL.0000000000000715

Woolley, D., and Campbell, N. K. (1962). Serotonin-like and antiserotonin properties of psilocybin and psilocin.

Science, 136(3518), 777–778. https://doi.org/10.1126/science.136.3518.777

Wu, B., Hussain, M., Zhang, W., et al. (2019). Current insights into fungal species diversity and perspective on naming the environmental DNA sequences of fungi. *Mycology, 10*(3), 127–140. https://doi.org/10.1080/21501203.2019.1614106

Yaden, D. B., Berghella, A. P., Regier, P. S., et al. (2021). Classic psychedelics in the treatment of substance use disorder: Potential synergies with twelve-step programs. *International Journal of Drug Policy, 98*, 103380. https://doi.org/10.1016/j.drugpo.2021.103380

Yaden, D. B., Johnson, M. W., Griffiths, R. R., et al. (2021). Psychedelics and consciousness: Distinctions, demarcations, and opportunities. *International Journal of Neuropsychopharmacology, 24*. https://doi.org/10.1093/ijnp/pyab026

Yale Center for Clinical Investigation. (n.d.). Efficacy of psilocybin in OCD: A double-blind, placebo-controlled study. Retrieved October 10, 2023, from https://medicine.yale.edu/ycci/trial/neural-correlates-of-the-effects-of-psilocybin-in-obsessive-compulsive-disorder/

Yano, J. M., Yu, K., Donaldson, G. P., et al. (2015). Indigenous bacteria from the gut microbiota regulate host serotonin biosynthesis. *Cell, 161*(2), 264–276. https://doi.org/10.1016/j.cell.2015.02.047

Yoo, H. J., Thayer, J. F., Greening, S., et al. (2018). Brain structural concomitants of resting state heart rate variability in the young and old: Evidence from two independent samples. *Brain Structure and Function, 223*(2), 727–737. https://doi.org/10.1007/s00429-017-1519-7

Zarrindast, M.-R., and Khakpai, F. (2015). The modulatory role of dopamine in anxiety-like behavior. *Archives of Iranian Medicine*, *18*(9), 591–603.

Zavala, A. (2023, September 8). California lawmakers OK magic mushrooms, natural psychedelics. KCRA. https://www.kcra.com/article/california-lawmakers-approve-magic-mushrooms/45042798

Zeidan, F. (2023). Behavioral and neural mechanisms supporting psilocybin-assisted therapy for phantom limb pain (Clinical Trial Registration NCT05224336). ClinicalTrials.gov. https://clinicaltrials.gov/study/NCT05224336

Zeifman, R. J., Wagner, A. C., Monson, C. M., and Carhart-Harris, R. L. (2023). How does psilocybin therapy work? An exploration of experiential avoidance as a putative mechanism of change. *Journal of Affective Disorders*, *334*, 100–112. https://doi.org/10.1016/j.jad.2023.04.105

Zhang, H., Hook, J. N., Hodge, A. S., et al. (2022). Nonreligious spirituality, mental health, and well-being. *Spirituality in Clinical Practice*, *9*(1), 60–71. https://doi.org/10.1037/scp0000279

Zhu, F., Tu, H., and Chen, T. (2022). The microbiota–gut–brain axis in depression: The potential pathophysiological mechanisms and microbiota combined antidepression effect. *Nutrients*, *14*(10), 2081. https://doi.org/10.3390/nu14102081

Zollikofer, C. P. E., Bienvenu, T., Beyene, Y., et al. (2022). Endocranial ontogeny and evolution in early *Homo sapiens*: The evidence from Herto, Ethiopia. *Proceedings of the National Academy of Sciences*, *119*(32), e2123553119. https://doi.org/10.1073/pnas.2123553119

Zoomies Canada. (2023, July 31). Golden Teacher mushrooms: The best strain for beginners. Retrieved October 12, 2023, from https://www.zoomiescanada.ca/exploring-why-golden-teacher-mushrooms-are-the-best-strain-for-beginners/

INDEX

Page numbers of illustrations appear in italics.